Ambulatory Anesthesia

Guest Editor

PETER S.A. GLASS, MB, ChB

ANESTHESIOLOGY CLINICS

www.anesthesiology.theclinics.com

Consulting Editor

LEE A. FLEISHER, MD, FACC

June 2010 • Volume 28 • Number 2

SAUNDERS an imprint of ELSEVIER, Inc.

W.B. SAUNDERS COMPANY
A Division of Elsevier Inc.

1600 John F. Kennedy Boulevard, Suite 1800 • Philadelphia, PA 19103-2899

http://www.theclinics.com

ANESTHESIOLOGY CLINICS Volume 28, Number 2
June 2010 ISSN 1932-2275, ISBN-13: 978-1-4377-1796-9

Editor: Rachel Glover

Developmental Editor: Theresa Collier

Anesthesiology Clinics (ISSN 1932-2275) is published quarterly by Elsevier Inc., 360 Park Avenue South, New York, NY 10010-1710. Months of issue are March, June, September, and December. Periodicals postage paid at New York, NY and at additional mailing offices. Subscription prices are $134.00 per year (US student/resident), $268.00 per year (US individuals), $328.00 per year (Canadian individuals), $417.00 per year (US institutions), $517.00 per year (Canadian institutions), $189.00 per year (Canadian and foreign student/resident), $372.00 per year (foreign individuals), and $517.00 per year (foreign institutions). To receive student and resident rate, orders must be accompanied by name of affiliated institution, date of term, and the *signature* of program/residency coordinator on institutions letterhead. Orders will be billed at individual rate until proof of status is received. Foreign air speed delivery is included in all *Clinics'* subscription prices. All prices are subject to change without notice. POSTMASTER: Send address changes to *Anesthesiology Clinics,* Elsevier Health Sciences Division, Subscription Customer Service, 3251 Riverport Lane, Maryland Heights, MO 63043. Customer Service (orders, claims, online, change of address): Elsevier Health Sciences Division, Subscription Customer Service, 3251 Riverport Lane, Maryland Heights, MO 63043. Tel: 1-800-654-2452 (U.S. and Canada); 314-447-8871 (outside U.S. and Canada). Fax: 314-447-8029. E-mail: journalscustomerservice-usa@elsevier.com (for print support); journalsonlinesupport-usa@elsevier.com (for online support).

Reprints. For copies of 100 or more of articles in this publication, please contact the Commercial Reprints Department, Elsevier Inc., 360 Park Avenue South, New York, NY 10010-1710. Tel.: 212-633-3812; Fax: 212-462-1935; E-mail: reprints@elsevier.com.

Anesthesiology Clinics, is also published in Spanish by McGraw-Hill Inter-americana Editores S. A., P.O. Box 5-237, 06500 Mexico D. F., Mexico.

Anesthesiology *Clinics*, is covered in *MEDLINE/PubMed (Index Medicus), Current Contents/Clinical Medicine, Excerpta Medica, ISI/BIOMED*, and *Chemical Abstracts*.

Printed and bound by CPI Group (UK) Ltd, Croydon, CR0 4YY

Transferred to Digital Print 2011

Contributors

CONSULTING EDITOR

LEE A. FLEISHER, MD, FACC
Robert D. Dripps Professor and Chair of Anesthesiology and Critical Care, University of Pennsylvania School of Medicine, Philadelphia, Pennsylvania

GUEST EDITOR

PETER S.A. GLASS, MB, ChB
Professor and Chairman, Department of Anesthesiology, School of Medicine, SUNY Stony Brook, Stony Brook, New York

AUTHORS

SHIREEN AHMAD, MD
Associate Professor; Associate Chair for Faculty Development, Department of Anesthesiology, Northwestern University Feinberg School of Medicine, Chicago, Illinois

DEBORAH A. AXELROD, MD
Clinical Instructor, Acute Pain and Regional Anesthesia Fellow, Department of Anesthesiology, University of Utah Orthopaedics Hospital, University of Utah, Salt Lake City, Utah

GLORIA S. CHENG, MD
Assistant Professor, Department of Anesthesiology, University of Utah Orthopaedics Hospital, University of Utah, Salt Lake City, Utah

FRANCES CHUNG, MD, FRCPC
Professor, Department of Anesthesia, University Health Network, University of Toronto, Toronto, Ontario, Canada

COREY E. COLLINS, DO, FAAP
Director, Department of Anesthesiology, Pediatric Anesthesia, Massachusetts Eye and Ear Infirmary; Instructor, Harvard Medical School, Boston, Massachusetts

THOMAS W. CUTTER, MD, MAEd
Professor; Associate Chairman, Department of Anesthesia and Critical Care, Pritzker School of Medicine, University of Chicago; Medical Director for Perioperative Services, University of Chicago Medical Center, Chicago, Illinois

JENNIFER J. DAVIS, MD
Associate Professor, Department of Anesthesiology; Director of Acute Pain Service, University of Utah Orthopaedics Hospital, University of Utah, Salt Lake City, Utah

JOHN A. DILGER, MD
Assistant Professor, Department of Anesthesiology, Mayo Clinic, Rochester, Minnesota

OFELIA LOANI ELVIR-LAZO, MD
Research Physician, Department of Anesthesiology, Cedars Sinai Medical Center, Los Angeles, California

LUCINDA L. EVERETT, MD, FAAP
Associate Professor, Harvard Medical School; Division Chief, Pediatric Anesthesia, Department of Anesthesiology, Critical Care and Pain Medicine, Massachusetts General Hospital, Boston, Massachusetts

TONG JOO GAN, MD, FRCA
Professor of Anesthesiology; Vice Chair for Clinical Research, Department of Anesthesiology, Duke University Medical Center, Duke University School of Medicine, Durham, North Carolina

PETER M. HESSION, MD
Resident in Anesthesiology, Department of Anesthesiology and Pain Management, University of Texas Southwestern Medical Center, Dallas, Texas

ADAM K. JACOB, MD
Assistant Professor, Department of Anesthesiology, Mayo Clinic, Rochester, Minnesota

GIRISH P. JOSHI, MBBS, MD, FFARCSI
Professor of Anesthesiology and Pain Management; Director of Perioperative Medicine and Ambulatory Anesthesia, Department of Anesthesiology and Pain Management, University of Texas Southwestern Medical Center, Dallas, Texas

MATT M. KURREK, MD, FRCP(C)
Assistant Professor, Department of Anesthesia, University of Toronto, Toronto, Ontario, Canada

JOHN J. LAUR, MD, MS
Medical Director, Ambulatory Surgery, University of Iowa Hospitals and Clinics, Iowa City, Iowa

TINA P. LE, BS
Department of Anesthesiology, Duke University Medical Center, Duke University School of Medicine, Durham, North Carolina

KATARZYNA LUBA, MD, MS
Assistant Professor, Department of Anesthesia and Critical Care, Pritzker School of Medicine, University of Chicago, Chicago, Illinois

DOUGLAS G. MERRILL, MD, MBA
Director, The Center for Perioperative Services; Medical Director, Outpatient Surgery, Dartmouth-Hitchcock Medical Center, Lebanon, New Hampshire

DEBORAH C. RICHMAN, MBChB, FFA(SA)
Assistant Professor of Clinical Anesthesiology, Department of Anesthesiology; Director of Preoperative Services, Stony Brook University Medical Center, Stony Brook, New York

EDWIN SEET, MBBS, MMed
Consultant Anesthesiologist, Department of Anesthesia, Alexandra Health Private Limited, Khoo Teck Puat Hospital, Singapore

JEFFREY D. SWENSON, MD
Professor, Department of Anesthesiology; Medical Director, University of Utah Orthopaedics Hospital, University of Utah, Salt Lake City, Utah

REBECCA S. TWERSKY, MD, MPH
Professor, Department of Anesthesiology; Medical Director, Ambulatory Surgery Unit, State University of New York Downstate Medical Center, Brooklyn, New York

MICHAEL T. WALSH, MD
Assistant Professor of Anesthesiology, Department of Anesthesiology, Mayo Clinic, Rochester, Minnesota

PAUL F. WHITE, PhD, MD, FANZCA
Professor and Margret Milam McDermott Distinguished Chair, Department of Anesthesiology and Pain Management, University of Texas Southwestern Medical Center, Dallas, Texas; Visiting Scientist and Professor, Cedars Sinai Medical Center, Los Angeles, California; Policlinico Abano, Leonardo Foundation, Abano Terme; Visiting Professor of Anesthesia, Pharma University, Parma, Italy; President, The White Mountain Institute, Los Altos, California

Contents

FORTHCOMING ISSUES

September 2010
Current Topics in Anesthesia for Head and Neck Surgery
Joshua H. Atkins, MD,
and Jeff E. Mandel, MD,
Guest Editors

December 2010
Quality in Anesthesia
Elizabeth A. Martinez, MD,
and Mark Neuman, MD,
Guest Editors

RECENT ISSUES

March 2010
Anesthesia for Patients Too Sick for Anesthesia
Benjamin A. Kohl, MD, and
Stanley H. Rosenbaum, MD,
Guest Editors

December 2009
Preoperative Medical Consultation: A Multidisciplinary Approach
Lee A. Fleisher, MD, FACC, and
Stanley H. Rosenbaum, MD,
Guest Editors

September 2009
Problems with Geriatric Anesthesia Patients
Jeffrey H. Silverstein, MD,
Guest Editor

Foreword
Ambulatory Anesthesia

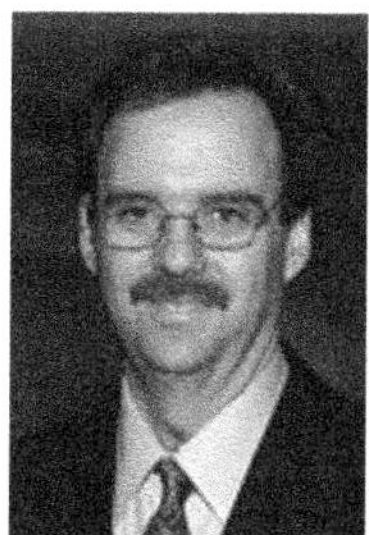

Lee A. Fleisher, MD
Consulting Editor

Over the past 40 years, there has been a marked increase in the percentage of patients having surgery in an ambulatory setting. This has been the result of multiple factors, including the development of new anesthetic and analgesic agents, new surgical techniques and technology, and an increased desire to reduce costs and improve patient convenience. This issue contains a series of articles highlighting some of the important questions related to delivery of ambulatory care and means of measuring and improving outcomes. It also highlights some of the issues related to a growing area of ambulatory practice—the office-based setting.

As Guest Editor for this issue, I am fortunate to have Peter Stanley Abraham Glass, MB, ChB, Professor and Chairman, Department of Anesthesiology at Stony Brook University Medical Center. He has authored 96 original articles and 40 book chapters. He has conducted many funded investigations related to delivery of anesthesia and analgesia in the outpatient setting. He has been President of the Society for Intravenous Anesthesia and is an active member and currently Secretary of the Society for Ambulatory Anesthesia. Given his research, education, and leadership roles, he has been able to assemble an outstanding group of contributors to this issue of *Anesthesiology Clinics*.

Lee A. Fleisher, MD
University of Pennsylvania School of Medicine
3400 Spruce Street, Dulles 680
Philadelphia, PA 19104, USA

E-mail address:
fleishel@uphs.upenn.edu

Anesthesiology Clin 28 (2010) xiii
doi:10.1016/j.anclin.2010.03.003
anesthesiology.theclinics.com

Preface

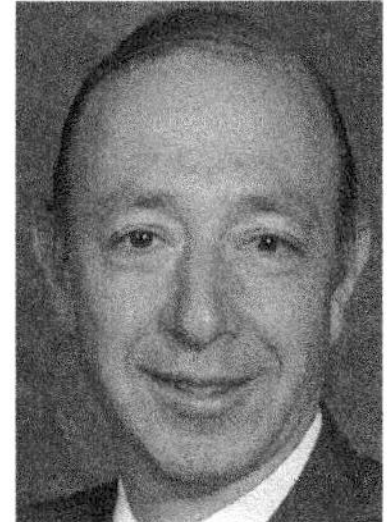

Peter S.A. Glass, MB, ChB
Guest Editor

This issue of *Anesthesiology Clinics* is devoted to ambulatory and office-based anesthesia. Outpatient/ambulatory or same-day surgery is not really new. James Nicoll documented the successful administration of 8,988 ambulatory anesthetics in England in a 10-year period from 1899 to 1908. Ralph Waters opened an outpatient facility in 1918 in Sioux City, Iowa. The successes of anesthesia and surgery led to a greater trend toward hospitalization. Despite occasional publications in the surgical literature, there was little organized effort to pursue outpatient surgery and anesthesia until the 1960s. In 1962, the University of California, Los Angeles, opened an outpatient surgical clinic within the hospital. In 1966, George Washington University Hospital opened its ambulatory surgical facility, and in 1970, Reed and Ford opened the Surgicenter in Phoenix, Arizona, the first ambulatory surgery center (ASC) that was not affiliated with an acute care hospital. Freestanding ASCs grew from 459 in 1985 to 1,381 in 1990. In 1974, national societies dedicated to the field began to appear. In 1984, the Society for Ambulatory Anesthesia was organized as the first and only specialty society within the American Society of Anesthesiologists dedicated to ambulatory anesthesia. Over the past more than 40 years, ambulatory surgery and its extension into the office has grown to approximately 70% of all surgical procedures performed in the United States. There have been several drivers that have facilitated this conversion from inpatient to outpatient surgery. These include enhanced quality of patient care with increasing patient satisfaction, financial incentives, pharmacologic and technical advances in anesthesia, and, lastly, major technical advances in surgical procedures.

Probably the most significant of these drivers has been a combination of economic advantages coupled with improved quality of care and patient satisfaction that ambulatory surgery provided. In the 1960s and 1970s, there was great pressure on surgical bed capacity and a national cry to reduce health care spending. Several studies have compared surgical procedures (such as simple cataract extraction and cholecystectomy) done in a hospital with those done in an ASC. All demonstrated little difference in adverse outcomes (largely a lower rate of infection in an ASC) with greater patient satisfaction. Enhanced patient satisfaction was improved by the far better efficiency

Anesthesiology Clin 28 (2010) xv–xviii
doi:10.1016/j.anclin.2010.03.002 **anesthesiology.theclinics.com**
1932-2275/10/$ – see front matter

obtained within an ASC. This greater efficiency also was important in driving down the cost of the episode of care. A study performed by Blue Shield/Blue Cross in 1977 estimated that a procedure performed in an ASC cost 47% less than if performed within the hospital. As the cost of care was reduced and patient satisfaction improved, Medicare began increasing the number of procedures covered in ASCs. Private insurers encouraged this trend and in the 1990s, Medicare actually cut back on reimbursement for a number of procedures that were performed in a hospital. This site of service differential has become the norm for private and government insurers, thereby solidifying the role of ambulatory surgery. The growth of ambulatory surgery has not been universal, with many European countries having 10% or fewer surgeries done on a same-day basis.

At the same time that economic incentives were at work, there were simultaneous advances in drugs available to anesthesiologists to provide anesthesia that enabled rapid recovery of patients from anesthesia. In addition, more effective drugs for the treatment of pain and anesthesia side effects, such as postoperative nausea and vomiting (PONV), were being released. Propofol probably has had the most significant impact on ambulatory anesthesia. As an induction and a maintenance agent, it enhanced the speed and quality of recovery. Probably the quality of recovery by creating awake patients without the feeling of a hangover and a marked reduction in the incidence of PONV (and the possible reduction in postoperative pain) played a significant role in the acceptability by patients of having their surgery on an ambulatory basis. The introduction of propofol also led to the enormous growth of providing moderate and deep sedation for minimally invasive or less-invasive surgeries and procedures done under local or regional anesthesia. Although sedation may seem an easier and safer technique than general anesthesia, review of the Medicare database as well as state audits have shown this is not true. Performing safe and effective deep sedation is an important skill that anesthesia providers need to acquire to work in an ASC environment. Drs Hession and Joshi provide the science and art of sedation.

At the same time, short-acting analgesics (fentanyl, alfentanil, and remifentanil) and neuromuscular blockers (atracurium, vecuronium, cisatracurium, and mivacurium) were introduced, making it easier for anesthesiologists to provide intense analgesia and profound neuromuscular blockade yet allowing patients to wake up within minutes and leave the ASC for their own home within an hour of completing a surgical procedure. This ability to titrate anesthetic drugs more precisely was enhanced by increasing knowledge of drug interactions during anesthesia and the development of brain function monitors.

As PONV was recognized as the most undesirable side effect of anesthesia, a greater effort was made in understanding its pathophysiology; at the same time, new drugs with fewer side effects became available (serotonin-3 antagonists). In this issue, one of the leaders in the field of PONV, Dr Gan and colleagues, provide a review of these advances and current management of PONV.

The management of postoperative pain presented an equal challenge to insuring the growth of ambulatory surgery. Again, increasing knowledge of pain pathophysiology, concepts of multimodal analgesia, and new compounds all contributed in making sure that patients had adequate pain control postoperatively. A major leader in the field of postoperative pain management has been Dr White. In this issue of *Anesthesiology Clinics*, he and Dr Elvir-Lazo provide an overview of current knowledge on how best to manage postoperative pain in the ambulatory environment.

In line with the increasing knowledge of multimodal analgesia, an increasing interest in regional analgesia occurred. Technological advances in ultrasound imaging further stimulated increasing use of regional anesthesia. At the same time, the advantages and safety of continuous regional catheters for patients discharged home became evident. Swenson and colleagues and Jacob and colleagues present 2 excellent articles that bring readers up to date with the use of regional anesthesia, ultrasound, and catheters for regional anesthesia blockade.

Another technological advance that has had a major impact on the practice of ambulatory anesthesia is the advent of the laryngeal mask airway. Although its development probably did not add to the actual growth of ambulatory surgery, it had a significant impact on how anesthesia is practiced in this environment as well as helping to minimize postoperative sore throat. Drs Luba and Cutter provide a complete overview of laryngeal mask airways presently available to anesthesia practitioners.

Probably the largest population that has embraced ambulatory surgery is doctors working with children. The whole concept of reduced anxiety, efficient care, and rapid return to a friendly environment makes ambulatory surgery ideal for pediatric patients. They present their own challenges for care in an ASC. Drs Collins and Everett provide an excellent review of how to take care of pediatric patients for ambulatory anesthesia.

As rapidly as the practice of anesthesia has changed to enhance ambulatory surgery, so has technology within surgery. Endoscopic equipment advances have almost paralleled the growth in ambulatory surgical volume. Advances in imaging, catheters, and minimally invasive techniques have combined to move procedures that were done in a hospital setting followed by days of recovery in a hospital bed to an ambulatory environment with recovery at home.

ASCs grew in number, size, and complexity. To this end, great emphasis has been placed on effective management of ASCs so that they can continue to provide the advantages that were evident in their initial evolution. Although ASCs are a social-based business, they still lend themselves well to management principles as Six Sigma or Toyota's lean production system. Drs Merrill and Laur provide readers with an excellent approach (based on their own ASC) to providing highly effective management in this environment.

With the increasing move to ambulatory surgery, patients were no longer available to be seen by an anesthesia provider the evening before surgery. Similarly, patients who were to be admitted to the hospital post surgery were also being admitted only on the morning of surgery. This led to the need for an alternative method of seeing patients and optimizing them before surgery and anesthesia. The preoperative clinic was established to accommodate this role. As preoperative clinics evolved, the question of what preoperative work-up was really needed began to be asked. Incorporated in this question was who needed to be seen and what preoperative testing was appropriate. Several articles appeared demonstrating that patients received excessive preoperative testing and that for some procedures (eg, lens extraction), no testing, even in the sickest of patients, is required. How much testing for ambulatory patients is needed is not yet fully resolved. Dr Richman provides the most recent evidence available to answer this question.

As time passes, old diseases become more prominent as knowledge of their cause and impact becomes more evident. A classic example of this is obstructive sleep apnea (OSA). The publication of the American Society of Anesthesiologists guidelines on the management of OSA generated much concern and consternation as to how these patients were to be evaluated preoperatively and how they were to be managed intraoperatively. This stimulated increasing research in this area. Frances Chung and her group in Toronto have published extensively and contributed significant new information on OSA and anesthesia. We are lucky to have her group provide an update on OSA and anesthetic management.

With the success of ambulatory surgery within ASCs, practitioners began to push the envelope further by performing low-risk procedures within an office setting. This is now the fastest growing market within ambulatory surgery. This environment has created the greatest challenge to anesthesia providers for a variety of reasons. Not only is the physical space limited, but also anesthesia equipment is rarely available and needs to be brought onto the premises each time surgery is scheduled; expectations of surgeons and patients are high. In addition, many states have not yet regulated office-based surgery and anesthesia, thus standards vary considerably across sites. Already, several disasters occurring with office-based surgery have been exposed in the lay press. Thus, it is important that anesthesia providers contemplating providing anesthesia in an office setting familiarize themselves with the pitfalls and minimum standards promulgated by the American Society of Anesthesiologists. Drs Kurrek and Twersky have been leaders in creating these standards and provide readers with an excellent overview of what is needed in setting up an office-based anesthesiology practice, whereas Dr Ahmad provides many practical approaches in providing anesthesia care in an office setting.

Peter S.A. Glass, MB, ChB
Department of Anesthesiology
School of Medicine
SUNY Stony Brook
HSC Level 4, Room 060
Stony Brook, NY 11794-8480, USA

E-mail address:
pglass@notes.cc.sunysb.edu

Ambulatory Surgery: How Much Testing Do We Need?

Deborah C. Richman, MBChB, FFA(SA)[a,b,*]

KEYWORDS

• Preoperative • Laboratory • Testing • Ambulatory
• Surgery • Assessment

Preoperative testing is done to predict risk, alter management, and improve outcomes. If this is the premise, then each test needs to be considered with one or all of these three aims in mind.

Currently more than two thirds of surgeries in the United States are done on an ambulatory basis. Apfelbaum predicts the growth of ambulatory surgeries to be close to 80% of all surgeries[1] in the United States within the next couple of years.

Patient selection is a major factor in running a successful ambulatory surgery unit with good patient outcomes. Different models of ambulatory surgery centers have different selection criteria. Some may offer full-service anesthesia and physically be part of the main hospital making admission a possibility, as part of the process. Others may not want the inefficiency of fiber-optic intubation for the difficult intubation and screen these patients out. Still others are free standing and admission is not an acceptable option, rather a complication and continuous quality improvement factor; consequently they have stricter selection criteria for appropriate patients.

Traditionally, preoperative testing has been part of the screening process for appropriate preoperative care and selection. Preoperative testing costs this country an estimated $18 billion annually. Ambulatory surgery is by definition low-risk surgery[2] and patients, who are usually American Society of Anesthesiologists (ASA) physical status 1 or 2, expect to be discharged home safely. Mortality risk in ASA 1 and 2 patients is 0.06% to 0.08% and 0.27% to 0.4%[3–5] in all surgeries, much lower in this low-risk category.

[a] Department of Anesthesiology, Stony Brook University Medical Center, Stony Brook, NY 11794-8480, USA
[b] Preoperative Services, c/o Department of Anesthesiology, Stony Brook University Medical Center, Stony Brook, NY 11794-8480, USA
* Department of Anesthesiology, Stony Brook University Medical Center, Stony Brook, NY 11794-8480.
E-mail address: drichman@notes.cc.sunysb.edu

Anesthesiology Clin 28 (2010) 185–197
doi:10.1016/j.anclin.2010.03.001 anesthesiology.theclinics.com

Measuring differences in outcomes, when poor outcomes are so rare, needs appropriately powered, randomized controlled studies. Many studies have been published since the late 1970s supporting selective testing. Although various organizations, including the ASA and the Society for Perioperative Assessment and Quality Improvement, and agencies, such as Centers for Medicare and Medicaid Services, have supported appropriate and minimal testing there is still confusion about what is appropriate and resultantly minimal buy in into these cost-saving and evidence-backed initiatives.

EVIDENCE

It has long been accepted that no routine testing is indicated. Preoperative tests without specific indications lack utility. Few abnormalities detected by nonspecific testing result in changes in management, even in the elderly, and rarely have such changes benefited patients or lack of testing affected safe anesthesia.[6] It has also been demonstrated that eliminating routine testing does not increase risk.[7–9] Although Schein's work is procedure specific (cataract), these findings can potentially be extrapolated to other low-risk surgeries.

Statistically normal results are defined as within two standard deviations of the mean, which means that 5% of normal people will have an abnormal result when just one test is performed. The more tests, the more abnormal results, but not necessarily the more abnormalities. The major impacts of unnecessary testing are patient anxiety, increased costs, delays while waiting for further tests and consults, and possible injury from unnecessary workups. The economic impact is a combination of added testing costs and impact on operating room schedule. There are also medico-legal implications of not following up on abnormal test results.[10–12] Abnormal test results can lead to injury[10] (1 in 2000) associated with further workup.

Routine testing has a frequency of abnormal results in 0.0% to 2.6% in multiple studies reviewed.[13] When selective testing is done, abnormal results are more frequent: 30% in a study by Charpak and colleagues.[14] These abnormal results are not unexpected and were more likely to change management.

Attempts have been made to introduce testing guidelines following evidence from the literature. These guidelines are not yet uniformly followed, despite more than 30 years of evidence and education. A recent retrospective chart review from Canada[15] found a big variance in compliance with ordering guidelines (5%–98%). Only 61.6% of all the tests performed were normal, but management was affected by only 2.6% of the tests. Katz and colleagues[16] found a similar magnitude of over ordering compared with local guidelines.

Kaplan and colleagues[11] in his study of 2000 subjects found that 60% of tests were not indicated, and only 0.22% of these abnormal results prompted some management change. Another study of 991 subjects older than 40 years of age, by Ajimura and colleagues[17] found 52.5% had some laboratory abnormality, but none lead to a change in management.

A recent pilot study from Canada advocates no preoperative testing in ambulatory patients. Chung and colleagues[8] showed no difference between the routine testing and no testing groups in ambulatory surgery patients with regard to adverse events at 7 and at 30 days. There were several limitations to the study. Exclusion criteria selected out subjects with significant medical issues, especially cardiac and respiratory. Because bad outcomes are rare, the sample size was not large enough. Noncompliance was allowed; subjects wishing to be tested crossed over in the study. Further studies need to be done before no testing becomes the new routine. But the importance of this study is again raising the lack of benefit in testing, and in the current health economic climate this fact cannot be ignored.

As the majority of ambulatory patients are ASA 1 and 2, the goal of assessing these healthier patients is to detect any previously unrecognized disease that may increase perioperative risk above baseline. Mortality is low.[18] Warner and colleagues[19] found a 1- to 30-day postoperative major morbidity and mortality of 0.08% (n = 33) in a group of 38,598 ambulatory surgery subjects. Four subjects died: two of myocardial infarcts and two of unrelated motor vehicle accidents.

Do patients who are not ASA class 1 or 2 need to be treated differently? Natof,[20] in a study of more than 13 000 subjects, found that well-controlled subjects who were ASA class 3 were at no higher risk for postoperative complications than those in ASA class 1 or 2.

SPECIFIC POPULATIONS

Age

Older age is another concern as a risk factor. Previously published work by Chung and Mezei[21,22] showed no increase in major cardiovascular complications in the elderly compared with younger subjects, and to their advantage, the older group had a lower incidence of postoperative nausea and vomiting.

Extremes of age may confer higher risk for postoperative admission especially in infants less than 55 to 60 weeks post-conceptual age and also in elderly patients older than 85 years of age.[18] Preoperative testing does not appear to play a role in decreasing this risk.

Generally, age is not considered a risk factor for adverse outcomes in ambulatory surgery,[23] but a systematic review by Smetana and colleagues[24] found that age greater than 60 (odds ratio [OR] 2.09) and greater than 70 (OR 3.04) to be an independent risk factor for the development of postoperative pulmonary complications in all surgeries. Again testing does not play a role in decreasing these complications, only identifying those at risk.

Obesity

Obesity is not a risk factor for major adverse outcomes.[25] The review by Smetana and colleagues[24] found one study where morbid obesity is a predictor of postoperative pulmonary complications, but this remains controversial. Obesity is however, an independent risk factor for deep vein thrombosis.[26]

So What Do We Do?

The preoperative history and physical (H&P) are the key elements in patient assessment, which is backed by legislation and professional society standards. Basic Joint Commission regulatory requirements for all patients include a history and physical performed within 30 days of the procedure.[27] In addition, ASA has standards and guidelines for preanesthesia care[28] that specifically state that no routine testing is indicated.

In the Australian Incident Monitoring Study,[29,30] inadequate preoperative evaluation and communication problems were shown to be sentinel contributing factors to preventable major adverse events (incidence 3.1%) including death and major morbidity. Laboratory testing or lack thereof was not implicated in these complications.

How preoperative assessment is achieved varies by institution. Some assess patients only on the day of surgery, others have all patients come through a preoperative evaluation clinic approximately 2 weeks before surgery. Some authors[31,32] have found the latter method to be cost effective in reducing day of surgery cancellations, even in the healthier ambulatory population.

No testing substitutes for a history and physical examination. An important component of the history is assessing self-reported exercise tolerance. Reilly and colleagues[33] showed that postoperative complications were inversely related to exercise ability. Although the study group was major surgeries, this can be extrapolated to ambulatory surgery.

Tests should only be ordered if the result will change the anesthetic or surgical plan or decrease the risk of the procedure. If medical condition is stable, then laboratory tests performed in the preceding 4 months[34] to 1 year[35] can be used.

The following tests are the minimum to be considered:

Tests

Type and screen

- Surgeries with anticipated blood loss
- Rhesus antibody result needed for possible Rhogam therapy.

Pregnancy

Beta human chorionic gonadotrophin (bHCG) assay is recommended but not mandated by the ASA, and policy is institution specific. Mandated testing will identify some previously undiagnosed pregnancies, and elective surgery is then postponed, but this testing comes with a cost. A study by Kahn and colleagues quantified this cost as $3273/ true positive pregnancy test.[36] Consider testing in all women of reproductive age, except after hysterectomy or oophorectomy. This testing can be done on the day of surgery but is recommended earlier if history suggests pregnancy is a possibility, as cancellations on the day of surgery have a bigger economic impact.

It is not clear what the extent of the risk of anesthesia is to the fetus, but current practice is not to do elective surgery in patients who are pregnant when it can be delayed, because there is risk to the fetus, especially in the first trimester, and increased risk for miscarriage.[37]

Hemoglobin

Anemia is a marker of perioperative mortality.[19,38] It is unclear if the increased risk is from the underlying causative disease or the anemia itself.

Hemoglobin preoperatively may be indicated in patients with symptoms of anemia, history of bleed, chemotherapy, radiotherapy, chronic renal failure, and clinical findings compatible with anemia. It is indicated as a baseline in surgery where significant blood loss (>500cc)[39] is expected.

Platelet count

Platelet count is indicated if patients have personal or family history of bleeding or bruising.

Coagulation studies

Coagulation studies are only done when patients have a personal or family history of bleeding or bruising, in the presence of liver disease or metastases, severe malnutrition, Vitamin K deficiency, and patients on anticoagulant therapy. Abnormal results by routine screening have not shown clear positive predictive value for operative bleeding.[40–43]

Electrocardiogram

Twenty million preoperative electrocardiograms (ECGs) are performed each year, but there is no consensus by practitioners about whom, if anyone, should get these tests.

Recent publications[7,44–46] have questioned the value of the routine preoperative ECG and prior publications that included the ECG as part of the perioperative risk assessment,[47–50] may no longer be valid in this respect.

The utility of the screening 12 lead ECG for assessing for perioperative risk has been questioned. It is also unclear when an abnormal ECG should alter management.[45,51] A meta-analysis[52] found the resting ECG to be a poor screening tool for coronary artery disease. One study by Tervahauta and colleagues[53] found that if evidence of CAD was present on screening ECG, there was higher mortality in this group, but the perioperative implications of this non-surgery–related work are not known. Van Klei and colleagues[46] found, in a prospective observational study in subjects older than 50 years of age having non-cardiac surgery, that 45% of subjects had an abnormality on preoperative ECG, and bundle branch blocks were associated with postoperative myocardial infarction and death, but had no added predictive value over recognized risk factors such as gender, age, and the components of the revised cardiac risk index[49] (high-risk surgery, history of one or more of the following: ischemic heart disease, congestive heart failure, chronic renal failure, cerebrovascular accident, insulin dependent diabetes).

Correll and colleagues found that age greater than 65 years was an independent predictor of preoperative electrocardiogram abnormalities[54] but any management change was already indicated by the H&P. Rabkin and Horne[55] showed new ECG changes caused no cancellations, only minor change in anesthesia technique in 1% of subjects, and no difference in outcome.

The specificity of an ECG abnormality in predicting postoperative cardiac adverse events is only 26% and a normal ECG does not exclude cardiac disease.[45]

An ECG should not be done simply because of age. Previous recommendations for age-based testing were derived from the high number of ECG abnormalities found on patients who were elderly. The Centers for Medicare and Medicaid Services do not reimburse for preoperative or age-based ECGs.[56]

The ASA Preoperative Evaluation Practice Advisory recognized that ECGs did not improve prediction beyond risk factors identified by patient history.[28]

The AHA makes the following recommendations for preoperative ECG.[2]

Class 1: Recommendations for resting ECG are in patients undergoing vascular surgery or in those undergoing intermediate risk procedures who have known coronary artery, cerebrovascular, or peripheral vascular disease. If we accept ambulatory surgery as low risk, then this does not apply to the ambulatory subset of patients. But what about the 3-hour shoulder repair? Orthopedic surgery is considered intermediate risk, or does the arthroscopic component of this procedure make it an endoscopic procedure and thus a low-risk procedure? This question causes controversy.

Class 2a: Patients for vascular surgery with no risk factors

Class 2b: Patients with one risk factor for intermediate risk surgery

Class 3: Patients for low risk surgery who are asymptomatic (ECG should not be performed because it is not helpful and may even be harmful).

These recommendations suggest that patients undergoing ambulatory surgery (low risk) should not get ECGs if they are asymptomatic. Patients with class 2 angina pectoris undergoing a knee arthroscopy are low risk and symptomatic; which class does this fall into? There is no doubt that there are still a lot of unknowns out there. Ideally, perhaps the annual ECG from the primary care physician (PCP) would be adequate if symptoms were stable over the interceding interval. Reading further into the text of the AHA guidelines and the primary article,[18] it is suggested that stable (not asymptomatic) ambulatory patients need not have ECGs because morbidity and mortality associated with these procedures is so low and risk is negligible.

Chemistry

A review by Smetana and Macpherson[13] found that only 1.8% of electrolyte tests affected management and most of these were predictable from patients' history of renal disease or diuretic use.

Electrolytes: Consider testing if there have been recent changes in medication known to affect electrolytes (eg, diuretics, steroids) or in patients on digoxin. Also consider checking potassium in end-stage renal disease.

Chronic renal failure with a creatinine greater than 2mg/dl is an independent risk factor for perioperative morbidity and mortality.[2,24] Creatinine is indicated if patients are to receive contrast media. If the test is abnormal renal protective strategies can be used or an alternative study can be performed. Consider for risk assessment if it will affect informed consent, and no recent testing results are available.

Glucose should be checked on admission in patients who are diabetic and hourly in procedures lasting longer than 1 hour. Presuming that patients who are diabetic have good routine care, including regular glucose checks; a HBA1C less than seven; and assessment for end organ damage,[57] specifically workup of cardiac symptoms or abnormal ECG and a serum creatinine, then it is not necessary to test further for minor surgery.

Urinalysis

Urinalysis (UA) is never indicated for anesthesia. For orthopedic surgery with hardware implants, a urinalysis is frequently ordered to decrease the risk for subsequent infection. It is rare that the organisms associated with asymptomatic bacteruria cause orthopedic infection, and the administration of preoperative prophylactic antibiotics, which is standard of care, is usually enough to prevent this anyway. However, the catastrophic outcome of an infected joint is cited by the surgeons as a reason to maintain the practice of ordering UAs. No difference was found in wound infections in knee surgery whether UA was normal or abnormal. It was estimated by Lawrence[58,59] that the cost of treating wound infections (non-implant) was 500 times less than the cost of screening urinalyses and so these tests are not recommended.

Liver function tests

Albumin is a marker of chronic disease and markedly low levels may affect wound healing. It was the only laboratory predictor of postoperative pulmonary complications in the review by Smetana.[24]

Patients with acute hepatitis should not undergo elective surgery. Child-Pugh[60] grade C should also not undergo elective surgery. Those assessed as grade B are at increased risk and may benefit from therapy to improve their score before surgery. Decisions to perform these tests are guided by significant findings on history and physical examination.

Chest X ray

Chest X-Ray (CXR) abnormalities increase with age. A review of studies of routine preoperative CXRs by Joo and colleagues[61] found that most abnormalities are predicted on history and physical examination. Only 10% of those investigated for an abnormal CXR had a change in management. CXR usually only confirms clinical findings and is not useful at reducing risk.[62]

CXRs should be considered in patients with new signs or symptoms, history of end-stage renal disease, or decompensated heart failure, if it will change management. Patients with the latter are rarely candidates for the ambulatory setting except for minor procedures like ophthalmologic surgeries.

Cardiac evaluation

Cardiac evaluation is indicated based on the presence of active cardiac conditions[2] and patients with these are not current candidates for elective ambulatory surgery. Patients with unexplained dyspnea on exertion may warrant an echocardiogram – Class 2a.[2]

Heart failure, compensated and decompensated, carries increased risk for cardiac complications, approximately 5% to 7% and 20% to 30% respectively, and an echocardiogram may be considered for quantifying degree and type if it will change management.[63]

Pulmonary function testing

Postoperative pulmonary complications (PPC) are a common event (incidence ranges from 0%–75%).[64,65] They are more frequently associated with the presence of pulmonary risk factors and certain surgical factors: surgical site and length of procedure. Thoracic and upper abdominal surgeries are the highest risk procedures. Laparoscopic procedures significantly decrease the risk,[66] so surgical site is not usually a predisposing factor in ambulatory surgery. Duration of surgery greater than 2.5 to 4 hours confers increased risk.[24]

Independent patient risk factors for PPCs include smoking; pulmonary hypertension; obstructive sleep apnea[67] (see later discussion); morbid obesity; moderate to severe chronic obstructive pulmonary disease; congestive heart failure; poor general health, including baseline functional status (physical and mental); and age.[24]

Well-controlled asthma[68] and upper respiratory tract infections (URIs) are not risk factors for PPCs in adults. Patients with an intercurrent bronchitis of bacterial etiology are at a higher risk for postoperative pneumonia, and antibiotic therapy administered preoperatively can decrease this risk.[64] History, and not testing, affects outcome here.

A detailed history of pulmonary symptoms, medication compliance, presence of productive cough, and physical examination is adequate in patients undergoing ambulatory surgery. Pulmonary function testing (PFTs) is usually reserved for patients undergoing major non-ambulatory surgeries. A possible exception is the assessment of poorly controlled asthma to differentiate between severe asthma (not usually a candidate for ambulatory surgery) and inadequately treated bronchospasm. No studies have shown PFTs to improve outcomes.

Arterial blood gases

Arterial blood gases are not indicated in the ambulatory settings are they are markers of severe disease and these patients are not ambulatory candidates.

Sleep consult/polysomnography

Obstructive sleep apnea (OSA) is common with 4% of women and 25% of men having some degree of the disease. It is more common in the obese population.[69,70] The majority are undiagnosed.

Patients should be screened for OSA. The STOP/BANG screen[69] is a useful validated tool that can easily identify those who may have OSA. These patients can then be assessed for the need for further preoperative testing. The ASA[71] has published Practice Guidelines for the Perioperative Management of Patients with OSA. It applies an OSA scoring system (**Table 1**). The score takes into account the severity of the OSA, the invasiveness of the surgery, and the need for postoperative opiates. To accurately ascertain this score, polysomnography (PSG) is necessary. It should be ordered when the result would change the decision about venue, type of anesthesia, or proceeding with surgery.

In surgeries performed under local with or without sedation, PSG is advised for patients concurrently for health maintenance and risk reduction, but the results are not superior to clinical assessment in changing perioperative management and this workup can be done after surgery by the PCP.

Those patients with an OSA score of 5 or 6 are not appropriate for free-standing ambulatory centers. Patients with a score of 4 should be assessed on a case by case basis, especially if surgery interferes with use of continuous positive airway pressure (CPAP) or other OSA treatment devices.[70,71]

Patients also need to be monitored in recovery longer than their non-OSA counterparts. Patients with OSA should be first case or early enough in the day, especially in facilities that are not open overnight.

Pediatrics

Routine diagnostic testing in children is traumatic and this stress often leads to an uncooperative child on the day of surgery. Preoperative hemoglobin is not indicated in healthy children[72] unless there is anticipated blood loss. It can be considered in ex-premature infants if clinically indicated or not recently tested. Coagulation tests do not predict surgical bleeding in healthy children with no history of bleeding tendency or family history of bleeding disorders.[73] Many pediatricians and pediatric surgeons still insist on coagulation studies in surgeries where hemostasis is vital, specifically tonsillectomies and neurosurgical procedures.

Table 1
Scoring of Obstructive Sleep Apnea patient for management decisions

(maximum possible score = 6)		
Choose the higher of the following 2 scores and add to OSA severity score below:		
Opiate Need	**or**	**Surgical Invasiveness**
0 = None		0 = none
1 = Low dose oral		1 = Superficial/local anesthesia
2 = High dose oral		2 = Peripheral/general anesthesia
3 = Parenteral/neuroaxial		3 = Airway/major/abdominal
OSA Severity by PSG Result:		
1 = Mild		
2 = Moderate		
3 = Severe		

SUMMARY

Routine testing is not the standard of care. **Table 2** provides a summary of indicated testing for Ambulatory Surgical procedures.

There is no doubt that we are still over-testing preoperatively. We know that testing rarely changes management, and rarely affects outcome. We need to base our testing decisions on a good history and physical and evaluation of effort tolerance, and then order only those tests which offer information about risk—needed for informed consent; and those where expected results would alter management or outcome. Testing may need to be individualized to level of patient medical care and patient compliance.

It is recommended that anesthesiologists should be doing the ordering as they do it more appropriately and with effective cost reduction.[74]

Pasternak,[75] in an editorial advocates judicious testing and a formal structure for preoperative assessment for better implementation of evidence based management of patients.

There is already three decades of evidence in the literature supporting less testing, but as adverse outcomes are rare, we need better powered more inclusive prospective studies to back our current expert opinion based decisions.

Table 2
Summary of tests and their indications for ambulatory surgery (low risk surgery)

Test	Indicated	Guidelines	Exceptions
ECG	No	Class 3 AHA	—
Complete blood count	No	—	Anemia Anticipated blood loss Premature infants
bHCG	Yes by history	Institution specific	—
Coagulation studies/platelets	No	—	Personal/family history of bleeding diathesis Anticoagulants Liver disease ? Tonsillectomy and neurosurgery - controversial
Liver function tests	No	—	Risk assessment –cirrhosis Acute history
Pulmonary Functions	No	—	Only as part of routine management of asthma
Arterial blood gases	No	—	—
UA	No	—	Insertion of hardware
PSG	No	ASA practice advisory	Diagnosis of severe OSA will change venue
CXR	No	—	—
Type and screen	—	—	Anticipated blood loss >500cc Rhogam
Electrolytes	No	—	Recent change in medications affecting potassium/electrolytes
Creatinine	No	—	Contrast dye study
Glucose	No	—	Morning of surgery

We must also remember that even with best evidence studies, circumstances vary at different institutions and testing needs to be locally customized to the individual variations and restrictions of the practice.

REFERENCES

1. Apfelbaum J. Current controversies in adult outpatient anesthesia. Proceedings of ASA refresher course 2009; Ambulatory anesthesia 2009;115.
2. Fleisher LA, Beckman JA, Brown KA, et al. ACC/AHA 2007 guidelines on perioperative cardiovascular evaluation and care for noncardiac surgery: a report of the American College of Cardiology/American Heart Association Task Force on Practice Guidelines (Writing Committee to Revise the 2002 Guidelines on Perioperative Cardiovascular Evaluation for Noncardiac Surgery): developed in collaboration with the American Society of Echocardiography, American Society of Nuclear Cardiology, Heart Rhythm Society, Society of Cardiovascular Anesthesiologists, Society for Cardiovascular Angiography and Interventions, Society for Vascular Medicine and Biology, and Society for Vascular Surgery. Circulation 2007;116(17):e418–499.
3. Davenport DL, Bowe EA, Henderson WG, et al. National Surgical Quality Improvement Program (NSQIP) risk factors can be used to validate American Society of Anesthesiologists Physical Status Classification (ASA PS) levels. Ann Surg 2006;243(5):636–41 [discussion: 641–4].
4. Lagasse RS. Anesthesia safety: model or myth? A review of the published literature and analysis of current original data. Anesthesiology 2002;97(6):1609–17.
5. Morgan GE Jr, Murray MJ, et al. The practice of anesthesia. In: Clinical anesthesiology. 2002. p. 1–14.
6. Dzankic S, Pastor D, Gonzalez C, et al. The prevalence and predictive value of abnormal preoperative laboratory tests in elderly surgical patients. Anesth Analg 2001;93(2):301–8.
7. Schein OD, Katz J, Bass EB, et al. The value of routine preoperative medical testing before cataract surgery. Study of Medical Testing for Cataract Surgery. N Engl J Med 2000;342(3):168–75.
8. Chung F, Yuan H, Yin L, et al. Elimination of preoperative testing in ambulatory surgery. Anesth Analg 2009;108(2):467–75.
9. Narr BJ, Warner ME, Schroeder DR, et al. Outcomes of patients with no laboratory assessment before anesthesia and a surgical procedure. Mayo Clin Proc 1997; 72(6):505–9.
10. Apfelbaum J. Preoperation evaluation, laboratory screening, and selection of adult surgical outpatients in the 1990s. Anesthesiol Rev 1990;17(Suppl 2):4–12.
11. Kaplan EB, Sheiner LB, Boeckmann AJ, et al. The usefulness of preoperative laboratory screening. JAMA 1985;253(24):3576–81.
12. Gandhi TK, Kachalia A, Thomas EJ, et al. Missed and delayed diagnoses in the ambulatory setting: a study of closed malpractice claims. Ann Intern Med 2006; 145(7):488–96.
13. Smetana GW, Macpherson DS. The case against routine preoperative laboratory testing. Med Clin North Am 2003;87(1):7–40.
14. Charpak Y, Blery C, Chastang C, et al. Usefulness of selectively ordered preoperative tests. Med Care 1988;26(2):95–104.
15. Bryson GL, Wyand A, Bragg PR. Preoperative testing is inconsistent with published guidelines and rarely changes management. Can J Anaesth 2006;53(3):236–41.

16. Katz RI, Barnhart JM, Ho G, et al. A study on the frequency of unnecessary laboratory testing for surgery. Abstract presented at ASA, 2008.
17. Ajimura FY, Maia AS, Hachiya A, et al. Preoperative laboratory evaluation of patients aged over 40 years undergoing elective non-cardiac surgery. Sao Paulo Med J 2005;123(2):50–3.
18. Fleisher LA, Pasternak LR, Herbert R, et al. Inpatient hospital admission and death after outpatient surgery in elderly patients: importance of patient and system characteristics and location of care. Arch Surg 2004;139(1):67–72.
19. Warner MA, Shields SE, Chute CG. Major morbidity and mortality within 1 month of ambulatory surgery and anesthesia. JAMA 1993;270(12):1437–41.
20. Natof H. Ambulatory surgery: patients with pre-existing medical problems. Ill Med J 1984;166(2):101.
21. Chung F, Mezei G. Factors contributing to a prolonged stay after ambulatory surgery. Anesth Analg 1999;89(6):1352–9.
22. Chung F, Mezei G, Tong D. Pre-existing medical conditions as predictors of adverse events in day-case surgery. Br J Anaesth 1999;83(2):262–70.
23. Meridy HW. Criteria for selection of ambulatory surgical patients and guidelines for anesthetic management: a retrospective study of 1553 cases. Anesth Analg 1982;61(11):921–6.
24. Smetana GW, Lawrence VA, Cornell JE. Preoperative pulmonary risk stratification for noncardiothoracic surgery: systematic review for the American College of Physicians. Ann Intern Med 2006;144(8):581–95.
25. Dindo D, Muller MK, Weber M, et al. Obesity in general elective surgery. Lancet 2003;361(9374):2032–5.
26. Ageno W, Becattini C, Brighton T, et al. Cardiovascular risk factors and venous thromboembolism: a meta-analysis. Circulation 2008;117(1):93–102.
27. Commission TJ. Joint Commission Standard: RC.02.01.03, PC.01.02.03, EP 5.
28. American Society of Anesthesiologists Task Force on Preanesthesia Evaluation. Practice advisory for preanesthesia evaluation: a report by the American Society of Anesthesiologists Task Force on Preanesthesia Evaluation. Anesthesiology 2002;96(2):485–96.
29. Kluger MT, Tham EJ, Coleman NA, et al. Inadequate pre-operative evaluation and preparation: a review of 197 reports from the Australian incident monitoring study. Anaesthesia 2000;55(12):1173–8.
30. Holland R, Webb RK, Runciman WB. The Australian Incident Monitoring Study. Oesophageal intubation: an analysis of 2000 incident reports. Anaesth Intensive Care 1993;21(5):608–10.
31. Ferschl MB, Tung A, Sweitzer B, et al. Preoperative clinic visits reduce operating room cancellations and delays. Anesthesiology 2005;103(4):855–9.
32. Correll DJ, Bader AM, Hull MW, et al. Value of preoperative clinic visits in identifying issues with potential impact on operating room efficiency. Anesthesiology 2006;105(6):1254–9 [discussion: 1256A].
33. Reilly DF, McNeely MJ, Doerner D, et al. Self-reported exercise tolerance and the risk of serious perioperative complications. Arch Intern Med 1999;159(18):2185–92.
34. Macpherson DS, Snow R, Lofgren RP. Preoperative screening: value of previous tests. Ann Intern Med 1990;113(12):969–73.
35. Roizen MF. More preoperative assessment by physicians and less by laboratory tests. N Engl J Med 2000;342(3):204–5.
36. Kahn RL, Stanton MA, Tong-Ngork S, et al. One-year experience with day-of-surgery pregnancy testing before elective orthopedic procedures. Anesth Analg 2008;106(4):1127–31.

37. Mazze RI, Kallen B. Reproductive outcome after anesthesia and operation during pregnancy: a registry study of 5405 cases. Am J Obstet Gynecol 1989;161(5): 1178–85.
38. Wu WC, Schifftner TL, Henderson WG, et al. Preoperative hematocrit levels and postoperative outcomes in older patients undergoing noncardiac surgery. JAMA 2007;297(22):2481–8.
39. Greenberg J. Preoperative laboratory testing. Proceedings of UCLA HealthCare 2004 (Fall);8. Available at: http://www.med.ucla.edu/modules/wfsection/article.php?articleid=28. Accessed March 4, 2010.
40. Suchman AL, Mushlin AI. How well does the activated partial thromboplastin time predict postoperative hemorrhage? JAMA 1986;256(6):750–3.
41. Sie P, Steib A. Central laboratory and point of care assessment of perioperative hemostasis. Can J Anaesth 2006;53(Suppl 6):S12–20.
42. Bushick JB, Eisenberg JM, Kinman J, et al. Pursuit of abnormal coagulation screening tests generates modest hidden preoperative costs. J Gen Intern Med 1989;4(6):493–7.
43. Macpherson CR, Jacobs P, Dent DM. Abnormal peri-operative haemorrhage in asymptomatic patients is not predicted by laboratory testing. S Afr Med J 1993;83(2):106–8.
44. Noordzij PG, Boersma E, Bax JJ, et al. Prognostic value of routine preoperative electrocardiography in patients undergoing noncardiac surgery. Am J Cardiol 2006;97(7):1103–6.
45. Liu LL, Dzankic S, Leung JM. Preoperative electrocardiogram abnormalities do not predict postoperative cardiac complications in geriatric surgical patients. J Am Geriatr Soc 2002;50(7):1186–91.
46. van Klei WA, Bryson GL, Yang H, et al. The value of routine preoperative electrocardiography in predicting myocardial infarction after noncardiac surgery. Ann Surg 2007;246(2):165–70.
47. Goldman L, Caldera DL, Nussbaum SR, et al. Multifactorial index of cardiac risk in noncardiac surgical procedures. N Engl J Med 1977;297(16):845–50.
48. Detsky AS, Abrams HB, Forbath N, et al. Cardiac assessment for patients undergoing noncardiac surgery. A multifactorial clinical risk index. Arch Intern Med 1986;146(11):2131–4.
49. Lee TH, Marcantonio ER, Mangione CM, et al. Derivation and prospective validation of a simple index for prediction of cardiac risk of major noncardiac surgery. Circulation 1999;100(10):1043–9.
50. Eagle KA, Berger PB, Calkins H, et al. ACC/AHA guideline update for perioperative cardiovascular evaluation for noncardiac surgery—executive summary a report of the American College of Cardiology/American Heart Association Task Force on Practice Guidelines (Committee to Update the 1996 Guidelines on Perioperative Cardiovascular Evaluation for Noncardiac Surgery). Circulation 2002;105(10):1257–67.
51. Dorman T, Breslow MJ, Pronovost PJ, et al. Bundle-branch block as a risk factor in noncardiac surgery. Arch Intern Med 2000;160(8):1149–52.
52. Sox HC Jr, Garber AM, Littenberg B. The resting electrocardiogram as a screening test. A clinical analysis. Ann Intern Med 1989;111(6):489–502.
53. Tervahauta M, Pekkanen J, Punsar S, et al. Resting electrocardiographic abnormalities as predictors of coronary events and total mortality among elderly men. Am J Med 1996;100(6):641–5.
54. Correll DJ, Hepner DL, Chang C, et al. Preoperative electrocardiograms: patient factors predictive of abnormalities. Anesthesiology 2009;110(6):1217–22.

55. Rabkin SW, Horne JM. Preoperative electrocardiography effect of new abnormalities on clinical decisions. Can Med Assoc J 1983;128(2):146–7.
56. CMS. Centers for Medicare and Medicaid Services. Federal Register / Vol. 66, No. 226 / Friday, November 23, 2001 / Rules and Regulations. Available at: http://www.cms.hhs.gov.
57. American Diabetes Association. Standards of medical care in diabetes–2009. Diabetes Care 2009;32(Suppl 1):S13–61.
58. Lawrence VA, Gafni A, Gross M. The unproven utility of the preoperative urinalysis: economic evaluation. J Clin Epidemiol 1989;42(12):1185–92.
59. Lawrence VA, Kroenke K. The unproven utility of preoperative urinalysis. Clinical use. Arch Intern Med 1988;148(6):1370–3.
60. Pugh RN, Murray-Lyon IM, Dawson JL, et al. Transection of the oesophagus for bleeding oesophageal varices. Br J Surg 1973;60(8):646–9.
61. Joo HS, Wong J, Naik VN, et al. The value of screening preoperative chest x-rays: a systematic review. Can J Anaesth 2005;52(6):568–74.
62. Lawrence VA, Cornell JE, Smetana GW. Strategies to reduce postoperative pulmonary complications after noncardiothoracic surgery: systematic review for the American College of Physicians. Ann Intern Med 2006;144(8):596–608.
63. Sweitzer B. Preoperative evaluation and preparation. Proceedings of ASA Refresher Course Fundamentals of Anethesia 310. 2009.
64. Mohr DN, Lavender RC. Preoperative pulmonary evaluation. Identifying patients at increased risk for complications. Postgrad Med 1996;100(5):241–4, 247-248, 251-242 passim.
65. Pedersen T, Eliasen K, Henriksen E. A prospective study of risk factors and cardiopulmonary complications associated with anaesthesia and surgery: risk indicators of cardiopulmonary morbidity. Acta Anaesthesiol Scand 1990;34(2):144–55.
66. McMahon AJ, Russell IT, Ramsay G, et al. Laparoscopic and minilaparotomy cholecystectomy: a randomized trial comparing postoperative pain and pulmonary function. Surgery 1994;115(5):533–9.
67. Hwang D, Shakir N, Limann B, et al. Association of sleep-disordered breathing with postoperative complications. Chest 2008;133(5):1128–34.
68. Warner DO, Warner MA, Barnes RD, et al. Perioperative respiratory complications in patients with asthma. Anesthesiology 1996;85(3):460–7.
69. Chung F, Yegneswaran B, Liao P, et al. STOP questionnaire: a tool to screen patients for obstructive sleep apnea. Anesthesiology 2008;108(5):812–21.
70. Mickelson SA. Preoperative and postoperative management of obstructive sleep apnea patients. Otolaryngol Clin North Am 2007;40(4):877–89.
71. Gross JB, Bachenberg KL, Benumof JL, et al. Practice guidelines for the perioperative management of patients with obstructive sleep apnea: a report by the American Society of Anesthesiologists Task Force on Perioperative Management of patients with obstructive sleep apnea. Anesthesiology 2006;104(5):1081–93 [quiz: 1117–8].
72. Baron MJ, Gunter J, White P. Is the pediatric preoperative hematocrit determination necessary? South Med J 1992;85(12):1187–9.
73. Burk CD, Miller L, Handler SD, et al. Preoperative history and coagulation screening in children undergoing tonsillectomy. Pediatrics 1992;89(4 Pt 2):691–5.
74. Finegan BA, Rashiq S, McAlister FA, et al. Selective ordering of preoperative investigations by anesthesiologists reduces the number and cost of tests. Can J Anaesth 2005;52(6):575–80.
75. Pasternak LR. Preoperative testing: moving from individual testing to risk management. Anesth Analg 2009;108(2):393–4.

Obstructive Sleep Apnea: Preoperative Assessment

Edwin Seet, MBBS, MMed[a], Frances Chung, MD, FRCPC[b,*]

KEYWORDS

- Anesthesia • Obstructive sleep apnea
- Preoperative assessment • Perioperative management
- Polysomnography

Upper airway patency is essential for normal respiratory function. The maintenance of a patent airway is dependent primarily on the pharyngeal structures. In some individuals, there is a loss of this airway patency from collapse of pharyngeal soft tissue, and interruption of airflow occurs during sleep. Obstructive sleep apnea (OSA) is caused by repetitive partial or complete obstruction of the upper airway, characterized by episodes of breathing cessation during sleep, which last 10 or more seconds.

From the anesthesiologists' standpoint, patients with OSA pose significant problems in the perioperative period, including difficult airways, sensitivity to anesthetic agents, and postoperative adverse events. OSA has been associated with an increase in postoperative complications,[1,2] and is an independent risk factor for increased morbidity and mortality.[3,4]

A recent retrospective matched cohort study in elective surgical patients with OSA showed that patients with OSA had an increased incidence of postoperative oxygen desaturation, with a hazard ratio of 2.[2] In addition, there is a growing body of literature showing that patients with OSA undergoing upper airway surgery,[5,6] joint replacement surgery,[7] and cardiac surgery[8] have an increased risk of postoperative complications.

Optimal patient care begins with a tailored preoperative assessment, to facilitate patient risk stratification and optimization, followed by formulation of an individualized perioperative management plan.

PREVALENCE

OSA is the most prevalent breathing disturbance during sleep,[9] with an incidence in the general population estimated in the range of 1 in 4 men and 1 in 10 women.[10]

[a] Department of Anesthesia, Alexandra Health Private Limited, Khoo Teck Puat Hospital, 90 Yishun Central, Postal Code 768828, Singapore
[b] Department of Anesthesia, University Health Network, University of Toronto, 399 Bathurst Street, McL 2-405, Toronto, ON, M5T 2S8, Canada
* Corresponding author.
E-mail address: Frances.Chung@uhn.on.ca

Anesthesiology Clin 28 (2010) 199–215
doi:10.1016/j.anclin.2010.02.002
anesthesiology.theclinics.com
1932-2275/10/$ – see front matter

Moderately severe OSA was present in twice as many men (11.4%) than women (4.7%).[11,12] Aside from male gender predominance, OSA is more prevalent in obese patients; there is a 7 in 10 risk of OSA in patients presenting for bariatric surgery.[13]

A significant proportion of patients with OSA are undiagnosed before surgery.[14] It is therefore increasingly recognized as a significant perioperative problem.

DIAGNOSIS OF OSA

The diagnosis of OSA is established by an overnight sleep study or polysomnography. The apnea hypopnea index (AHI) is the number of abnormal respiratory events per hour of sleep. Classically, the accepted minimal clinical diagnostic criteria for OSA are an AHI of 10 plus symptoms of excessive daytime sleepiness (American Academy of Sleep Medicine Task Force 1999). The United States Medicare guidelines diagnose OSA with an AHI of 15, or an AHI of 5 with 2 comorbidities. Canadian Thoracic Society guidelines stipulate the diagnostic criteria for OSA as having daytime sleepiness not explained by other factors, or at least 2 other symptoms of OSA (choking/gasping during sleep, recurrent awakenings from sleep, unrefreshing sleep, daytime fatigue, impaired concentration), with an AHI of 5 or more on polysomnography.[15]

AHI cutoffs have been frequently used to describe the severity of OSA. The American Academy of Sleep Medicine defines mild OSA as AHI between 5 and 15, moderate OSA as AHI between 15 and 30, and severe OSA as AHI more than 30.[16] Clinicians should be cognizant that different published standards of hypopnea definitions might lead to differences in AHI.[17]

Some other factors used in the evaluation of OSA severity include duration of oxygen desaturation, rate of desaturation, adequacy of ventilation recovery, and level/stability of arousal threshold.

COMORBIDITIES AND PREDISPOSING FACTORS ASSOCIATED WITH OSA

OSA is associated with several comorbidities (**Table 1**): cardiovascular disease,[18] including acute myocardial infarction,[19] heart failure,[20] arrhythmias,[21] hypertension,[22] cerebrovascular disease,[23] metabolic syndrome,[24] obesity, and gastroesophageal reflux.[25]

Certain patient profiles (male, >50 years old, neck circumference >40 cm), endocrine disorders (Cushing disease, hypothyroidism), connective tissue disorders (Marfan syndrome), lifestyle habits (alcohol, smoking), and anatomic abnormalities may predispose to OSA.[26]

Upper airway obstruction occurs when the negative pressure generated by the inspiratory muscles exceeds the capacity of dilator muscles of the upper airway to maintain airway patency.[27] Obesity, with fatty deposits in the tongue and upper airway, or altered upper airway anatomy (craniofacial abnormalities, macroglossia, retrognathia) reduce lumen diameter, increasing the propensity for episodic airway obstruction. Because of the close correlation of obesity and OSA, it has been suggested that screening for OSA and polysomnography be recommended for patients undergoing bariatric surgery.[28]

During the preoperative assessment, the anesthesiologist should be aware of these predisposing factors and comorbidities, to have a heightened index of suspicion when managing patients suspected of having OSA.

PRACTICAL SCREENING OF PATIENTS WITH SUSPECTED OSA IN THE PREOPERATIVE CLINIC

A large number of surgical patients with OSA are undiagnosed when they present for surgery and anesthesia. Polysomnographic diagnosis of OSA is prohibitive as it is

Table 1
Comorbidities associated with OSA

Category	Condition	Prevalence (%)
Cardiac	Treatment-resistant hypertension	63–83
	Congestive heart failure	76
	Ischemic heart disease	38
	Atrial fibrillation	49
	Dysrhythmias	58
Respiratory	Asthma	18
	Pulmonary hypertension	77
Neurologic	First-ever stroke	71–90
Metabolic	Type II diabetes mellitus	36
	Metabolic syndrome	50
	Hypothyroidism	45
	Morbid obesity	50–90
Surgical	Bariatric surgery	71
	Intracranial tumor surgery	64
	Epilepsy surgery	33
Others	Gastroesophageal reflux disease	60
	Nocturia	48
	Alcoholism	17
	Primary open-angle glaucoma	20
	Head and neck cancer	76

costly and resource-intensive. Therefore, anesthesiologists are in need of a practical preoperative screening tool to identify patients more likely to have true OSA. For safety reasons, the screening tool should have a high degree of sensitivity, at the expense of lower specificity.

In a preoperative survey of elective surgeries, 24% of patients were identified as having a high risk of OSA using the Berlin questionnaire.[29] In another study screening more than 2000 patients, 27.5% of them were classified as being at high risk of OSA when the STOP questionnaire was used.[30] In the preoperative anesthesia assessment, a high index of suspicion for OSA is important.

Snoring is the premier symptom of OSA, and is 100% sensitive. However, it is not specific and its positive predictive value is low. Several questionnaire-based screening tools have been successfully developed. The Berlin questionnaire is a 10-item self-report instrument validated initially in the primary care setting.[31] It consists of 5 questions on snoring, 3 questions on excessive daytime sleepiness, 1 question on sleepiness while driving, and 1 question inquiring about a history of hypertension. Details pertaining to age, gender, weight, height, and neck circumference are also recorded. A study screening preoperative patients using the Berlin questionnaire determined that it had a sensitivity of 69% and a specificity of 56% in surgical patients.[32] The drawback of the Berlin questionnaire is the complicated scoring system and the large number of questions.

In 2006, the American Society of Anesthesiologists (ASA) taskforce on OSA developed a tool to assist anesthesiologists in identifying patients with OSA. The tool comprises a 14-item checklist categorized into physical characteristics, history of apparent airway obstruction during sleep, and complaints of somnolence.[33] The sensitivity of the ASA checklist was 79% and 87% at AHI cutoff level of 15 or more and 30 or more.[32]

Subsequently, a more concise and easy-to-use clinical screening tool for anesthesiologists was developed (**Box 1**): the STOP questionnaire (S, snore loudly; T, daytime tiredness; O, observed to stop breathing during sleep; P, high blood pressure). The sensitivity of the STOP questionnaire with AHI of 15 or more and 30 or more as cutoffs was 74% and 80%, respectively, and the specificity 53% and 49%, respectively.[30] When incorporating 4 additional variables with the acronym Bang (B, body mass index [BMI, calculated as weight in kilograms divided by the square of height in meters] >35 kg/m^2; A, more than 50 years old; N, neck circumference greater than 40 cm; G, male gender), the STOP-Bang questionnaire (see **Box 1**) improved the sensitivity to 93% and 100% at AHI cutoffs of 15 or more and 30 or more, respectively.[30] The specificity of the STOP-Bang was 43% and 37%, respectively.

There was no significant difference in the predictive parameters of the Berlin questionnaire, the ASA checklist, and the STOP questionnaire. All the questionnaires showed a moderately high level of sensitivity for OSA screening (**Table 2**). The sensitivities of the Berlin questionnaire, the ASA checklist, and STOP questionnaire were similar: 69% to 87%, 72% to 87%, and 66% to 80% at different AHI cutoffs.[30,32]

A recent meta-analysis of clinical screening tests for OSA identified 26 different clinical prediction tests, with 8 in the form of questionnaires, and 18 algorithms, regression models, or neural networks.[34] As a preoperative screening test, the summary recommendation based on ease of use, false-negative rate, and test accuracy stated that the STOP-Bang questionnaire was a user-friendly and excellent method to predict severe OSA (AHI >30) with a diagnostic odds ratio of 142.[34] The linear scale and the simple acronym make the STOP-Bang practical and easy to use in the preoperative setting.

Several other simple screening modalities have been described and may add value to predicting the patient with OSA in the preoperative period. The modified Mallampati score assesses the relative tongue size in the oral cavity. A class 3 or 4 modified Mallampati score suggests possible anatomic obstruction and the presence of OSA.[35] Waist circumference of 102 cm (40 inches) or more also correlated well with increased AHI.[36]

NOCTURNAL OXIMETRY AND HOME SLEEP TESTING

Nocturnal oximetry may be a sensitive and specific tool to detect OSA in surgical patients. The authors' recent research found that there was a strong correlation between oxygen desaturation index (ODI) from nocturnal oximetry and the AHI from polysomnography.[37] ODI greater than 5, ODI greater than 15, and ODI greater than 30 were sensitive and specific predictors for surgical patients with AHI greater than 5, AHI greater than 15, or AHI greater than 30, respectively. The sensitivity was found to be 75% to 95% and the specificity 67% to 97%.[37]

Multichannel home sleep testing is another modality that is easy to use and may be accurately performed. It improves access and may be an excellent diagnostic tool for OSA.[38]

EVALUATION OF PATIENTS WITH SUSPECTED OSA IN THE PREOPERATIVE CLINIC

A patient is at high risk of OSA if 2 items or more score positive on the STOP questionnaire, or 3 items or more score positive on the STOP-Bang questionnaire (see **Box 1**, **Fig. 1**). Urgent or emergent surgery should not be delayed for the detailed evaluation of suspected OSA. Based on recent research, expert opinion, and the collation of various departmental protocols on OSA, a flow diagram for the suggested preoperative evaluation of a suspected OSA patient is outlined in **Fig. 1**.

Box 1
OSA screening tools

STOP questionnaire

1. Snoring: do you snore loudly (loud enough to be heard through closed doors)?

   Yes/No

2. Tired: do you often feel tired, fatigued, or sleepy during daytime?

   Yes/No

3. Observed: has anyone observed you stop breathing during your sleep?

   Yes/No

4. Blood pressure: do you have or are you being treated for high blood pressure?

   Yes/No

High risk of OSA: answering yes to 2 or more questions.
Low risk of OSA: answering yes to fewer than 2 questions.

STOP-Bang scoring model

1. Snoring: do you snore loudly (loud enough to be heard through closed doors)?

   Yes/No

2. Tired: do you often feel tired, fatigued, or sleepy during daytime?

   Yes/No

3. Observed: has anyone observed you stop breathing during your sleep?

   Yes/No

4. Blood pressure: do you have or are you being treated for high blood pressure?

   Yes/No

5. BMI: BMI more than 35 kg/m^2?

   Yes/No

6. Age: age more than 50 years old?

   Yes/No

7. Neck circumference: neck circumference greater than 40 cm?

   Yes/No

8. Gender: male?

   Yes/No

High risk of OSA: answering yes to 3 or more items.
Low risk of OSA: answering yes to fewer than 3 items.
Adapted from Chung F, Yegneswaran B, Liao P, et al. STOP questionnaire: a tool to screen patients for obstructive sleep apnea. Anesthesiology 2008;108:812–21; with permission.

If the high-risk patient is presenting for major elective surgery and has comorbidities suggestive of long-standing severe OSA, the anesthesiologist could consider a preoperative referral to the sleep physician. Subsequently, a formal polysomnography or a multichannel home sleep test may be performed if resources permit. These comorbidities include uncontrolled hypertension, heart failure, arrhythmias, cerebrovascular disease, morbid obesity, and metabolic syndrome. A timely and early consult is helpful so that the sleep physician has adequate time to prepare a perioperative management

Table 2
Screening questionnaires for OSA

Berlin Questionnaire	ASA Checklist	STOP Questionnaire	STOP-Bang Questionnaire
Netzer et al 2003[31]	Gross et al 2006[33]	Chung et al 2008[30]	Chung et al 2008[30]
Clinician-administered	Clinician-administered	Self-administered	Clinician-administered
Validated in primary care setting and perioperative setting	Validated in perioperative setting	Validated in perioperative setting	Validated in perioperative setting
10-item	14-item	4-item	8-item
3 categories: snoring, daytime sleepiness, driving	3 categories: predisposing characteristics, symptoms of OSA, complaints	No categories	No categories
High risk if 2 or more categories score positive	High risk if 2 or more categories score positive	High risk if 2 or more items score positive	High risk if 3 or more items score positive
For AHI >30 Sensitivity 87% Specificity 46% PPV 32% NPV 93%	For AHI >30 Sensitivity 87% Specificity 36% PPV 28% NPV 91%	For AHI >30 Sensitivity 80% Specificity 49% PPV 30% NPV 90%	For AHI >30 Sensitivity 100% Specificity 37% PPV 31% NPV 100%
For AHI >15 Sensitivity 79% Specificity 51% PPV 51% NPV 78%	For AHI >15 Sensitivity 79% Specificity 37% PPV 45% NPV 73%	For AHI >15 Sensitivity 74% Specificity 53% PPV 51% NPV 76%	For AHI >15 Sensitivity 93% Specificity 43% PPV 52% NPV 90%
Complicated scoring procedure	Clinician required to complete checklist	Concise, easy to use	Improve sensitivity compared with the STOP questionnaire

Abbreviations: NPV, negative predictive value; PPV positive predictive value.

plan, which may include positive airway pressure (PAP) treatment.[33] Major elective surgery may have to be deferred in patients with a high clinical suspicion of severe OSA with systemic complications.

The specificity of these screening tests is in the range of 37% to 53% for severe OSA. Therefore there is a high false-positive rate. The decision for further preoperative testing (eg, polysomnography) should depend on the clinical judgment and expertise of the attending physician, taking into account the patient-specific and logistical considerations.

On the other hand, there may be patients who are at high risk on the OSA screening questionnaires, but who are otherwise without significant comorbidities. These patients may be scheduled to undergo minor surgery. In addition, some of them may have had uneventful general anesthesia in the past. These at-risk patients may represent false-positives on screening, or represent patients with mild OSA with AHI less than 15. Screening positive on the OSA questionnaires would raise the awareness of the anesthesia health care team so that perioperative precautions for possible OSA

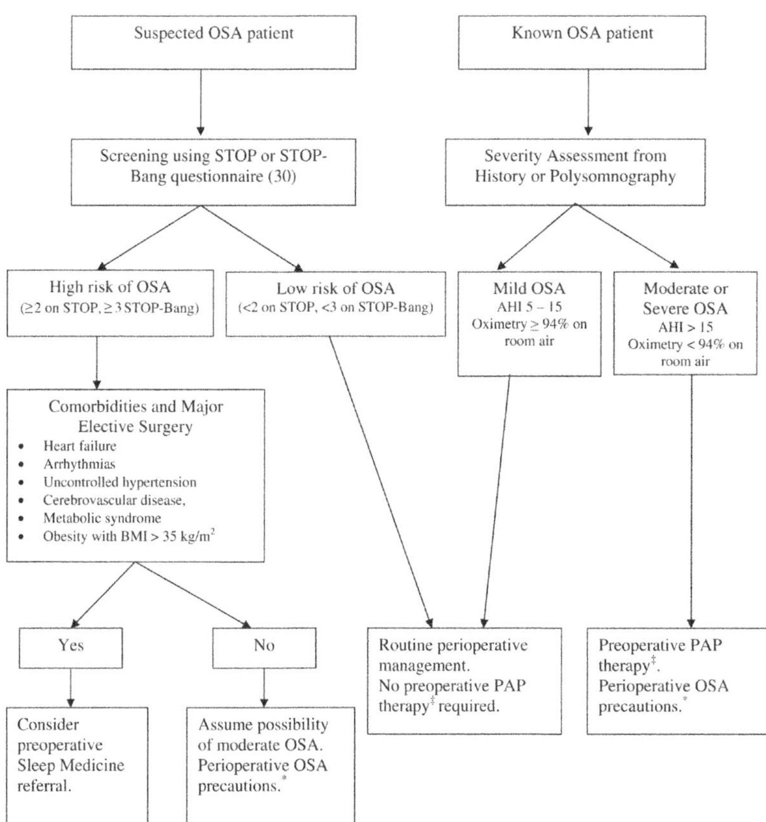

Fig. 1. Preoperative evaluation of the patient with known or suspected OSA in the anesthesia clinic *Perioperative OSA precautions include anticipating possible difficult airway, use of short-acting anesthetic agents, opioid avoidance, verifying full neuromuscular block reversal, and extubation in a nonsupine position. ‡PAP therapy: continuous PAP, bilevel PAP, or autotitrating PAP.

might be undertaken (**Table 3**). These patients can be assumed to have mild/moderate OSA. If subsequent intraoperative (difficult airway) or postoperative events (postanesthesia care unit [PACU] recurrent respiratory events) suggest a higher probability of OSA, a polysomnography and a sleep physician referral after surgery may be indicated. More research is needed to define the optimal clinical pathways for these surgical patients with increased OSA risk.

Because of the high sensitivity and negative predictive value of the OSA screening tools, the incidence of false-negatives would be low. Therefore patients who are at low risk of OSA (<2 on STOP or <3 on STOP-Bang) would not likely have OSA. These patients may be managed with routine perioperative care (see **Fig. 1**).

EVALUATION OF PATIENTS WITH KNOWN OSA IN THE PREOPERATIVE CLINIC

In patients who are known to have OSA, the severity of the sleep disorder may be assessed from the patient history or from previous polysomnography results (see **Fig. 1**). Long-standing OSA may have systemic complications, which should be ascertained. These complications include hypoxemia, hypercarbia, polycythemia, and cor

Table 3
Perioperative anesthetic management of the patient with OSA

Phase	Anesthetic Concern	Principles of Management
Preoperative period	Cardiac arrhythmias and unstable hemodynamic profile	Indirect evidence advocating the usefulness of PAP to reduce cardiac arrhythmias, stabilize variable blood pressure, and decrease myocardial oxygen consumption
	Multisystemic comorbidities	Preoperative risk stratification and patient optimization Individualized intraoperative anesthetic management tailored to comorbidities
	Sedative premedication	α_2-adrenergic agonist (clonidine, dexmedetomidine) premedication may reduce intraoperative anesthetic requirements and have an opioid-sparing effect
	OSA risk stratification, evaluation and optimization	Preoperative anesthesia consults for symptom evaluation, airway assessment, polysomnography if indicated, and formulation of anesthesia management
Intraoperative period	Difficult intubation (8 times more prevalent)	Sniffing position Ramp from scapula to head Adequate preoxygenation ASA difficult airway algorithm
	Opioid-related respiratory depression	Opioid avoidance or minimization Use of short-acting agents Regional and multimodal analgesia (nonsteroidal antiinflammatory drugs, acetaminophen, tramadol, ketamine, gabapentin, pregabalin, dexamethasone)
	Carry-over sedation effects from longer-acting intravenous sedatives and inhaled anesthetic agents	Use of propofol for maintenance of anesthesia Use of insoluble potent anesthetic agents (desflurane)
	Excessive sedation in monitored anesthetic care	Use of capnography for intraoperative monitoring
Reversal of anesthesia	Postextubation airway obstruction and desaturations	Verification of full reversal of neuromuscular blockade Ensure patient fully conscious and cooperative before extubation Semiupright posture for recovery
Immediate postoperative period	Suitability for day-case surgery	Lithotripsy, superficial, or minor orthopedic surgeries using local or regional techniques may be considered for day surgery No requirement for high-dose postoperative opioids Transfer arrangement to inpatient facility should be available
	Postoperative respiratory event in known and suspected high risk patients with OSA	Longer monitoring in the PACU Continuous oximetry monitoring and PAP therapy may be necessary if recurrent PACU respiratory events occur (desaturation, apnea, bradypnea, pain-sedation mismatch)

pulmonale. A simple screening tool in the preoperative clinic may be pulse oximetry. In the authors' opinion, an oxygen saturation value of less than 94% in room air in the absence of other causes should be a red flag for severe long-standing OSA. The presence of comorbidities such as uncontrolled hypertension, arrhythmias, cerebrovascular disease, heart failure, metabolic syndrome, and obesity should be determined. A detailed list of associated comorbidities is found in **Table 1**. The use of continuous PAP or other PAP devices and the compliance with PAP therapy should be assessed for the subgroup of patients who have been prescribed with PAP therapy.

Patients with a known diagnosis of OSA, who have been lost to sleep medicine follow-up, have had recent exacerbation of OSA symptoms, have undergone OSA-related airway surgery, or have been noncompliant with PAP treatment may have to be referred to the sleep physician for reassessment preoperatively. Due consideration should be given to the reinitiation of preoperative PAP in the noncompliant patient, although evidence is lacking in this preoperative context.

Patients with moderate and severe OSA who have been on PAP therapy should continue PAP therapy in the preoperative period.[33] Perioperative OSA precautions should be taken (see **Table 3**). These measures include anticipating possible difficult airways, the use of short-acting anesthetic agents, opioid avoidance or minimization if possible, full reversal before endotracheal extubation, and extubation in a nonsupine position. It is unclear from the current literature if mild OSA (AHI >5–15) is a significant disease entity. In the authors' opinion, patients with mild OSA would not require preoperative PAP therapy. Patients with mild OSA, without respiratory events in the PACU, may be managed with routine perioperative care.

For all patients with known OSA, there should also be a focus on airway assessment, Mallampati scoring,[35] and formulation of a perioperative management plan. Patient-specific comorbidities should be assessed and optimized. The anesthesiologist should engage the patient to explore the various anesthetic options and discuss patient-specific risks pertaining to OSA. Sedative premedication should be avoided.

PREOPERATIVE PAP THERAPY

Conventional PAP therapy acts as an airway stent and is the primary treatment of patients with OSA. There are several kinds of PAP devices: continuous PAP, autotitrating PAP, and bilevel PAP. PAP therapy has been shown to alleviate undesirable symptoms of OSA.[39] PAP has the potential to reduce cardiac rhythm abnormalities,[40] stabilize variability of blood pressure,[41] and improve the hemodynamic profile.[42] One week of PAP treatment has been shown to improve pharyngeal collapsibility and increase pharyngeal cross-sectional area.[43] In an 18-year follow-up cohort study, PAP was found to be protective against cardiovascular death and improved survival.[3]

However, high level of evidence is lacking in the perioperative context. It is still unclear if the use of PAP therapy reduces adverse events attributed to OSA in rigorous randomized controlled trials. Only 1 study of 53 patients with severe OSA undergoing uvulopalatopharyngoplasty with preoperative PAP therapy showed reduction in the surgical risk and perioperative complications.[44]

Taking into account the low level of invasiveness of PAP therapy, its short-term use immediately preoperatively may be considered, particularly in patients with severe OSA.[33] Based on consensus opinion, patients already on treatment with PAP should be advised to continue the treatment perioperatively, and to bring the PAP device to the hospital on admission. Further research in this area is warranted.

Anesthesiologists should be aware that asymptomatic patients might not easily accept PAP therapy. Appropriate timing for surgery should be a joint decision made by the anesthesiologist, the surgeon, and the patient, weighing the risks of delaying the surgery and the benefits of preoperative OSA investigation and PAP treatment.

OSA AND DIFFICULT AIRWAYS

Upper airway abnormalities, which predispose to OSA, share a similar etiologic pathway with difficult airways: mask ventilation and tracheal intubation. Snoring and OSA were found to be independent risk factors for difficult or impossible mask ventilation.[45] In a retrospective matched case-control study of 253 patients, difficult intubations was found to occur 8 times as often in the patients with OSA versus the control group (21.9% vs 2.6%, $P<.05$). OSA therefore is a risk factor for difficult endotracheal intubation.[46] In another study of more than 1500 patients, OSA, but not the magnitude of the BMI, was associated with a higher incidence of difficult laryngoscopy.[47] In patients undergoing uvulopalatopharyngoplasty, an AHI greater than 40 was a predictor for difficult intubation.[48]

In support of the strong association between OSA and a difficult airway, the corollary is also true: patients with difficult intubations have a higher risk of being diagnosed with OSA.[49] In a prospective study looking at the correlation between OSA and difficult intubations, the authors found that 66% of patients with unexpected difficult intubation were later diagnosed with OSA by polysomnography. Patients with difficult intubation are at high risk for OSA and should be screened for signs and symptoms of sleep apnea and may have to be referred for sleep studies.[50]

There are several clinical features that the anesthesiologist associates with difficult intubations, which are likewise linked with the propensity for obstruction in the unsupported upper airway during sleep and anesthesia. These features include obesity, increased neck circumference,[51] limited neck extension, nasal obstruction, a crowded oropharynx (including decreased pharyngeal width, a high Mallampati score, decreased retrolingual airway size,[52] an enlarged tongue or tonsils), dental abnormalities, limited mouth opening, hypoplasia of the maxilla or mandible, decreased thyromental distance, and increased mandibular angle. A detailed airway assessment should be performed in the preoperative clinic in anticipation of possible difficult airways.

Adequate intraoperative preparation is recommended for the airway management of the patient with OSA. Patients should be in the optimal "sniffing" position before the induction of general anesthesia. Proper position for ventilation and laryngoscopy aligns the ear with the sternal notch in a straight line. A ramp may be built under the patient from the scapula to the head. This strategy is prudent, particularly in morbidly obese patients with OSA. To achieve this, blankets or other devices like the Troop Elevation Pillow (Mercury Medical, FL, USA) may be placed under the patient's head and shoulders.[53] Oropharyngeal and nasal airways may be useful to bypass the upper airway obstruction and should be readily available when mask ventilation is difficult. Videolaryngoscopy techniques may also be useful and improve intubating conditions in these patients.[54]

Full preoxygenation should be performed with the patient breathing an F_{IO_2} of 1.0 for 3 minutes via a tightly fitted mask. The application of PAP at induction may also improve oxygenation and prevent airway obstruction.[55] Gastroesophageal reflux is common in patients with OSA with hypotonia of the lower esophageal sphincter.[56] Rapid sequence induction and cricoid pressure may be considered in this context.

A variety of airway adjuncts and skilled anesthesia assistance should be made available in advance for dealing with the possible difficult airway. ASA practice guidelines for the management of the difficult airway may be used as a roadmap to assist the anesthesiologist.[57]

PLANNING FOR LOCAL, REGIONAL, OR GENERAL ANESTHESIA

The use of local and regional blocks (neuroaxial or peripheral nerve blocks) as a sole anesthetic without sedation may potentially be beneficial to the patient with OSA as it circumvents the issue of upper airway patency in the perioperative period. Based on expert opinion and consensus by consultants, ASA guidelines recommend regional anesthesia rather than general anesthesia for peripheral surgery.[33] The ASA guidelines, however, remain equivocal regarding whether combined regional and general anesthetics techniques are useful.

PLANNING FOR POSTOPERATIVE ANALGESIA

Optimal intraoperative management encompasses knowledge of the problems associated with OSA, and taking measures to minimize the aggravating effects of anesthesia. Patients with OSA are sensitive to the respiratory depressant effects of anesthetic drugs, in particular opioid analgesic agents. This sensitivity is largely a result of the propensity of airway collapse, sleep deprivation, and blunting of the physiologic response to hypercarbia and hypoxia. Therefore avoidance or minimization of the use of longer-acting anesthetic drugs should be recommended.

The dangers of opioid use in patients with evidence of a compromised upper airway have been highlighted in several case reports. The use of morphine in patients with OSA has been associated with severe respiratory depression and even death.[58,59] Postoperative oxygen desaturations were 12 to 14 times more likely to occur in patients with OSA receiving oral or parenteral opioids after surgery versus nonopioid analgesic agents.[60]

A multimodal approach for analgesia is therefore advocated,[61] where a combination of analgesics from different classes is used. Medications such as nonsteroidal antiinflammatory drugs, acetaminophen, tramadol, ketamine, gabapentin, pregabalin, clonidine, and dexamethasone are used to alleviate the opioid-related adverse effects of respiratory depression in susceptible patients with OSA. Dexmedetomidine has been purported in several case reports to have beneficial effects in patients with OSA because of the lack of respiratory depression and opioid-sparing effects in the perioperative period.[62–65]

The postoperative use of nerve-block catheters or epidural catheters with local anesthetics obviates systemic opioid analgesics. This system potentially reduces the risk of sedation and upper airway obstruction. However, this is not the case if neuroaxial opioids are administered. The occurrence of sudden postoperative respiratory arrests from epidural opioids has been reported in a case series of 3 patients with OSA.[66] Likewise, if postoperative systemic strong opioid analgesics are administered after a regional anesthetic, the patient with OSA is at increased risk for respiratory complications.[67]

PLANNING FOR AMBULATORY SURGERY

Controversy exists as to whether patients with OSA should be treated on an ambulatory basis. ASA guidelines highlighted that superficial surgeries or minor orthopedic surgery using local or regional techniques and lithotripsy may be performed on an ambulatory basis.[33] Considerations include the types of surgeries, the comorbidities, patient age, status (treated vs untreated) and severity of OSA, use of postoperative opioids, type of anesthesia, and the level of home care.[33]

Based on expert opinion, in the absence of moderate to severe OSA, recurrent PACU respiratory events (apnea, bradypnea, desaturation),[68] and the need for strong postoperative opioids for analgesia, patients may be discharged home at the discretion of the attending anesthesiologist (**Fig. 2**). Ambulatory surgical facilities managing patients with OSA should have transfer arrangements to an inpatient facility, and be equipped to handle the problems (eg, difficult airway, postoperative respiratory depression) associated with the patient with OSA.

PLANNING FOR INPATIENT SURGERY

Depending on the severity of the OSA, the extent of the surgery, and the type of anesthetics administered, and postoperative analgesics required, the patient may shift to the higher end of the risk continuum, increasing the need for step-down care (see

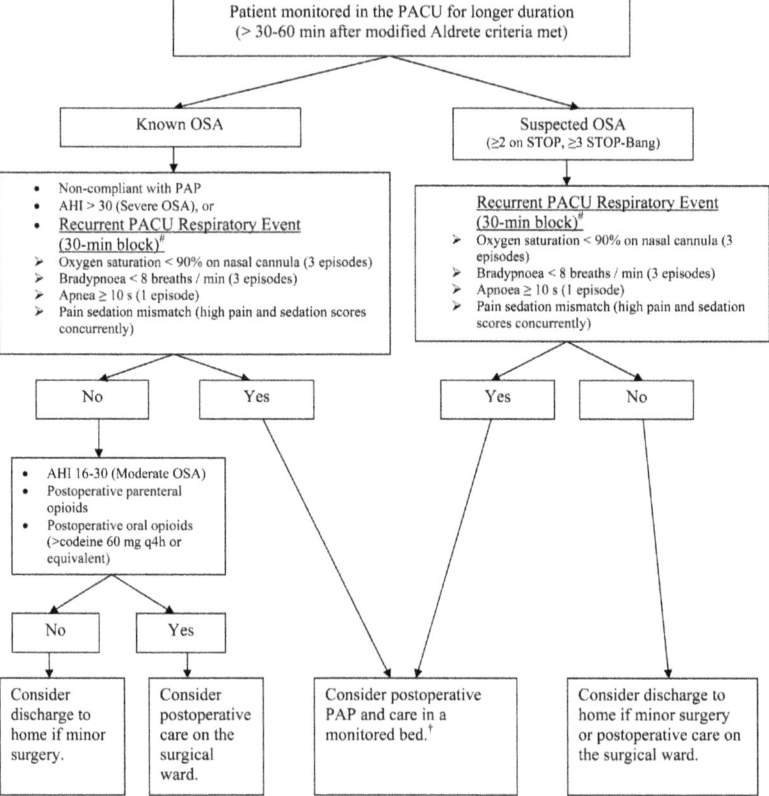

Fig. 2. Postoperative management of the patient with known or suspected OSA after general anesthesia. #Recurrent PACU respiratory event: any event occurring more than once in each 30-minute evaluation period (it does not have to be the same event). (*Data from* Gali B, Whalen FX, Schroeder D, et al. Identification of patients at risk for postoperative respiratory complications using a preoperative obstructive sleep apnea screening tool and postanesthesia care assessment. Anesthesiology 2009;110:869–77.) †Monitored bed: environment with continuous oximetry and the possibility of early nursing intervention (eg, step-down unit, general surgical ward near nursing station, or remote pulse oximetry with telemetry in surgical ward).

Fig. 2). The anesthesiologist should ensure that a postoperative monitored bed is available for a patient with a high AHI undergoing major surgery or airway surgery. A monitored bed refers to an environment with continuous oximetry with the possibility of early nursing intervention (eg, step-down unit, or general surgical ward near the nursing station, or remote continuous oximetry with telemetry).

After general anesthesia, the authors recommend that all patients with known OSA or patients with suspected OSA (positive on screening with STOP or STOP-Bang) should be observed in PACU with continuous pulse oximetry for a longer period than a patient without OSA.[33]

The decision of whether the patient requires postoperative inpatient monitoring is dependent on the judgment and discretion of the attending anesthesiologist. Based on expert opinion and a collation of various departmental protocols on OSA, **Fig. 2** presents a simple algorithm to guide the anesthesiologist in making the decision regarding the postoperative disposition of the patient with OSA. For all patients with known OSA or patients with suspected OSA ($\geq$2 criteria on STOP, or $\geq$3 criteria on STOP-Bang) who have undergone general anesthesia, the authors propose an extended PACU observation of at least 30 to 60 minutes in an unstimulated environment after the patient has met the modified Aldrete criteria for discharge.

To determine whether the patient with known OSA or the patient with suspected OSA requires continuous postoperative monitoring, observation of recurrent PACU respiratory events can be used as a second-phase approach to guide further management. A single PACU respiratory event occurs when a patient has apnea for 10 seconds or more (1 episode needed for yes), bradypnea of less than 8 breaths per minute (3 episodes needed for yes), pain-sedation mismatch, or desaturation to less than 90% with nasal cannula (3 episodes needed for yes). Recurrent PACU respiratory events occur when any 1 of the PACU respiratory events occurs in 2 separate 30-minute time blocks (it does not have to be the same event).[68]

Patients who are at high risk of OSA on the screening questionnaires, and have recurrent PACU respiratory events, are associated with higher postoperative respiratory complication.[68] It may be prudent to place these patients in a monitored bed postoperatively. Depending on the degree of desaturation, these patients may also require postoperative PAP therapy (see **Fig. 2**).

Patients with known OSA who have been noncompliant with PAP therapy or have severe OSA (AHI > 30) may have to be fitted with postoperative PAP therapy and cared for in a monitored environment with oximetry, especially if there has been a recurrent PACU respiratory event (see **Fig. 2**). Patients with moderate OSA (AHI 16–30) requiring postoperative parenteral opioids or higher dose oral opioids (>60 mg codeine every 4 hours or equivalent), and without recurrent PACU respiratory events can be managed postoperatively on the surgical ward with continued periodic monitoring (see **Fig. 2**). It may also be expedient to place patients requiring postoperative parenteral opioids on supplemental oxygen.[69] Patients with mild OSA who have undergone minor surgery, without recurrent PACU respiratory events, and without the need for higher dose of oral opioids, may be discharged home (see **Fig. 2**).

Newer remote pulse oximetry monitoring devices enable data from a bedside monitor to be continuously streamed wirelessly to a central observation station (eg, Oxinet III telemetry, Nellcor, CO, USA) or paging system. This technology may be useful in the context of postoperative monitoring of patients with OSA. However, studies are lacking in this area. This technology potentially allows patients with OSA to be cared for postoperatively in the surgical ward instead of the step-down unit, thus lessening caregiver burden.

Recently our research found that patients with OSA have more profound increases in AHI after surgery, with a peak on night 3 and returning to preoperative level only on night 7.[70] Therefore monitoring the patient with OSA overnight may not safeguard against all respiratory events in the first postoperative week. Further research on the postoperative management of patients with OSA is essential.

SUMMARY

In the perioperative setting, OSA is underappreciated, with a high proportion of patients being undiagnosed. Patients with OSA have a plethora of comorbid conditions, and may be associated with less favorable postoperative outcomes. Surgical patients with OSA are vulnerable to the aggravating effects of sedation and opioid analgesia. Adverse outcomes such as episodic sleep-related desaturations and cardiorespiratory arrest may result in extreme cases.

The patient with OSA poses special challenges to the anesthesiologist in the perioperative period. Preoperative evaluation through vigilant screening and formulation of an anesthesia management plan may ameliorate the perioperative morbidity associated with patients with OSA.

ACKNOWLEDGMENTS

The authors wish to thank Dr Terence Davidson (San Diego Health Care System University of California, San Diego, CA, USA), Dr Janet Van Vlymen (Kingston General Hospital, Kingston, ON, Canada), Dr Stephen Cohen (Beth Israel Daeconess Medical Center, Boston, MA, USA), Dr Norman Bolden (MetroHealth Medical Center, Cleveland, OH, USA), Dr Michael Bishop (University of California, San Diego, San Diego, CA, USA), and Dr Gregory Bryson (The Ottawa Hospital, Ottawa, ON, Canada) for sharing with us their expert opinion and for allowing us to peruse their institutional OSA protocols and policies.

REFERENCES

1. Hwang D, Shakir N, Limann B, et al. Association of sleep-disordered breathing with postoperative complications. Chest 2008;133:1128–34.
2. Liao P, Yegneswaran B, Vairavanathan S, et al. Postoperative complications in patients with obstructive sleep apnoea: a retrospective matched cohort study. Can J Anesth 2009;56:819–28.
3. Young T, Finn L, Peppard PE, et al. Sleep disordered breathing and mortality: eighteen-year follow-up of the Wisconsin sleep cohort. Sleep 2008;31:1071–8.
4. Marshall NS, Wong KKH, Liu PY, et al. Sleep apnea as an independent risk factor for all-cause mortality: the Busselton Health Study. Sleep 2008;31:1079–85.
5. Kim JA, Lee JJ, Jung HH. Predictive factors of immediate postoperative complications after uvulopalatopharyngoplasty. Laryngoscope 2005;115:1837–40.
6. Pang KP. Identifying patients who need close monitoring during and after upper airway surgery for obstructive sleep apnea. J Laryngol Otol 2006;120:655–60.
7. Gupta RM, Parvizi J, Hanssen AD, et al. Postoperative complications in patients with obstructive sleep apnea syndrome undergoing hip or knee replacement: a case-control study. Mayo Clin Proc 2001;76:897–905.
8. Kaw R, Golish J, Ghamande S, et al. Incremental risk of obstructive sleep apnea on cardiac surgical outcomes. J Cardiovasc Surg (Torino) 2006;47:683–9.
9. Kryger MH. Diagnosis and management of sleep apnea syndrome. Clin Cornerstone 2000;2:39–47.

10. Young T, Evans I, Finn I, et al. Estimation of the clinically diagnosed proportion of sleep apnea syndrome in middle-aged men and women. Sleep 1997;20:705–6.
11. Bixler EO, Vgontzas AN, Ten Have T, et al. Effects of age on sleep apnea in men: I. Prevalence and severity. Am J Respir Crit Care Med 1998;157:144–8.
12. Bixler EO, Vgontzas AN, Lin HM, et al. Prevalence of sleep-disordered breathing in women: effects of gender. Am J Respir Crit Care Med 2001;163:608–13.
13. Frey WC, Pilcher J. Obstructive sleep-related breathing disorders in patients evaluated for bariatric surgery. Obes Surg 2003;13:678–83.
14. Chung F, Ward B, Ho J, et al. Preoperative identification of sleep apnea risk in elective surgical patients using the Berlin questionnaire. J Clin Anesth 2007;19:130–4.
15. Fleetham J, Ayas N, Bradley D, et al. Canadian Thoracic Society guidelines: diagnosis and treatment of sleep disordered breathing in adults. Can Respir J 2006; 13:387–92.
16. Iber C, Ancoli-Israel S, Cheeson A, et al. The AASM manual for the scoring of sleep and associated events, rules, terminology and technical specifications. Westchester (IL): American Academy of Sleep Medicine; 2007.
17. Ruehland WR, Rochford PD, O'Donoghue FJ, et al. The new AASM criteria for scoring hypopneas: impact on the apnea hypopnea index. Sleep 2009;32:150–7.
18. Peker Y, Kraiczi H, Hedner J, et al. An independent association between obstructive sleep apnoea and coronary artery disease. Eur Respir J 1999;14:179–84.
19. Kuniyoshi FH, Garcia-Touchard A, Gami AS, et al. Day-night variation of acute myocardial infarction in obstructive sleep apnea. J Am Coll Cardiol 2008;52: 343–6.
20. Sin DD, Fitzgerald F, Parker JD, et al. Relationship of systolic BP to obstructive sleep apnea in patients with heart failure. Chest 2003;123:1536–43.
21. Mehra R, Benjamin EJ, Shahar E, et al. Association of nocturnal arrhythmias with sleep-disordered breathing: the Sleep Heart Health Study. Am J Respir Crit Care Med 2006;173:910–6.
22. Ohayon MM, Guilleminault C, Priest RG, et al. Is sleep-disordered breathing an independent risk factor for hypertension in the general population (13,057 subjects)? J Psychosom Res 2000;48:593–601.
23. Arzt M, Young T, Finn L, et al. Association of sleep-disordered breathing and the occurrence of stroke. Am J Respir Crit Care Med 2005;172:1447–51.
24. Coughlin SR, Mawdsley L, Mugarza JA, et al. Obstructive sleep apnoea is independently associated with an increased prevalence of metabolic syndrome. Eur Heart J 2004;25:735–41.
25. Mickelson SA. Preoperative and postoperative management of obstructive sleep apnea patients. Otolaryngol Clin North Am 2007;40:877–89.
26. Chung F, Elsaid H. Screening for obstructive sleep apnea before surgery: why is it important? Curr Opin Anaesthesiol 2009;22:405–11.
27. McNicholas WT, Ryan S. Obstructive sleep apnoea syndrome: translating science to clinical practice. Respirology 2006;11:136–44.
28. Hallowell PT, Stellato TA, Schuster M, et al. Potentially life-threatening sleep apnea is unrecognized without aggressive evaluation. Am J Surg 2007;193: 364–7.
29. Chung S, Yuan H, Chung F. A systematic review of obstructive sleep apnea and its implications for anesthesiologists. Anesth Analg 2008;107:1543–63.
30. Chung F, Yegneswaran B, Liao P, et al. STOP Questionnaire: a tool to screen patients for obstructive sleep apnea. Anesthesiology 2008;108:812–21.
31. Netzer NC, Hoegel JJ, Loube D, et al. Prevalence of symptoms and risk of sleep apnea in primary care. Chest 2003;124:1406–14.

32. Chung F, Yegneswaran B, Liao P, et al. Validation of the Berlin questionnaire and American Society of Anesthesiologist checklist as screening tools for obstructive sleep apnea in surgical patients. Anesthesiology 2008;108:822–30.
33. Gross JB, Bachenberg KL, Benumof JL, et al. Practice guidelines for the perioperative management of patients with obstructive sleep apnea: a report by the American Society of Anesthesiologists Task Force on Perioperative Management of patients with obstructive sleep apnea. Anesthesiology 2006;104:1081–93.
34. Ramachandran SK, Josephs LA. A meta-analysis of clinical screening tests for obstructive sleep apnea. Anesthesiology 2009;110:928–39.
35. Nuckton TJ, Glidden DV, Browner WS, et al. Physical examination Mallampati score as an independent predictor of obstructive sleep apnea. Sleep 2006;29:903–8.
36. Davidson T, Patel M. Waist circumference and sleep disordered breathing. Laryngoscope 2008;118:339–47.
37. Chung F, Liao P, Sun F, et al. Nocturnal oximeter: a sensitive and specific tool to detect the surgical patients with moderate and severe OSA. Anesthesiology 2009;111:A480.
38. Patel MR, Davidson TM. Home sleep testing in the diagnosis and treatment of sleep disordered breathing. Otolaryngol Clin North Am 2007;40:761–84.
39. Yamamoto H, Akashiba T, Kosaka N, et al. Long-term effects nasal continuous positive airway pressure on daytime sleepiness, mood and traffic accidents in patients with obstructive sleep apnoea. Respir Med 2000;94:87–90.
40. Becker H, Brandenburg U, Peter JH, et al. Reversal of sinus arrest and atrioventricular conduction block in patients with sleep apnea during nasal continuous positive airway pressure. Am J Respir Crit Care Med 1995;151:215–8.
41. Bonsignore MR, Parati G, Insalaco G, et al. Baroreflex control of heart rate during sleep in severe obstructive sleep apnoea: effects of acute PAP. Eur Respir J 2006;27:128–35.
42. Kaye DM, Mansfield D, Naughton MT. Continuous positive airway pressure decreases myocardial oxygen consumption in heart failure. Clin Sci Lond 2004;106:599–603.
43. Corda L, Redolfi S, Montemurro LT, et al. Short- and long-term effects of PAP on upper airway anatomy and collapsibility in OSAH. Sleep Breath 2009;13:187–93.
44. Li RH, Zeng Y, Wang YJ, et al. [Perioperative management of severe obstructive sleep apnea hypopnea syndrome]. Nan Fang Yi Ke Da Xue Xue Bao 2006;26:661–3 [in Chinese].
45. Kheterpal S, Han R, Tremper KK, et al. Incidence and predictors of difficult and impossible mask ventilation. Anesthesiology 2006;105:885–91.
46. Siyam MA, Benhamou D. Difficult endotracheal intubation in patients with sleep apnea syndrome. Anesth Analg 2002;95:1098–102.
47. Ezri T, Medallion B, Weisenberg M, et al. Increased body mass index per se is not a predictor of difficult laryngoscopy. Can J Anesth 2003;50:179–83.
48. Kim JA, Lee JJ. Preoperative predictors of difficult intubation in patients with obstructive sleep apnea syndrome. Can J Anesth 2006;53:393–7.
49. Hiremath AS, Hillman DR, James AL, et al. Relationship between difficult tracheal intubation and obstructive sleep apnoea. Br J Anaesth 1998;80:606–11.
50. Chung F, Yegneswaran B, Herrera F, et al. Patients with difficult intubation may need referral to sleep clinics. Anesth Analg 2008;107:915–20.
51. Gonzalez H, Minville V, Delanoue K, et al. The importance of increased neck circumference to intubation difficulties in obese patients. Anesth Analg 2008;106:1132–6.

52. Barkdull G, Kohl C, Davidson T. Computed tomography imaging of patients with obstructive sleep apnea. Laryngoscope 2008;118:1486–92.
53. Rao SL, Kunselman AR, Schuler HG, et al. Laryngoscopy and tracheal intubation in the head-elevated position in obese patients: a randomized, controlled, equivalence trial. Anesth Analg 2008;107:1912–8.
54. Marrel J, Blanc C, Frascarolo P, et al. Videolaryngoscopy improves intubation conditions in morbidly obese patients. Eur J Anaesthesiol 2007;24:1045–9.
55. Rusca M, Proietti S, Schnyder P, et al. Prevention of atelectasis formation during induction of general anesthesia. Anesth Analg 2003;97:1835–9.
56. Sabate JM, Jouet P, Merrouche M, et al. Gastroesophaegeal reflux in patients with morbid obesity: a role of obstructive sleep apnea syndrome? Obes Surg 2008;18:1479–84.
57. American Society of Anesthesiologists Task Force on Management of Difficult Airway. Practice guidelines for management of the difficult airway: an updated report by the American Society of Anesthesiologists task force on management of the difficult airway. Anesthesiology 2003;98:1269–77.
58. Lofsky A. Sleep apnea and narcotic postoperative pain medication: a morbidity and mortality risk. APSF Newsletter 2002;17:24–5.
59. Byard RW, Gilbert JD. Narcotic administration and stenosing lesions of the upper airway – a potentially lethal combination. J Clin Forensic Med 2005;12: 29–31.
60. Bolden N, Smith CE, Auckley D, et al. Perioperative complications during use of an obstructive sleep apnea protocol following surgery and anesthesia. Anesth Analg 2008;105:1869–70.
61. White PF. The changing role of non-opioid analgesic techniques in the management of postoperative pain. Anesth Analg 2005;101:5–22.
62. Hofer RE, Sprung J, Sarr MG, et al. Anesthesia for a patient with morbid obesity using Dexmedetomidine without narcotics. Can J Anesth 2005;52:176–80.
63. Ramsay MA, Saha D, Hebeler RF. Tracheal resection in the morbidly obese patient: the role of Dexmedetomidine. J Clin Anesth 2006;18:452–4.
64. Bamgbade OA, Alfa JA. Dexmedetomidine anaesthesia for patients with obstructive sleep apnoea undergoing bariatric surgery. Eur J Anaesthesiol 2009;26: 176–7.
65. Plunkett AR, Shields C, Stojadinovic A, et al. Awake thyroidectomy under local anesthesia and dexmedetomidine infusion. Mil Med 2009;174:100–2.
66. Ostermeier AM, Roizen MF, Hautkappe M, et al. Three sudden postoperative respiratory arrests associated with epidural opioids in patients with sleep apnea. Anesth Analg 1997;85:452–60.
67. Yegneswaran B, Chung F. The importance of screening for obstructive sleep apnea before surgery. Sleep Med 2009;10:270–1.
68. Gali B, Whalen FX, Schroeder D, et al. Identification of patients at risk for postoperative respiratory complications using a preoperative obstructive sleep apnea screening tool and postanesthesia care assessment. Anesthesiology 2009;110: 869–77.
69. Blake DW, Chia PH, Donnan G, et al. Preoperative assessment for obstructive sleep apnoea and the prediction of postoperative respiratory obstruction and hypoxaemia. Anaesth Intensive Care 2008;36:379–84.
70. Chung F, Liao P, Fazel H, et al. Evolution of sleep pattern and sleep breathing disorders during first seven nights after surgery – a pilot study. Sleep 2009;32: 0667.

Postoperative Pain Management After Ambulatory Surgery: Role of Multimodal Analgesia

Ofelia Loani Elvir-Lazo, MD[a], Paul F. White, PhD, MD, FANZCA[b,c,d,e,f,*]

KEYWORDS

- Ambulatory surgery • Multimodal analgesia • Opioid analgesics
- Nonopioid analgesics

Postoperative pain remains a challenging problem, which requires a proactive approach using a variety of treatment modalities to obtain an optimal outcome with respect to enhancing patient comfort and facilitating the recovery process. Multimodal (or balanced) analgesia represents an increasingly popular approach to preventing postoperative pain. The approach involves administering a combination of opioid and nonopioid analgesics that act at different sites within the central and peripheral nervous systems in an effort to improve pain control while eliminating opioid-related side effects.[1–5] The adaptation of multimodal (or balanced) analgesic techniques as the standard approach for the prevention of pain in the ambulatory setting is one of the keys to improving the recovery process after day-case surgery.[1,6]

Poorly controlled pain is a major factor contributing to a delayed discharge after ambulatory surgery.[2,4] Improving postoperative pain control accelerates the ability of patients to resume their activities of daily living.[5] Many patients undergoing ambulatory surgery continue to experience unacceptably high levels of pain after their operation.[2–4] Despite recent advances in our knowledge of multimodal analgesic therapies[1] and progress in our understanding of the pathophysiologic basis of acute pain, there remains a need for clinicians to implement evidence-based, procedure-specific

[a] Department of Anesthesiology, Cedars Sinai Medical Center, Los Angeles, CA, USA
[b] Department of Anesthesiology and Pain Management, University of Texas Southwestern Medical Center, Dallas, TX, USA
[c] Cedars Sinai Medical Center, Los Angeles, CA, USA
[d] Policlinico Abano, Leonardo Foundation, Abano Terme, Italy
[e] Pharma University, Parma, Italy
[f] The White Mountain Institute, 144 Ashby Lane, Los Altos, CA 94022, USA
* Corresponding author. The White Mountain Institute, 144 Ashby Lane, Los Altos, CA 94022.
E-mail address: whitemountaininstitute@hotmail.com

Anesthesiology Clin 28 (2010) 217–224
doi:10.1016/j.anclin.2010.02.011 **anesthesiology.theclinics.com**
1932-2275/10/$ – see front matter

multimodal analgesic protocols, which are modified to meet the needs of individual patients and to enhance the quality of postoperative pain management.[6]

The armamentarium of analgesic drugs and techniques for the management of postoperative pain continues to grow at a rapid rate. However, there seems to be a significant disconnect between the publication of analgesic studies in the peer-reviewed literature, demonstrating approaches to improving acute pain management and the application of these concepts in clinical practice. A part of the problem relates to the increasing number and complexity of elective operations that are being performed on an ambulatory (or short-stay) basis in which the use of conventional opioid-based intravenous patient controlled analgesia and central neuraxial (spinal and epidural) analgesia techniques are simply not practical for acute pain management. This rapidly expanding patient population requires an aggressive perioperative analgesic regimen that provides effective pain relief, has minimal side effects, is intrinsically safe, and can be managed by the patient and their family members away from a hospital or surgical center.

One of the most important factors in determining when a patient can be safely discharged from a surgical facility, and that also has a major influence on the patient's ability to resume their normal activities of daily living, is the adequacy of postoperative pain control.[3,7] Perioperative analgesia has traditionally been provided using potent opioid (narcotic) analgesics. However, extensive reliance on opioid medication for acute pain management is associated with a variety of perioperative complications (eg, drowsiness and sedation, postoperative nausea and vomiting (PONV), pruritus, urinary retention, ileus, constipation, ventilatory depression), which can contribute to a delayed hospital discharge and resumption of normal activities of daily living.[8] Anesthesiologists are increasingly using a combination of nonopioid analgesic medications as the first line of therapy for the prevention of pain in the postoperative period. However, opioid analgesics will likely remain the primary treatment option for patients who require rescue analgesic therapy in the postoperative period until more potent and rapid-acting nonopioid analgesics become available for routine clinical use.

In 2000, the Joint Commission on Accreditation of Healthcare Organizations (JCAHO) introduced new standards that mandated pain assessment and treatment as part of routine patient care in an attempt to improve control of acute pain. Many medical institutions have misinterpreted this mandate as requiring that the treatment of pain must be guided by patient reports of pain intensity indexed to a numerical pain scale.[5] After the implementation of a routine numeric pain scoring system in the recovery room, Frasco and colleagues[9] reported a significant increase in the use of opioid analgesics. Vila and colleagues[10] reported that as a result of the JCAHO-mandated policy for pain management, the incidence of opioid-related adverse reactions increased from 11 to 25 per 100,000 inpatient days at their medical center. Most adverse drug reactions were preceded by a documented decrease in the patient's level of consciousness due to opioid-related sedation. In the ambulatory setting, the primary factor responsible for postdischarge nausea and vomiting is the use of oral opioid-containing analgesics.[11] Raeder and colleagues[12] reported that the use of ibuprofen after ambulatory surgery was associated with fewer gastrointestinal side effects (eg, PONV, constipation) when compared with the use of an oral combination of acetaminophen and codeine.

Early studies evaluating approaches to facilitating the recovery process have demonstrated that the use of multimodal analgesic techniques can improve early recovery as well as other clinically meaningful outcomes after ambulatory surgery.[13,14] These benefits have been confirmed in more recent studies[15,16] and are currently the recommended practice in most fast-track clinical care plans.[5] It is clear that the reliance on a single nonopioid analgesic modality (eg, local analgesics, nonsteroidal antiinflammatory drugs [NSAIDs], and/or acetaminophen) will not suffice to control moderate to severe postoperative pain, and excessive reliance on opioid analgesics produces undesirable side effects.[8,17] The short- and long-term benefits of using multimodal analgesia regimens to reduce opioid-related side effects remain controversial, because the definition of multimodal analgesia is not uniform in the anesthesia and surgery literature.[1] In some contexts, multimodal analgesia refers to systemic administration of analgesic drugs with different mechanisms of action, whereas in other situations it refers to concurrent application of analgesic pharmacotherapy in combination with regional analgesia.

A deficiency in the design of many of the published studies involving multimodal analgesic therapies is that the drug regimens were not continued into the postdischarge period.[18] For example, only immediate pre- and postoperative administration of the cyclooxygenase 2 (COX-2) inhibitor rofecoxib as part of a multimodal analgesic regimen in outpatients undergoing inguinal hernia repair provided limited benefits beyond the early postoperative period.[19] However, when the COX-2 inhibitors are administered for 3 to 5 days after ambulatory surgery,[15,16] the greater benefits were achieved with respect to clinically relevant patient outcomes (eg, resumption of normal activities) and improvements in pain control. While opioid analgesics continue to play an important role in the acute treatment of moderate to severe pain in the early postoperative period, nonopioid analgesics will likely assume a greater role as preventative analgesics in the future as the number of minimally invasive (keyhole) surgery cases continues to expand.

Nonopioid analgesics are increasingly being used as adjuvants before, during, and after surgery to facilitate the recovery process after ambulatory surgery because of their anesthetic- and analgesic-sparing effects and their ability to reduce postoperative pain (with movement), opioid analgesic requirement, and side effects, thereby shortening the duration of the hospital stay. The use of traditional NSAIDs, COX-2 inhibitors, acetaminophen,[20–23] ketamine,[24,25] dexmedetomidine,[26,27] dextromethorphan, alpha2-agonists, gabapentin,[28–30] pregabalin,[31–34] β-blockers,[35–39] and glucocorticoid steroids can provide beneficial effects when administered in appropriate doses as part of a multimodal analgesic regimen in the perioperative setting.[1,8,40] Dexamethasone when used as an adjuvant decreases oxycodone consumption and helps to reduce postoperative pain.[41–43] Recent studies have confirmed that a rational combination of different nonopioid analgesics when given as part of multimodal analgesia reduces postoperative pain.[32,44,45]

The potential beneficial effects of administering local anesthetics via alternative routes of administration for improving the perioperative outcomes continue to be investigated. The administration of intranasal lidocaine in combination with naphazoline decreased both intra- and postoperative pain and reduced rescue analgesic requirements in the postoperative period.[46] Although intra-abdominal administration of levobupivacaine was alleged to produce satisfactory analgesia in patients undergoing abdominal hysterectomy procedures, the study was flawed due to the failure to include a placebo control group.[47] However, other studies have demonstrated the effectiveness of the intravenous infusion of lidocaine in reducing postoperative pain and facilitating the recovery process.[48–51] Yardeni and colleagues[52] suggested that perioperative administration of intravenous lidocaine could improve early postoperative pain control and reduce surgery-induced immune alterations.

The use of continuous local anesthetic techniques (eg, for perineural blocks or wound infiltration) has become increasingly popular due to their ability to control moderate to severe pain after major ambulatory orthopedic surgery procedures.[53–57] The availability of disposable local anesthetic infusion systems and the encouraging results from these early studies have led to the increasing popularity of these techniques for pain control in the postdischarge period. However, the clear benefits of these approaches for managing pain after ambulatory surgery must be balanced against the cost of the equipment and the resources needed to safely manage these systems outside the hospital environment.

Topical capsicum has also been found to produce prolonged analgesic effects because of its ability to alter nociceptive input at the peripheral nerve ending.[58] The use of transcutaneous electrical nerve stimulation and acupoint stimulation has also been reported to improve postoperative pain management. Because these techniques cause no adverse effects, their use as an adjunct to conventional pharmaceutical approaches could be considered, particularly for patients in whom conventional analgesic techniques fail and/or are accompanied by severe medication-related adverse events.[59,60]

Preemptive analgesic techniques have been postulated to provide superior analgesia by preventing the establishment of central sensitization.[61] However, this approach does not seem to offer any clinically significant advantages over so-called preventative multimodal analgesic regimens when an effective pro-active approach to pain management is initiated in the early postoperative period and extended into the postdischarge period.[62]

Of importance for improving the quality of pain control and facilitating recovery in the future is the need to educate patients and their family members (caregivers) about the importance of continuing their analgesic medications after the patient leaves the hospital or day-surgery center. It is also important to emphasize the need for collaboration between the various health care providers involved in the patient's perioperative care (eg, anesthesiologists, surgeons, nurses, and physiotherapists) to integrate improved perioperative pain management strategies with the recently described fast-track recovery paradigms.[5] This type of multi-disciplinary approach has been documented to improve the quality of the recovery process and reduce the hospital stay and postoperative morbidity, leading to a shorter period of convalescence after surgery.[63]

A critical assessment of the peer-reviewed literature regarding the optimal analgesic therapies for outpatient laparoscopic cholecystectomy by Bisgaard[64] concluded that a multimodal analgesic regimen consisting of a preoperative single dose of dexamethasone, incisional local anesthetics (at the beginning and/or end of surgery), and continuous treatment with NSAIDs (or COX-2 inhibitors) during the first 3 to 4 days provided the best clinical outcome. It was further suggested that elimination of opioid-based analgesia would be highly desirable in the future. These important findings have been confirmed by White and colleagues.[15] In a prospective, placebo-controlled study, involving the administration of celecoxib on the day of surgery and subsequently for 3 days after outpatient laparoscopic surgery as part of a multimodal analgesic regimen, it was found that celecoxib-treated patients not only experienced less pain and reduced need for opioid-containing oral analgesics but also (more importantly) were able to resume normal activities of daily living 1 to 2 days earlier.

With the more widespread use of multimodal perioperative analgesic regimens, involving both opioid and nonopioid analgesic therapies, physicians and nurses are becoming increasingly aware of the important role that these techniques play in facilitating the recovery process and improving patient satisfaction. Although many factors, in addition to pain, must be carefully controlled to minimize postoperative morbidity and facilitate the recovery process after elective surgery (eg, PONV, hydration status), the adequacy of pain control should remain a major focus of health care providers, caring for patients undergoing ambulatory surgical procedures.[17,19]

With the changes in health care dictated by economic pressures, there has been a realization that the duration of the hospital stay can be reduced without compromising the quality of patient care. Advances in surgical technology and anesthetic drugs and techniques have made an impact on the way perioperative care is currently being delivered to patients undergoing ambulatory surgery. Multidisciplinary fast-track or accelerated recovery processes encompass many aspects of anesthesia and analgesic care,[5] optimizing not only the preoperative preparation and prehabilitation but also the intraoperative attenuation of surgical stress and postoperative pain control and rehabilitation procedures.[65]

Current evidence suggests that these improvements in patient outcome related to pain control can best be achieved by using a combination of preventative analgesic techniques involving both central and peripheral-acting analgesic drugs as well as novel approaches to administering drugs in locations remote from the hospital setting. It is of critical importance for clinical investigators to return to the hard work of performing prospective, randomized clinical trials on a procedure-specific basis to evaluate the use of different analgesic combinations as part of multimodal analgesic treatment regimens in the postoperative period.[63,66] Improving recovery after ambulatory surgery by optimizing anesthetic and analgesic techniques will benefit patients, health care providers, and society-at-large in the future.[67]

REFERENCES

1. White PF. Multimodal pain management - the future is now! Curr Opin Investig Drugs 2007;8:517–8.
2. Pavlin DJ, Chen C, Penazola DA, et al. Pain as a factor complicating recovery and discharge after ambulatory surgery. Anesth Analg 2002;95:627–34.
3. Chung F, Ritchie E, Su J. Postoperative pain in ambulatory surgery. Anesth Analg 1997;85:808–16.
4. Brennan F, Carr DB, Cousins M. Pain management: a fundamental human right. Anesth Analg 2007;105:205–21.
5. White PF, Kehlet H, Neal JM, et al. Role of the anesthesiologist in fast-track surgery: from multimodal analgesia to perioperative medical care. Anesth Analg 2007;104:1380–96.
6. Schug S, Chong C. Pain management after ambulatory surgery. Curr Opin Anaesthesiol 2009;22:738–43.
7. Kavanagh T, Hu P, Minogue S. Daycase laparoscopic cholecystectomy: a prospective study of postdischarge pain, analgesic and antiemetic requirements. Ir J Med Sci 2008;177:111–5.
8. White PF. The changing role of non-opioid analgesic techniques in the management of postoperative pain. Anesth Analg 2005;101:S5–22.
9. Frasco PE, Sprung J, Trentman TL. The impact of the joint commission for accreditation of healthcare organizations pain initiative on perioperative opiate consumption and recovery room lengths of stay. Anesth Analg 2005;100:162–8.
10. Vila H Jr, Smith RA, Augustyniak MJ, et al. The efficacy and safety of pain management before and after implementation of hospital-wide pain management standards: is patient safety compromised by treatment based solely on numerical pain ratings? Anesth Analg 2005;101:474–80.
11. White PF. Prevention of nausea and vomiting: a multimodal solution to a persistent problem. N Engl J Med 2004;350:2511–2.

12. Raeder JC, Steine S, Vatsgar TT. Oral ibuprofen versus paracetamol plus codeine for analgesia after ambulatory surgery. Anesth Analg 2001;92:1470–2.
13. Michaloliakou C, Chung F, Sharma S. Preoperative multimodal analgesia facilitates recovery after ambulatory laparoscopic cholecystectomy. Anesth Analg 1996;83:44–51.
14. Eriksson H, Tenhunen A, Korttila K. Balanced analgesia improves recovery and outcome after outpatient tubal ligation. Acta Anaesthesiol Scand 1996;40:151–5.
15. White PF, Sacan O, Tufanogullari B, et al. Effect of short-term postoperative celecoxib administration on patient outcome after outpatient laparoscopic surgery. Can J Anaesth 2007;54:342–8.
16. Gan TJ, Joshi GP, Viscusi E, et al. Preoperative parenteral parecoxib and follow-up oral valdecoxib reduce length of stay and improve quality of patient recovery after laparoscopic cholecystectomy surgery. Anesth Analg 2004;98:1665–73.
17. White PF, Kehlet H. Improving pain management: are we jumping from the frying pan into the fire? [editorial]. Anesth Analg 2007;105:10–2.
18. Ma H, Tang J, White PF, et al. Perioperative rofecoxib improves early recovery after outpatient herniorrhaphy. Anesth Analg 2004;98:970–5.
19. White PF, Kehlet H. Postoperative pain management and patient outcome: time to return to work! [editorial]. Anesth Analg 2007;104:487–90.
20. Mitchell A, van Zanten SV, Inglis K, et al. A randomized controlled trial comparing acetaminophen plus ibuprofen versus acetaminophen plus codeine plus caffeine after outpatient general surgery. J Am Coll Surg 2008;206:472–9.
21. Gorocs TS, Lambert M, Rinne T, et al. Efficacy and tolerability of ready-to-use intravenous paracetamol solution as monotherapy or as an adjunct analgesic therapy for postoperative pain in patients undergoing elective ambulatory surgery: open, prospective study. Int J Clin Pract 2009;63:112–20.
22. Api O, Unal O, Ugurel V, et al. Analgesic efficacy of intravenous paracetamol for outpatient fractional curettage: a randomised, controlled trial. Int J Clin Pract 2009;63:105–11.
23. Ohnesorge H, Bein B, Hanss H, et al. Paracetamol versus metamizol in the treatment of postoperative pain after breast surgery: a randomized, controlled trial. Eur J Anaesthesiol 2009;26:648–53.
24. Viscomi CM, Friend A, Parker C, et al. Ketamine as an adjuvant in lidocaine intravenous regional anesthesia: a randomized, double-blind, systemic control trial. Reg Anesth Pain Med 2009;34:130–3.
25. Suzuki M. Role of N-methyl-D-aspartate receptor antagonists in postoperative pain management. Curr Opin Anaesthesiol 2009;22:618–22.
26. Lin TF, Yeh YC, Lin FS, et al. Effect of combining dexmedetomidine andmorphine for intravenous patient-controlled analgesia. Br J Anaesth 2009;102:117–22.
27. Salman N, Uzun S, Coskun F, et al. Dexmedetomidine as a substitute for remifentanil in ambulatory gynecologic laparoscopic surgery. Saudi Med J 2009;30:77–81.
28. Gilron I, Orr E, Tu D, et al. A randomized, double-blind, controlled trial of perioperative administration of gabapentin, meloxicam and their combination for spontaneous and movement-evoked pain after ambulatory laparoscopic cholecystectomy. Anesth Analg 2009;108:623–30.
29. Srivastava U, Kumar A, Saxena S, et al. Effect of preoperative gabapentin on postoperative pain and tramadol consumption after minilap open cholecystectomy: a randomized double-blind, placebo-controlled trial. Eur J Anaesthesiol 2010;27:331–5.
30. Sen H, Sizlan A, Yanarates O, et al. A comparison of gabapentin and ketamine in acute and chronic pain after hysterectomy. Anesth Analg 2009;109:1645–50.

31. Agarwal A, Gautam S, Gupta D, et al. Evaluation of a single preoperative dose of pregabalin for attenuation of postoperative pain after laparoscopic cholecystectomy. Br J Anaesth 2008;101:700–4.
32. Mathiesen O, Jacobsen LS, Holm HE, et al. Pregabalin and dexamethasone for postoperative pain control: a randomized controlled study in hip arthroplasty. Br J Anaesth 2008;101:535–41.
33. Buvanendran A. Perioperative oral pregabalin reduces chronic pain after total knee arthroplasty: a prospective, randomized controlled trial. Anesth Analg 2010;110:199–207.
34. White PF, Tufanogullari B, Taylor J, et al. The effect of pregabalin on preoperative anxiety and sedation levels: a dose-ranging study. Anesth Analg 2009;108: 1140–5.
35. Collard V, Mistraletti G, Taqi A, et al. Intraoperative esmolol infusion in the absence of opioids spares postoperative fentanyl in patients undergoing ambulatory laparoscopic cholecystectomy. Anesth Analg 2007;105:1255–62.
36. Coloma M, Chiu J, White P, et al. The use of esmolol as an alternative to remifentanil during desflurane anesthesia for fast-track outpatient gynecologic laparoscopic surgery. Anesth Analg 2001;92:352–7.
37. White PF, Wang BG, Tang J, et al. The effect of intraoperative use of esmolol and nicardipine on recovery after ambulatory surgery. Anesth Analg 2003;97:1633–8.
38. Chia YY, Chan MH, Ko NH, et al. Role of β-blockade in anaesthesia and postoperative pain management after hysterectomy. Br J Anaesth 2004;93:799–805.
39. Ozturk T, Kaya H, Aran G, et al. Postoperative beneficial effects of esmolol in treated hypertensive patients undergoing laparoscopic cholecystectomy. Br J Anaesth 2008;100:211–4.
40. Salerno A, Hermann R. Efficacy and safety of steroid use for postoperative pain relief. Update and review of the medical literature. J Bone Joint Surg Am 2006;88: 1361–72.
41. Kardash KJ, Sarrazin F, Tessler MJ, et al. Single-dose dexamethasone reduces dynamic pain after total hip arthroplasty. Anesth Analg 2008;106:1253–7.
42. Jokela RM, Ahonen JV, Tallgren MK, et al. The effective analgesic dose of dexamethasone after laparoscopic hysterectomy. Anesth Analg 2009;109:607–15.
43. Vieira PA, Pulai I, Tsao GC, et al. Dexamethasone with bupivacaine increases duration of analgesia in ultrasound-guided interscalene brachial plexus blockade. Eur J Anaesthesiol 2010;27:285–8.
44. Mathiesen O, Rasmussen ML, Dierking G, et al. Pregabalin and dexamethasone in combination with paracetamol for postoperative pain control after abdominal hysterectomy. A randomized clinical trial. Acta Anaesthesiol Scand 2009;53: 227–35.
45. Rasmussen ML, Mathiesen O, Dierking O, et al. Multimodal analgesia with gabapentin, ketamine and dexamethasone in combination with paracetamol and ketorolac after hip arthroplasty: a preliminary study. Eur J Anaesthesiol 2010;27: 324–30.
46. Granier M, Dadure C, Bringuier S, et al. Intranasal lidocaine plus naphazoline nitrate improves surgical conditions and perioperative analgesia in septorhinoplasty surgery. Can J Anaesth 2009;56:102–8.
47. Perniola A, Gupta A, Crafoord K, et al. Intraabdominal local anaesthetics for postoperative pain relief following abdominal hysterectomy: a randomized, double-blind, dose-finding study. Eur J Anaesthesiol 2009;26:421–9.
48. Kaba A, Laurent SR, Detroz BJ, et al. Intravenous lidocaine infusion facilitates acute rehabilitation after laparoscopic colectomy. Anesthesiology 2007;106:11–8.

49. Lauwick S, Kim DJ, Michelagnoli G, et al. Intraoperative infusion of lidocaine reduces postoperative fentanyl requirements in patients undergoing laparoscopic cholecystectomy. Can J Anaesth 2008;55:754–60.
50. Herroeder S, Pecher S, Schonherr ME, et al. Systemic lidocaine shortens length of hospital stay after colorectal surgery: a double-blinded, randomized, placebo-controlled trial. Ann Surg 2007;246:192–200.
51. Groudine SB, Fisher HA, Kaufman RP Jr, et al. Intravenous lidocaine speeds the return of bowel function, decreases postoperative pain, and shortens hospital stay in patients undergoing radical retropubic prostatectomy. Anesth Analg 1998;86:235–9.
52. Yardeni IZ, Beilin B, Mayburd E, et al. The effect of perioperative intravenous lidocaine on postoperative pain and immune function. Anesth Analg 2009;109: 1464–9.
53. White PF, Issioui T, Skrivanek GD, et al. Use of a continuous popliteal sciatic nerve block for the management of pain after major podiatric surgery: does it improve quality of recovery? Anesth Analg 2003;97:1303–9.
54. Ilfeld BM, Enneking FK. Continuous peripheral nerve blocks at home: a review. Anesth Analg 2005;100:1822–33.
55. Capdevilla X, Dadure C, Bringuier S, et al. Effect of patient-controlled perineural analgesia on rehabilitation and pain after ambulatory orthopaedic surgery: a multicenter randomised trial. Anesthesiology 2006;105:566–73.
56. Liu SS, Richman JM, Thirlby R, et al. Efficacy of continuous wound catheters delivering local anesthetic for postoperative analgesia a quantitative and qualitative systematic review of randomized controlled trials. J Am Coll Surg 2006;203: 914–32.
57. Ilfeld BM, Le LT, Ramjohn J, et al. The effects of local anesthetic concentration and dose on continuous infraclavicular nerve blocks: a multicenter, randomized, observermasked, controlled study. Anesth Analg 2009;108:345–50.
58. Kim KS, Nam YM. The analgesic effects of capsicum plaster at the Zusanli point after abdominal hysterectomy. Anesth Analg 2006;103:709–13.
59. Wang B, Tang J, White PF, et al. Effect of the intensity of transcutaneous acupoint electrical stimulation on the postoperative analgesic requirement. Anesth Analg 1997;85:406–13.
60. Usichenko TI, Kuchling S, Witstruck T, et al. Auricular acupuncture for pain relief after ambulatory knee surgery: a randomized trial. CMAJ 2007;176:179–83.
61. Moiniche S, Kehlet H, Dahl JB. A qualitative and quantitative systematic review of preemptive analgesia for postoperative pain relief. Anesthesiology 2002;96: 725–41.
62. Sun T, Sacan O, White PF, et al. Perioperative vs postoperative celecoxib on patient outcome after major plastic surgery procedures. Anesth Analg 2008; 106:950–8.
63. White PF, Kehlet H. Improving postoperative pain management: what are the unresolved issues? Anesthesiology 2010;112:220–5.
64. Bisgaard T. Analgesic treatment after laparoscopic cholecystectomy: a critical assessment of the evidence. Anesthesiology 2006;104:835–46.
65. Baldini G, Carli F. Anesthetic and adjunctive drugs for fast-track surgery. Curr Drug Targets 2009;10(8):667–86.
66. White PF, Kehlet H, Liu S. Perioperative analgesia: what do we still know? Anesth Analg 2009;108:1364–7.
67. White PF. Facilitating the recovery process: who really benefits? Anesth Analg 2010;110:273–5.

Update on the Management of Postoperative Nausea and Vomiting and Postdischarge Nausea and Vomiting in Ambulatory Surgery

Tina P. Le, BS, Tong Joo Gan, MD, FRCA*

KEYWORDS

- Ambulatory surgery • Antiemetic • Multimodal prevention
- Postoperative nausea and vomiting
- Postdischarge nausea and vomiting • Prophylaxis

Over the past several decades, as the risk of major mortality due to surgery has decreased, attention has shifted to addressing factors that negatively influence patient morbidity and patient satisfaction, such as postoperative nausea and vomiting (PONV). Since the previous article on PONV in this publication,[1] several developments have aided in the prevention and management of this complication of surgical anesthesia. The 5-hydroxytryptamine type 3 (5-HT_3) receptor antagonists continue to be the mainstay of antiemetic therapy, but newer approaches, such as neurokinin-1 antagonists, a longer-acting serotonin receptor antagonist, multimodal management, and novel techniques for managing high-risk patients, are gaining prominence.

PONV continues to be one of the most common complaints following surgery, occurring in more than 30% of surgeries, or as high as 70% to 80% in certain high-risk populations without prophylaxis.[2] Though generally nonfatal and self-limited, PONV may lead to rare but serious medical consequences, including dehydration and electrolyte imbalance, venous hypertension, bleeding, hematoma formation, suture dehiscence, esophageal rupture,[3,4,5] blindness,[6] and aspiration.[7] PONV also has a profound impact on patient satisfaction, quality of life, and estimated health

Department of Anesthesiology, Duke University Medical Center, Duke University School of Medicine, Box 3094, Durham, NC 27710, USA
* Corresponding author.
E-mail address: gan00001@mc.duke.edu

Anesthesiology Clin 28 (2010) 225–249
doi:10.1016/j.anclin.2010.02.003 anesthesiology.theclinics.com
1932-2275/10/$ – see front matter

care costs as a result of delayed discharge, prolonged nursing care, and unanticipated hospital admissions.[8,9] PONV is often cited as one of the postsurgical complications patients would most like to avoid, and patients have reported being willing to pay between $56 and $100 out of pocket for an effective antiemetic.[10]

Nausea and vomiting due to surgery may also occur beyond the immediate postoperative period. Although not as well studied as PONV, the related problem of postdischarge nausea and vomiting (PDNV) has received increasing attention from health care providers, especially because patients who experience no PONV immediately after surgery may develop PDNV after discharge. In one study, approximately 36% of patients who experience PDNV had not experienced any nausea or vomiting before discharge.[11] Surveys of patients following ambulatory surgery have found PDNV to range between approximately 20% and 50%, resulting in increased difficulty in performing activities of daily living and longer recovery times before resuming normal activity.[11–14]

The issues of PONV and PDNV are especially significant in the context of ambulatory surgeries, which comprise more than 60% of the combined 56.4 million ambulatory and inpatient surgery visits in the United States.[15] Although the incidence of PONV and PDNV in ambulatory surgeries may be slightly lower than that of inpatient surgeries, it is believed to be underreported, given the limited amount of time that ambulatory surgery patients spend under direct medical care.[16] Yet because of this relatively brief period that ambulatory patients spend in health care facilities, it is particularly important to prevent and treat PONV and PDNV swiftly and effectively.

MECHANISM OF EMESIS

Much of our current understanding of the basic neuroanatomy and physiology of emesis comes from the work of Wang and Borison in the 1950s.[17,18] The central coordinating site for nausea and vomiting is located in an ill-defined area of the lateral reticular formation in the brainstem (**Fig. 1**).[18] This "vomiting center," as it is traditionally called, is not so much a discrete center of emetic activity as it is a "central pattern generator" (CPG) that sets off a specific sequence of neuronal activities throughout the medulla to result in vomiting.[19] Multiple inputs may arrive from areas such as

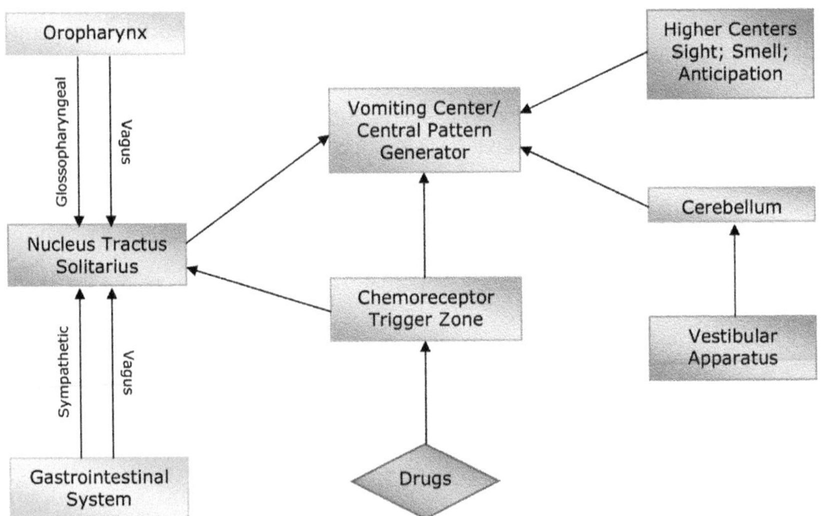

Fig. 1. Mechanism of nausea and vomiting.

the higher cortical centers, cerebellum, vestibular apparatus, vagal, and glossopharyngeal nerve afferents to trigger the complex motor response of emesis; direct electrical stimulation of the CPG also causes emesis.[20] A particularly important afferent is the chemoreceptor trigger zone (CTZ), located at the base of the fourth ventricle in the area postrema and outside the blood-brain barrier, which plays a role in detecting emetogenic agents in the blood and cerebrospinal fluid (CSF).[21] Although direct electrical stimulation of the CTZ does not cause vomiting, the CTZ communicates with the adjacent nucleus tractus solitarius (NTS), which in turn projects into the CPG.[22] Signals between these anatomic areas are mediated through a variety of neurotransmitter receptor systems, including serotonergic, dopaminergic, histaminergic, cholinergic, and neurokininergic; antiemetic prophylaxis or therapies block one or more of the associated receptors, including serotonin 5-HT_3, dopamine D_2, histamine H_1, muscarinic cholinergic, and neurokinin NK_1.[23]

RISK FACTORS AND PROTECTIVE FACTORS FOR PONV AND PDNV

Assessment of patient risk factors is a key component in guiding antiemetic prevention and management strategies. A variety of surgical, anesthetic, and patient factors have been investigated as predictors of patient risk for PONV, the most significant of which are listed in **Table 1**. However, according to the 2007 Society for Ambulatory Anesthesia (SAMBA) Guidelines for the Management of PONV, only a few baseline risk factors occur with enough consistency to be validated as independent predictors for PONV.[24] Several predictive models have been developed to stratify risk for PONV, but a simplified scoring system by Apfel and colleagues[25,26] continues to be one of the most popular and compares favorably against other scoring systems. In a 2-center inpatient study, Apfel and colleagues[27] identified 4 highly predictive risk factors for PONV: female gender, history of motion sickness or PONV, nonsmoker, and use of perioperative opioids. The presence of 0, 1, 2, 3, or 4 of these factors corresponded to a PONV incidence of 10%, 21%, 39%, 61%, and 79%, respectively. The Apfel score may be used to guide antiemetic strategies for high-risk patients, and in at least 2 studies, prophylaxis based on Apfel scores has led to a significant decrease the incidence of PONV.[28,29]

The use of risk scores in predicting postoperative vomiting (POV) has also been extended to the pediatric population with the POstoperative VOmiting in Children score (POVOC score).[30] The incidence of POV in pediatric patients is estimated to

Table 1
Risk factors for PONV and PDNV

Patient Factors	Anesthetic Factors	Surgical Factors
Female	Use of perioperative opioids	Duration of surgery
Nonsmoker	Use of volatile anesthetics	Type of surgery, including:
History of motion sickness or previous PONV	Nitrous oxide	Abdominal
Family history of motion sickness or PONV (pediatric)		Ear, nose, and throat
Age ≥3 y (pediatric)		Gynecologic
		Laparoscopic
		Ophthalmologic
		Orthopedic
		Plastic
		Strabismus (pediatric)

be about between 9% and 42% overall, and as high as 80% for specific types of surgery.[31] However, it should be noted that nausea is often not recorded, as it is often difficult to assess in this younger patient population. To develop the POVOC score, Eberhart and colleagues[30] compiled data from 1257 pediatric surgeries at 4 institutions and identified 4 independent risk factors for POV: duration of surgery 30 minutes or longer, age 3 years or older, strabismus surgery, and a positive history of POV in the child or POV/PONV in relatives (mother, father, or siblings). Similar to the Apfel score, the incidence of POV was 9%, 10%, 30%, 55%, and 70% for 0, 1, 2, 3, and 4 risk factors present, respectively. To date, there has only been one external validation study, which found that a modified POVOC score (excluding strabismus surgery) accurately predicted POV in pediatric patients, at a level comparable to the Apfel score for adults.[32]

The 1999 study by Sinclair and colleagues,[33] spanning 3 years and involving more than 17,000 patients, continues to be the most comprehensive examination of PONV risk factors specifically in ambulatory surgery patients. In addition to the 4 factors identified by Apfel and colleagues, duration of anesthesia longer than 30 minutes, general anesthesia, and type of surgery were also cited as independent predictors of PONV. However, it should be noted that while certain types of surgeries (particularly plastic, ophthalmologic, and orthopedic surgeries) appear to be correlated with higher rates of PONV, there is conflicting evidence as to whether other independent risk factors associated with type of surgery are actually responsible for the increased rates of PONV.[24] Other studies, not confined specifically to ambulatory surgery patients, have also pointed to the use of volatile anesthetics, use of nitrous oxide, and administration of intraoperative and postoperative opioids as significant risk factors for PONV.[24,34–37]

Risk factors for PDNV have mainly been studied in the context of risk factors for PONV. However, a recent study by White and colleagues[38] suggests that while higher Apfel scores correlate to a greater incidence of PONV symptoms in the early (0–24 hours) postoperative period, it appears to have little predictive value for emetic symptoms occurring in the late (24–72 hours) postoperative/postdischarge period. Nevertheless, the few studies attempting to identify specific PDNV risk factors have found them to be similar to those typically associated with PONV. Mattila and colleagues[14] evaluated postdischarge symptoms in 2754 adult and pediatric ambulatory surgery patients, and found that the odds ratios (ORs) of postdischarge vomiting were 0.23 and 0.26 for local and spinal anesthesia, respectively, when compared with general anesthesia. Female gender was also a risk factor for PDNV, with ORs of 2.74 and 2.79 for nausea and vomiting, respectively. Duration of surgery longer than 30 minutes increased the risk for nausea only, with a 56% increase in incidence of postdischarge nausea for surgeries 30 to 59 minutes' duration, and a 64% increase for surgeries 60 minutes or longer. However, type of surgical procedure had no impact.

In the same study, no specific risk factors for postdischarge vomiting could be identified in the pediatric population, although use of general anesthesia, age 3 years or older, and duration of surgery 30 minutes or longer correlated with an increased risk of postdischarge nausea.[14] Other studies have suggested that PDNV in children may be correlated to factors such as emetic symptoms prior to discharge, increased age, duration of journey home after discharge, pain at home, and use of postoperative opioids, but these associations need further study.[24,39,40]

ANTIEMETICS IN CLINICAL PRACTICE

Most antiemetic agents act on one or more of the neurotransmitter receptor types found in the anatomic sites responsible for emesis. To date, no single agent has been found to block all receptor types, nor is there any single drug that is completely effective against PONV in all cases. Thus, appropriate prevention and management of PONV and PDNV require familiarity with a broad range of drug classes. In comparing various antiemetics and the evidence for or against them, it is helpful to determine the number needed to treat (NNT), or the number of patients that must be exposed to a particular intervention in order for one patient to benefit over receiving placebo or no treatment. The number needed to harm (NNH) is an estimate of the frequency of drug-related adverse effects. A list of common antiemetics, typical dosages, and NNT are listed in **Table 2**.

Serotonin Antagonists

Since their introduction in the early 1990s to treat chemotherapy-induced nausea and vomiting,[41] serotonin antagonists have become one of the cornerstones of modern antiemetic prophylaxis and therapy, particularly in the setting of PONV. Serotonin is found in high levels in the enterochromaffin cells of the gastrointestinal tract, as well as in the central nervous system, and may be released to stimulate either the vagal afferent neurons or the CTZ to activate the vomiting center.[42] Although there are multiple serotonin receptor types, the 5-HT_3 subtype appears in its greatest concentration in the NTS, area postrema, and the dorsal motor nucleus of the vagus nerve, which all play a significant role in coordinating the vomiting reflex.[43] The 5-HT_3 receptor antagonists (5-HT_3 RAs), which include ondansetron, granisetron, dolasetron, ramosetron, tropisetron, and most recently palonosetron, act by inhibiting the action of serotonin in 5-HT_3 receptor-rich areas of the brain.

Ondansetron (Zofran), granisetron (Kytril), dolasetron (Anzemet), and palonosetron (Aloxi) are all approved for use in PONV by the Food and Drug Administration (FDA) (ramosetron and tropisetron are not available in the United States). In general, all of the 5-HT_3 RAs are safe, effective, and have similar side effect profiles. Side effects are usually short term and of mild to moderate intensity, with the most common being headache, dizziness, constipation, and diarrhea.[44–47] However, the differing chemical

Table 2
Number needed to treat (NNT) for common prophylactic antiemetic regimens

	NNT		
Agent or Strategies	**Nausea**	**Vomiting**	**PONV**
Ondansetron 4 mg IV[53]	4.6	6.4	4.4
Dexamethasone 8 mg IV or 10 mg PO (adults)[75]	Early 5.0 Late 4.3	Early 3.6 Late 4.3	
Dexamethasone 1–1.5 mg/kg IV (children)[75]		Early 10 Late 3.1	
Transdermal scopolamine 1.5 mg patch[82]	4.3	5.6	3.8
Droperidol 0.625–1.25 mg IV[85]	5	7	
Haloperidol 0.5–4 mg IM/IV[92]	3.2–4.5	3.9–5.1	
Metoclopramide 10 mg IV[100]	No significant effect	Early 9.1 Late 10	
Propofol infusion[105]	8.6 (Postdischarge 12.5)	11.2 (Postdischarge 10.3)	
Acupuncture[123]	30% baseline risk 11 70% baseline risk 5	30% baseline risk 11 70% baseline risk 5	

structures of each drug may explain slight differences in receptor binding affinity, dose response, and duration of action.[23] Most available data suggest that 5-HT_3 RAs are most effective when administered at the end of surgery,[48–50] but at least one study has suggested that dolasetron may be administered around the time of induction of anesthesia, with little effect on efficacy.[51]

All of the 5-HT_3 RAs are equally effective for the treatment of PONV.[52] Ondansetron, as the prototypical 5-HT_3 RA, has been the most studied. In a quantitative systematic review of placebo-controlled trials of ondansetron, Tramèr and colleagues[53] found that ondansetron, 4 mg had an NNT of about 4.6 for the prevention of vomiting, 6.4 for the prevention of nausea, and 4.4 for the prevention of both in the first 48 hours postoperatively. Risk of severe side effects was generally low, with an NNH of 36 for headache, 31 for elevated liver enzymes, and 23 for constipation. This study and others have also suggested that ondansetron is slightly more effective against vomiting than nausea.[52,53] However, a recent study by Jokela and colleagues[54] found that 4 mg ondansetron reduced the incidence of nausea by 26% over placebo, and vomiting by 33%, a difference that the investigators concluded was not of statistical significance. While not commenting on the antinausea versus antivomiting properties of ondansetron, a Cochrane systematic review found that ondansetron reduces the relative risk of nausea and vomiting by 32% and 45% over placebo, respectively.[55] The review also evaluated 5 studies of ondansetron and reported no evidence that the risk of PONV differed for groups based on timing of administration. Controversy also exists as to whether ondansetron offers greater benefit for PONV prophylaxis greater than 4 mg,[56–59] and a study in ferrets has found that the dose-response curve for ondansetron is unique in that it has better antiemetic efficacy at low (<50 μg/kg subcutaneously) and high (>100 μg/kg subcutaneously) doses.[60] However, for the purposes of clinical practice the usual recommended dose of ondansetron in humans is 4 mg intravenously (IV), administered at the end of surgery.[24]

Unlike ondansetron, the other 5-HT_3 RAs exhibit linear dose-response curves, with increasing doses achieving greater clinical effect until the maximal effective dose is reached.[61] The dose recommended for PONV prophylaxis with granisetron is 0.35 to 1.5 mg IV (5–20 μg/kg).[24,62,63] In a multicenter, dose-ranging study, Taylor and colleagues[64] found that intravenous doses as low as 0.1 mg given at the first symptoms of nausea or vomiting were effective in increasing the percentage of patients experiencing no vomiting in the first 24 hours to 38%, compared to 20% of patients with no vomiting on placebo. The recommended dose for dolasetron is 12.5 mg IV,[24] based on a trial demonstrating that single-dose dolasetron 12.5 mg administered before the end of surgery resulted in a greater than 50% increase in complete response (CR; no emesis and no rescue medication for 24 hours) over placebo, with no significant increase in CR at 25- or 50-mg doses.[65]

Palonosetron is the newest 5-HT_3 RA and has recently been approved in the United States for PONV. Unlike other drugs in its class, which exhibit simple bimolecular binding, palonosetron exhibits positive cooperativity in binding to its receptor; moreover, its molecular structure does not mimic that of serotonin and it therefore does not bind at the serotonin binding site of the 5-HT_3 receptor.[66] As a result, palonosetron may bind more tightly to the receptor, allow multiple palonosetron molecules to bind to a single receptor, and make it less likely to be displaced by serotonin molecules.[67] Furthermore, some data suggest that palonosetron may promote internalization of the 5-HT_3 receptor as an inverse agonist (similar to some G-protein coupled receptor antagonists), decreasing the function of the receptor in the absence of agonist exposure.[66] Thus, receptor internalization may contribute to palonosetron's relatively long duration of action.

A large, randomized, placebo-controlled study by Candiotti and colleagues[68] found that 43% of patients given palonosetron 0.075 mg before induction exhibited CR in the 0 to 24 hours postoperatively, compared with 20% of patients who received placebo. Moreover, patients receiving palonosetron reported less severe nausea and decreased interference in postoperative function due to PONV. A separate study of European patients by Kovac and colleagues[69] found similar results for palonosetron, 0.075 mg in increasing CR rates, and the investigators also noted continued efficacy of palonosetron over placebo for 24 to 72 hours. It has been suggested that the long half-life of palonosetron may confer an antiemetic effect for several days after administration, which would be particularly useful in minimizing PDNV following ambulatory surgery; however, further studies are necessary to confirm any advantage over other serotonin antagonists.

Few studies have examined 5-HT_3 RAs for the prevention of PDNV. A systematic review by Gupta and colleagues[13] found that ondansetron 4 mg resulted in a relative risk reduction of 23% and 37% for postdischarge nausea and vomiting, respectively. However, it should be noted that the NNT was 12.9 for nausea and 13.6 for vomiting. Ondansetron, granisetron, and dolasetron are available as intravenous medications or oral tablets; palonosetron is currently only available as an intravenous medication. Ondansetron is also available as an orally disintegrating tablet (ODT), which seems to be as effective as the intravenous form.[70] Some studies suggest that providing patients with the ODT before discharge may be particularly helpful in reducing the incidence of PDNV at home. In a study of pediatric patients, Davis and colleagues[71] found that only 14.5% of children who received 5 at-home doses of ondansetron ODT experienced postdischarge vomiting, compared with 32% of children receiving placebo. A small study by Gan and colleagues[72] found a decreased incidence of PDNV and PDNV severity in patients receiving ondansetron ODT following ambulatory surgery.

A relatively new but growing field in 5-HT_3 RA research is that of pharmacogenomics. The 5-HT_3 RAs are metabolized by cytochrome P450 in the liver, and differences in the activity or levels of the CYP2D6 isoform of the enzyme appear to have an effect on the pharmacokinetics and clinical efficacy of the drug in certain individuals.[23] Candiotti and colleagues[73] have reported that patients with 3 copies of the CYP2D6 gene or who have certain genetic polymorphisms in the CYP2D6 gene are ultrarapid metabolizers of ondansetron and are more likely to experience ondansetron failure for POV. Another recent study by Rueffert and colleagues[74] analyzed DNA from 95 patients who had suffered from POV and matched them with 94 controls. The researchers found that variations in the genes of the serotonin receptor subunits, HTR3A and HTR3B, were associated with increased individual risk of developing POV. Although pharmacogenomic research is still in its early stages and it is currently of limited use in actual clinical practice, it may provide greater insights into assessing individual patient risk for PONV in the future.

Steroids

Dexamethasone has been shown to be useful in the management of PONV. The mechanism of its antiemetic activity has not been fully elucidated, but it is believed that corticosteroids act centrally to inhibit prostaglandin synthesis or to control endorphin release.[75] Dexamethasone may also be particularly effective when used in combination with 5-HT_3 receptor antagonists, as it may (1) reduce levels of serotonin by depleting its precursor tryptophan, (2) prevent release of serotonin in the gut, and (3) sensitize the 5-HT_3 receptor to other antiemetics.[75]

According to a study by Wang and colleagues,[76] dexamethasone is most effective for PONV prophylaxis when administered at induction rather than at the end of surgery. A systematic review and meta-analysis of 17 trials by Karanicolas and colleagues[77] found that dexamethasone reduced the incidence of postoperative nausea (PON) by 41%, POV by 59%, and nausea or vomiting by 45% relative to placebo, with the incidences of headache and dizziness being similar between the 2 groups. These results are similar to an earlier quantitative systematic review, which reported an NNT of 7.1 for the prevention of early vomiting in adults and children, and 3.8 for the prevention of late vomiting.[75] Karanicolas and colleagues[77] also reported that doses of 8 to 16 mg were significantly more effective at reducing PONV than doses of 2 to 5 mg, consistent with an earlier study by Elhakim and colleagues concluding that a dose of 8 mg dexamethasone provided maximal PONV prophylaxis when combined with ondansetron.[78] However, the SAMBA guidelines recommend a prophylactic dose of dexamethasone 4 to 5 mg IV at induction, which seems to be as effective as ondansetron 4 mg IV in preventing PONV.[24]

Cholinergic Antagonists

The anticholinergic agents are among the oldest antiemetics. Both scopolamine (hyoscine) and atropine block muscarinic cholinergic emetic receptors in the cerebral cortex and the pons.[79] However, atropine has weaker antiemetic effects than scopolamine[80] and is generally not used in the postoperative period because of its cardiovascular effects.[1]

Most studies of scopolamine for use in PONV have investigated transdermal scopolamine (TDS) patch, designed to release 1.5 mg of scopolamine over 3 days. In a double-blind sham and placebo-controlled study of 150 patients, White and colleagues[81] compared preoperative transdermal scopolamine (TDS) 1.5 mg patch to intravenous ondansetron 4 mg or droperidol 1.25 mg administered before the end of surgery. The investigators found that premedication with TDS was as effective as ondansetron or droperidol in the prevention of both early and late PONV/PDNV, but also noted that TDS was associated with a greater risk of dry mouth. These findings correlate with an earlier quantitative systematic review by Kranke and colleagues,[82] which found that although TDS is an effective antiemetic and has an NNT of 5.6 for the prevention of POV, the NNH is 5.6 for visual disturbances, 12.5 for dry mouth, and 50 for dizziness. Thus, the high rate of anticholinergic side effects of scopolamine may limit its use as a stand-alone antiemetic agent.

Scopolamine may be most useful as an adjunct to other antiemetics. In a trial of outpatient plastic surgery patients at high risk for PONV, Sah and colleagues[83] found that those who received a preoperative TDS patch in addition to intraoperative ondansetron had a statistically significant reduction in PON between 8 and 24 hours in comparison with those who received a placebo patch and ondansetron only. However, a similar, larger, multicenter trial found that a combination TDS and ondansetron reduced PONV as compared with ondansetron alone 24 hours after surgery, but not at 48 hours.[84] This study also noted that the incidence of adverse effects, including anticholinergic effects was not statistically different between the 2 groups, while patient satisfaction in the TDS group was significantly higher, suggesting that scopolamine might be a safe and effective adjunct in the management of PONV, especially when used in combination with ondansetron.

Dopamine Antagonists

The dopamine receptor antagonists act at the D_2 receptors in the CTZ and area postrema to suppress nausea and vomiting. There are 3 types of dopamine antagonists commonly used as antiemetics: butyrophenones, benzamides, and phenothiazines.

Butyrophenones

In addition to their strong D_2 receptor antagonism, the butyrophenones are α-blockers, contributing to their adverse effects of sedation and extrapyramidal symptoms, although the latter are rare at the low doses given for PONV.[80] The 2 primary antiemetic agents in this group are haloperidol and droperidol. The clinical efficacy of droperidol 0.625 to 1.25 mg IV before the end of surgery has been well established,[85,86] and until recently it had been widely used in the prevention and management of PONV as a cost-effective antiemetic. The IMPACT trial, a factorial trial of more than 5000 patients, found that droperidol is as effective as ondansetron and dexamethasone in reducing the risk of PONV.[2] A meta-analysis by Leslie and Gan[87] examining the safety of the 5-HT_3 antagonists with dexamethasone or droperidol found that all were generally well tolerated and had comparable safety profiles, even when used in combination.

However, in 2001 the FDA issued a "black box" warning for droperidol, citing reports of severe cardiac arrhythmias (eg, torsades de pointes) and rare cases of sudden cardiac death associated with the use of droperidol.[88] Although the use of droperidol has declined precipitously since then, many experts and anesthesia providers still believe that the warning was not justified, and that droperidol remains a safe, effective, and economical antiemetic.[88–90] Nevertheless, the warning, along with the FDA's recommendation that all elective surgery patients receiving droperidol be placed on continuous electrocardiographic monitoring for 2 to 3 hours following administration, has limited its use in the ambulatory setting.

Accordingly, there has been an increased interest in haloperidol as an antiemetic. Haloperidol has been used primarily as a potent antipsychotic since the 1960s.[91] Haloperidol has a faster onset of antiemetic action and has a longer half-life than droperidol, but its effect does not last as long, most likely because it has a weaker binding affinity than droperidol for the D_2 receptors in the CTZ and area postrema.[80] In a meta-analysis of published and unpublished trials from 1962 to 1988, Buttner and colleagues[92] found that haloperidol 0.5 to 4 mg was effective for established PONV over placebo, with an NNT of 3.2 to 5.1 over the first 24 hours postoperatively, although some of the trials included had flaws in design or data reporting. A small study of 90 nonsmoking, female patients in Taiwan found that haloperidol 2 mg IV was as effective as ondansetron 4 mg IV in preventing PONV for the first 24 hours, with no QTc prolongation observed.[92] A similar study also did not observe QTc prolongation and found that haloperidol 1 mg IV was similar to ondansetron 4 mg IV, but both medications were only effective antiemetics relative to placebo in the early postoperative phase (0–2 hours).[93] More recent studies by Rosow and colleagues[94,95] have demonstrated the antiemetic efficacy of haloperidol over placebo and increased efficacy of haloperidol with ondansetron over ondansetron alone. However, additional studies are necessary to determine optimal dosing, timing, and safety profile before haloperidol may be used in regular clinical practice, either as prophylaxis or treatment.

Phenothiazines

The phenothiazines, which include promethazine, chlorpromazine, prochlorperazine, perphenazine, and thiethylperazine, are some of the most commonly used antiemetics in the world. However, their use has fallen out of favor due to their high incidence of adverse effects, such as sedation, restlessness, diarrhea, agitation, and central nervous system depression, and more rarely, extrapyramidal effects, hypotension, neuroleptic syndrome, and supraventricular tachycardia.[23] Promethazine 12.5 to 25 mg IV given at the induction of surgery,[96] and prochlorperazine 5 to 10 mg IV given at the end of surgery[97] have both been shown to have antiemetic efficacy when combined with ondansetron. A retrospective review has also suggested that promethazine 6.25 mg, a dose low enough to limit most adverse effects, may be more effective than ondansetron for treating PONV in patients who have failed previous ondansetron prophylaxis.[98] However, strong data are lacking and phenothiazines are currently not recommended as first-line antiemetic agents.[24]

Benzamides

The most commonly used antiemetic in this group is metoclopramide, a procainimide derivative that blocks D_2 receptors both centrally at the CTZ and area postrema, and peripherally in the gastrointestinal tract.[80] Metoclopramide increases lower esophageal tone and promotes gastric motility, which may make it useful in preventing the delayed gastric emptying caused by opioids.[99] A quantitative systematic review of 66 studies using various regimens of metoclopramide found no significant antinausea effect, an NNT of 9.1 to prevent early vomiting in adults, and an NNT of 10 to prevent late vomiting in the same population.[100] In children, the NNT to prevent early vomiting was 5.8, with no significant late antivomiting effect. The review also noted that the best documented doses of metoclopramide were 10 mg IV for adults and 0.25 mg/kg IV for children. A more recent double-blind study in children undergoing tonsillectomy failed to show equivalence between metoclopramide 0.5 mg/kg and ondansetron 0.1 mg/kg, and in fact showed that ondansetron was superior for control of POV.[101] Given the lack of evidence showing antiemetic efficacy, metoclopramide is not recommended for PONV at this time.

Antihistamines

The antiemetic properties of antihistamines such as diphenhydramine, dimenhydrinate, cyclizine, doxylamine, and promethazine are derived from their blockade of the histamine H_1 receptor in the NTS, at the vomiting center, and vestibular system; they have little or no direct action at the CTZ.[42] However, their anticholinergic activity is responsible for their most common side effects of sedation, dry mouth, blurred vision, and urinary retention. Although generally inexpensive and readily available, the use of antihistamines in PONV has not been well studied. In a meta-analysis of 18 controlled trials, Kranke and colleagues[102] reported that prophylactic dimenhydrinate (classified there to include both dimenhydrinate and the related diphenhydramine) reduces PONV in adults and children up to 48 hours after surgery, with a recommended dose of 1 mg/kg IV. There have been few studies of dimenhydrinate that specifically compare it with other antiemetics, and dose, timing, and side effect profiles have not been fully established. Doxylamine in combination with pyridoxine (Diclectin) has been shown to reduce the incidence of POV in women undergoing laparoscopic tubal ligation. Although doxylamine is available in the United States, the combination with pyridoxine is only approved in Canada.[103]

Propofol

The mechanism of antiemetic activity using propofol is unclear, but it has been observed that patients who receive propofol for induction tend to have less PONV.[104] This observation has been supported by several meta-analyses, including one that examined postoperative outcomes under inhaled and intravenous anesthetic techniques.[105] Gupta and colleagues found that maintenance with a propofol infusion resulted in a decreased incidence of PONV and PDNV over inhaled anesthetics, with an NNT of 8.6 and 11.2 for PON and POV, respectively, and an NNT of 12.5 and 10.3 for postdischarge nausea and vomiting, respectively. A clinical trial of 2010 surgical patients in the Netherlands found that propofol total intravenous anesthesia (TIVA) resulted in a significant reduction of PONV compared with isoflurane-nitrous oxide anesthesia, with an NNT of 6.[106]

Recent studies have suggested that TIVA alone may not be an optimal strategy for PONV prophylaxis. In a small randomized trial, White and colleagues[107] found that although there were no significant differences in early PONV outcomes between patients given dolasetron prophylaxis and those given propofol-based TIVA, PDNV was significantly more common for patients in the TIVA group. The investigators suggest that although TIVA may be similar in efficacy to dolasetron for early PONV, its effects may be too short-lived to offer protection against PDNV.

Over the past several years, particularly as experience with the technique has increased and costs have decreased, the use of TIVA with propofol has become more popular for ambulatory surgery. One of the greatest limiting factors for increased use of TIVA continues to be cost, as economic analyses have suggested that routine use of TIVA for PONV prophylaxis is generally not cost-effective.[106,108,109] Nevertheless, propofol-based TIVA is still a reasonable option for high-risk patients, especially as part of a multimodal management strategy (see *Combination Therapies and Multimodal Prevention,* below).

NOVEL ANTIEMETIC THERAPIES

Neurokinin-1 Antagonists

The neurokinin-1 receptor antagonists (NK_1 RAs) are a new class of antiemetic drugs that competitively inhibit the binding of substance P, a neuropeptide released from enterochromaffin cells.[110] Substance P plays an important role in emesis as a ligand for neurokinin-1 receptors, which are located in the gastrointestinal tract and the area postrema.[23] The NK_1 RAs are believed to suppress nausea and vomiting by acting centrally on the neurotransmission between the NTS and CPG.[111] These agents may also act peripherally to block NK_1 receptors in the vagal terminals of the gut to decrease the intensity of the emetogenic signals sent to the CPG.[112]

The first NK_1 RA to be approved by the FDA was aprepitant (Emend), for chemotherapy-induced nausea and vomiting.[113] The first clinical trial to study the efficacy of aprepitant in PONV was a multicenter, double-blind study of 805 patients conducted by Gan and colleagues,[114] who found that preoperative aprepitant, both 40 mg and 125 mg orally were equivalent to preoperative ondansetron 4 mg IV in terms of CR rates, nausea control, and use of rescue antiemetics. However, the study also found that aprepitant was superior for prevention of vomiting in the first 24 and 48 hours, with no vomiting in 90% of patients in the aprepitant 40 mg group, 95% of the aprepitant 125 mg group, and 74% of the ondansetron group in the first 24 hours. A follow-up study by the same group in an international population confirmed that aprepitant was superior to ondansetron for incidences of no vomiting in the first 24 and 48 hours, and also found that peak nausea scores were lower in patients receiving either dose of aprepitant.[115] A post hoc analysis of the pooled data from both studies found that in the 24 hours after surgery, aprepitant 40 mg was slightly more effective than ondansetron in terms of no significant nausea (56.4% vs 48.1%), no nausea (39.6% vs 33.1%), no vomiting (86.7% vs 72.4%), no nausea and no vomiting

(38.3% vs 31.4%), and no nausea, vomiting, and no use of rescue antiemetics (37.9% vs 31.2%).[116] The study group also noted that the 125-mg dose was similar or even slightly less effective than the lower dose, leading to the recommended and approved preoperative dose of 40 mg for PONV prophylaxis.

NK_1 RAs are safe and well tolerated, with the most common side effects being asthenia, diarrhea, dizziness, and hiccups.[117] Although further studies are needed to establish their place in clinical practice, the NK_1 RAs offer many potential benefits for the management of PONV, especially as an alternative to patients who have failed treatment or prophylaxis with antiemetics in other classes. Aprepitant may be particularly useful in the ambulatory setting, as it comes in both a convenient oral form and a recently approved intravenous form (fosaprepitant) that may be useful for established PONV,[113] although clinical trials with the intravenous formulation have not been conducted in the PONV setting.

Opioid Antagonists

Perioperative opioid use has long been known to increase the risk of PONV by decreasing gastric motility and delaying gastric emptying via the inhibition of central μ-opioid receptors.[118] Thus, the use of centrally acting opioid receptor antagonists, such as naloxone, may have antiemetic efficacy. Preliminary studies have found that low-dose naloxone (0.25 μg/kg/h) is effective in reducing the incidence of PONV compared with placebo in both adults[119] and children.[120] A recent small study of 50 patients undergoing knee replacement surgery found that epidural sufentanil containing low-dose naloxone was effective in reducing PONV compared with sufentanil without naloxone.[121] However, there is a paucity of clinical data about the use of opioid receptor antagonists in PONV, and further study is necessary.

NONPHARMACOLOGIC TECHNIQUES

Given that no single pharmacologic therapy is completely effective for PONV prophylaxis, nonpharmacologic techniques have become a reasonable adjunct to antiemetic drugs. Of all the nonpharmacologic techniques, acupuncture is one of the most well studied and accepted forms of treatment of PONV. The mechanism of acupuncture in the prevention of nausea and vomiting is not entirely clear; it may activate A-β and A-δ fibers to influence neurotransmission in the dorsal horn or other centers, influence the release of endogenous opioids, or inhibit gastric acid secretion and normalize gastric dysrrhythmia.[122]

Most data about acupuncture in PONV have examined the use of the acupuncture point pericardium 6, or P6, located 4 cm proximal from the wrist crease between the tendons of the palmaris longus and flexor carpi radialis muscles. A recently revised Cochrane database review of 40 randomized controlled trials determined that acupoint stimulation of P6 is effective in the prevention of PONV, with few side effects.[123] The NNTs were reported based on the baseline risk of nausea. At a control event rate of 30% (the estimated overall incidence of PONV), the NNT was 11 for both nausea and vomiting. At a baseline risk of 70% (estimate for high-risk populations), the NNT was 5 for both nausea and vomiting.

There are several comparable variations on traditional acupuncture, including acupressure and acupressure wristbands, acustimulation using transcutaneous electrical stimulation, acupuncture injections, and electroacupuncture.[122] These techniques may be of particular benefit in the ambulatory setting, as many of them can be performed rapidly and do not require special training. Another benefit of acupuncture is its favorable side effect profile compared with pharmacologic techniques, making it a reasonable adjunct to antiemetic drugs. In a large prospective survey of doctors and physiotherapists, there were no serious adverse events due to acupuncture and the risk of adverse events was 14 per 10,000 treatments, with the most common being mild, including fainting, exacerbation of symptoms, and lost or forgotten needle.[124]

THERAPIES LACKING SUFFICIENT EVIDENCE

In addition to some of the antiemetic agents mentioned previously, several other therapies that have been previously explored lack sufficient evidence or fail to demonstrate significant effect to be recommended for routine use in the management of PONV and PDNV.

Although earlier studies reported on the use of supplemental oxygen to reduce the incidence of PONV,[125,126] their findings have not been confirmed by subsequent studies. A systematic review of 10 trials by Orhan-Sungur and colleagues[127] reported that the relative risk of overall PONV in patients receiving 80% FiO_2 was 0.91, and concluded that supplemental oxygen did not reduce the incidence of PONV. Another recent randomized trial of 304 women receiving ambulatory gynecologic laparoscopy found that there were no significant differences in PONV or antiemetic use between women receiving 80% supplemental oxygen and those in the 30% oxygen control group.[128]

The use of cannabinoids, including dronabinol, tetrahydrocannabinol, and nabilone, in PONV has not been well studied, and clinical data are lacking. Tramèr and colleagues[129] conducted a systematic review of 30 trials evaluating cannabinoids in the setting of chemotherapy-induced nausea and vomiting, and found that dronabinol had superior antiemetic activity to phenothiazines. However, the analysis failed to demonstrate statistically significant improvement in antiemetic efficacy between dronabinol and placebo, and between nabilone and phenothiazines, although the investigators did cite a "clinically significant difference" in favor of the cannabinoids and urged further study. Nevertheless, given the common and often unpleasant side effects of most cannabinoids, which include dysphoria, depression, and hallucinations, they are unlikely to be used in regular clinical practice.[129]

Despite its long history of use in traditional Chinese and Indian medicine, ginger (*Zingiber officinale*) does not appear to be effective for PONV. A systematic review of 6 randomized controlled trials by Ernst and Pittler was unable to draw a conclusion about the efficacy of ginger.[130] Since then, there have been few additional studies, with one placebo-controlled trial of 180 patients finding that ginger failed to reduce the incidence of PONV after gynecologic laparoscopy.[131]

MANAGEMENT STRATEGY

As no single intervention can completely prevent or treat PONV, it is important to formulate multimodal approaches to maximize clinical efficacy while minimizing risks to the patient. While there is no clear formula for the prevention and management of PONV, an effective management strategy should consider (1) assessment of risk for developing PONV and baseline risk reduction, (2) prophylaxis and cost-effectiveness, (3) combination therapy, and (4) rescue treatment. **Fig. 2** shows a recommended management strategy based on patient risk.

Assessment of Risk and Baseline Risk Reduction

As discussed earlier, the Apfel score may be a useful clinical tool in assessing patient risk. After taking these patient factors into consideration along with the surgical risk

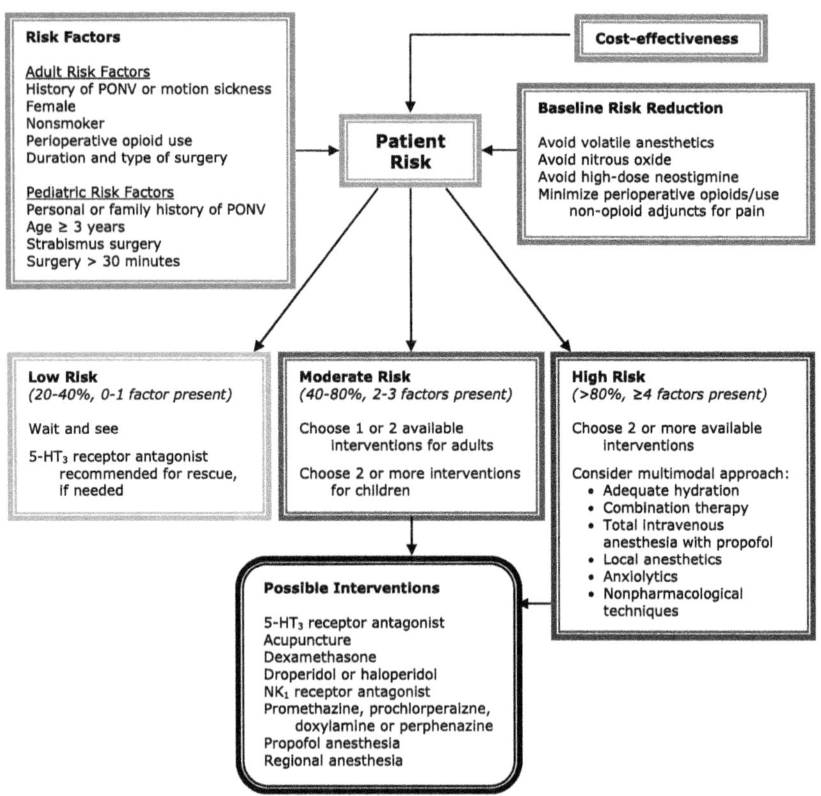

Fig. 2. Antiemetic management strategies based on patient risk.

factors for PONV, the patient's overall risk for PONV should be determined, and the anesthesia technique should be tailored to minimize the patient's baseline risk.

When appropriate, the use of regional anesthesia over general anesthesia can significantly reduce a patient's risk of PONV.[33] In high-risk patients, avoidance of volatile anesthetics and nitrous oxide through the use of TIVA with propofol may be appropriate. Two meta-analyses by Tramèr and colleagues[132,133] have found that avoidance of nitrous oxide reduces the risk of PONV, with an NNT of 13 to prevent early and late vomiting. It should be noted, however, that in studies with higher than average baseline risks of PONV, the investigators found that the NNT was about 5, whereas in studies in which the risk was lower than average, omitting nitrous oxide had no effect on outcome. This observation emphasizes the importance of assessing a patient's individual risk factors before formulating an approach for the management of PONV. A separate systematic review by Tramèr and Fuchs-Buder[134] found that high-dose neostigmine (>2.5 mg) is associated with increased risk of PONV, suggesting reduction or avoidance of neostigmine as another strategy to decrease PONV risk. Baseline risk reduction may also be achieved by minimizing the use of intraoperative and postoperative opioids with nonopioid adjuncts, such as nonsteroidal anti-inflammatory drugs, cyclooxygenase-2 inhibitors, and local anesthetics.[24]

Prophylaxis and Cost-Effectiveness

The cost-effectiveness of PONV prophylaxis is an important consideration in formulating a management strategy. Unfortunately, it is often difficult to gauge and compare the cost-effectiveness of many antiemetic therapies, as cost-effectiveness analyses vary widely in terms of the antiemetic regimens they choose to evaluate, the costs they take into account, and the criteria they use in drawing a conclusion. A cost-effectiveness study by Hill and colleagues[9] compared ondansetron 4 mg, droperidol 0.625 mg, droperidol 1.25 mg, and placebo, and determined that the use of antiemetic prophylaxis was more cost-effective and achieved higher satisfaction rates compared with placebo in high-risk patients. Frighetto and colleagues[135] used a decision-analysis model to determine that prophylactic antiemetic therapy with dolasetron or droperidol was more cost-effective than no prophylaxis followed by subsequent rescue therapy. However, other studies have suggested that treatment of PONV may be more cost-effective than prophylaxis for patients at both low (30%) and high (60%) risk, due to the high efficacy of ondansetron for the treatment of established PONV.[136]

Despite these conflicting data, it seems that studies comparing antiemetic therapy with placebo tend to find that using an antiemetic is more effective than placebo and preferable to no prophylaxis.[137] Still, it remains unclear which antiemetic therapies are most cost-effective, what doses of medication are most cost-effective, and whether PONV prophylaxis is cost-effective for all patients or only for those at higher risk. Future studies have been encouraged to follow established guidelines for cost-effectiveness studies, such as reporting cost-effectiveness as a ratio of resource use to value of health consequences.[138–140]

Combination Therapies and Multimodal Prevention

Because there are no single antiemetic agents that are completely effective in preventing or treating PONV, the concept of combination therapy using multiple agents has become particularly appealing. As noted earlier, the IMPACT trial found that ondansetron 4 mg IV, dexamethasone 4 mg IV, and droperidol 1.25 mg IV are equally effective as single agents for the prevention of PONV.[2] Due to their established efficacy and widespread use, these 3 agents are the most commonly studied antiemetics used in combination therapy. The IMPACT trial examined the effect of various combinations of the 3 therapies, and determined that each of the 3 antiemetics acted independently, such that combinations of any 2 or 3 of them would reduce the risk of PONV in an additive manner. These findings are similar to those of various meta-analyses and systematic reviews, which have reported that combinations of 5-HT_3 RAs and either droperidol or dexamethasone are equally safe and effective in reducing PONV.[75,87,141] A cost-effectiveness analysis by Pueyo and colleagues[142] compared each of the possible 2-drug combinations of ondansetron, droperidol, and dexamethasone. The investigators found that ondansetron and droperidol is less expensive than, and as effective as, ondansetron and dexamethasone, while being more effective than droperidol and dexamethasone—albeit at a slightly increased cost. Regardless, the evidence would suggest that combination therapy using any of these 3 drugs would be a reasonable strategy for decreasing PONV risk.[24]

In general, combination therapy is recommended for patients at moderate risk for PONV. For patients at high risk of PONV, combination antiemetic therapy can be used in conjunction with other pharmacologic and nonpharmacological techniques to further reduce the risk of PONV. This approach is often labeled "multimodal management" or "balanced antiemesis," as it combines multiple therapeutic options to maximize antiemetic efficacy. Scuderi and colleagues[143] reported on the use of a multimodal approach that included preoperative anxiolysis, aggressive hydration, supplemental oxygen, droperidol and dexamethasone at induction, ondansetron at the end of surgery, TIVA with propofol and remifentanil, and ketorolac, with no use of nitrous oxide or neuromuscular blockade. The multimodal approach achieved a 98% CR rate, compared with 76% with antiemetic monotherapy using ondansetron 4 mg, and a 59% CR rate on placebo. However, the researchers did note that patient satisfaction scores were similar between the multimodal approach and monotherapy, although they were both higher than those for patients receiving placebo and rescue antiemetic therapy only.

Habib and colleagues[144] have compared 3 regimens: a multimodal management strategy, which included TIVA with propofol, ondansetron, and droperidol; a combination therapy with ondansetron and droperidol, and receiving isoflurane and nitrous oxide (no TIVA); and TIVA with propofol only. The CR rates at 24 hours were 80% for the multimodal approach, 63% for the combination therapy group, and 43% for the TIVA-only group. In slight contrast to the study by Scuderi and colleagues, patient satisfaction scores were found to be highest for the multimodal approach, over both combination therapy with inhaled anesthetics or TIVA only.

Rescue Treatment and Management of PDNV

Even with baseline risk reduction and antiemetic prophylaxis, some patients will inevitably experience PONV or PDNV.[16] Before initiating rescue antiemetic drugs, other factors that may contribute to PONV should be considered and addressed, such as pain, concomitant use of opioids or other medications, or mechanical reasons (eg, blood in the throat, abdominal obstruction, and so forth). In general, patients who have not previously received antiemetic prophylaxis should be given a 5-HT_3 RA, while patients who have already received prophylaxis should be given a rescue antiemetic from a different treatment class than the prophylactic drug.[24] Unlike PONV prophylaxis, there are relatively few trials that have studied treatment options for established PONV. However, a systematic review by Kazemi-Kjellberg and colleagues[52] has evaluated several different antiemetic regimens and found that the NNT of 5-HT_3 RAs for established PONV is about 4 to 5. Treatment doses of 5-HT_3 RAs for established PONV are generally smaller than those needed for prophylaxis: ondansetron 1 mg, dolasetron 12.5 mg (similar to the recommended prophylactic dose), and granisetron 0.1 mg. Although ondansetron 1 mg has been shown to be as effective as ondansetron 4 mg for antiemetic rescue, most clinicians tend to use the 4-mg dose in practice. It should also be noted that in patients who received a 5-HT_3 RA for prophylaxis, no further benefit is achieved from repeat doses in the 6 hours after the initial dose.[145] In such cases, alternatives to 5-HT_3 RAs are recommended and include dexamethasone 2 to 4 mg, droperidol 0.625 mg, or promethazine 6.25 to 12.5 mg, although dexamethasone and transdermal scopolamine are not recommended for emetic episodes that occur more than 6 hours postoperatively, because of their longer duration of action.[24]

SUMMARY

Although awareness has greatly increased over the past several decades and the number of available treatment options has also increased, PONV and PDNV remain a common problem of ambulatory surgery. Appropriate management of PONV begins with an assessment of risk and baseline risk reduction, followed by consideration of antiemetic prophylaxis and, if necessary, rescue treatment. In patients who are at increased risk, combination therapy or multimodal approaches is recommended in preventing PONV and PDNV. Given the brief period of time that ambulatory surgery patients are under direct medical care, it is particularly important to recognize these problems and appropriately administer longer-acting antiemetics to prevent negative medical consequences, maximize patient satisfaction and return to normal activity, and minimize health care costs.

REFERENCES

1. Cameron D, Gan TJ. Management of postoperative nausea and vomiting in ambulatory surgery. Anesthesiol Clin N Am 2003;21(2):347–65.
2. Apfel CC, Korttila K, Abdalla M, et al. A factorial trial of six interventions for the prevention of postoperative nausea and vomiting. N Engl J Med 2004;350(24):2441–51.
3. Atallah FN, Riu BM, Nguyen LB, et al. Boerhaave's syndrome after postoperative vomiting. Anesth Analg 2004;98(4):1164–6.
4. Eroglu A, Kurkcuoglu C, Karaoglanoglu N, et al. Spontaneous esophageal rupture following severe vomiting in pregnancy. Dis Esophagus 2002;15(3):242–3.
5. Komenaka IK, Gandhi SG, deGraft-Johnson JB, et al. Postoperative vomiting causing esophageal rupture after antiemetic use. A case report. J Reprod Med 2003;48(2):124–6.
6. Zhang GS, Mathura JR Jr. Images in clinical medicine. Painless loss of vision after vomiting. N Engl J Med 2005;352(17):e16.
7. Nanji GM, Maltby JR. Vomiting and aspiration pneumonitis with the laryngeal mask airway [see comment]. Can J Anaesth 1992;39(1):69–70.
8. Williams KS. Postoperative nausea and vomiting. Surg Clin N Am 2005;85(6):1229–41.
9. Hill RP, Lubarsky DA, Phillips-Bute B, et al. Cost-effectiveness of prophylactic antiemetic therapy with ondansetron, droperidol, or placebo. Anesthesiology 2000;92(4):958–67.
10. Gan T, Sloan F, Dear Gde L, et al. How much are patients willing to pay to avoid postoperative nausea and vomiting? Anesth Analg 2001;92(2):393–400.
11. Carroll NV, Miederhoff P, Cox FM, et al. Postoperative nausea and vomiting after discharge from outpatient surgery centers. Anesth Analg 1995;80(5):903–9.
12. Wu CL, Berenholtz SM, Pronovost PJ, et al. Systematic review and analysis of postdischarge symptoms after outpatient surgery. Anesthesiology 2002;96(4):994–1003.
13. Gupta A, Wu CL, Elkassabany N, et al. Does the routine prophylactic use of antiemetics affect the incidence of postdischarge nausea and vomiting following ambulatory surgery? A systematic review of randomized controlled trials. Anesthesiology 2003;99(2):488–95.
14. Mattila K, Toivonen J, Janhunen L, et al. Postdischarge symptoms after ambulatory surgery: first-week incidence, intensity, and risk factors. Anesth Analg 2005;101(6):1643–50.
15. Cullen KA, Hall MJ, Golosinskiy A. Ambulatory surgery in the United States, 2006. Natl Health Stat Report 2009;11:1–25.
16. Gan TJ. Postoperative nausea and vomiting—can it be eliminated? JAMA 2002;287(10):1233–6.
17. Wang SC, Borison HL. A new concept of organization of the central emetic mechanism: recent studies on the sites of action of apomorphine, copper sulfate and cardiac glycosides. Gastroenterology 1952;22(1):1–12.
18. Wang SC, Borison HL. The vomiting center; a critical experimental analysis. Arch Neurol Psychiatry 1950;63(6):928–41.
19. Hornby PJ. Central neurocircuitry associated with emesis. Am J Med 2001;111(Suppl 8A):106S–12S.

20. Watcha MF, White PF. Postoperative nausea and vomiting. Its etiology, treatment, and prevention. Anesthesiology 1992;77(1):162–84.
21. Borison HL. Area postrema: chemoreceptor circumventricular organ of the medulla oblongata. Prog Neurobiol 1989;32(5):351–90.
22. Leslie RA. Neuroactive substances in the dorsal vagal complex of the medulla oblongata: nucleus of the tractus solitarius, area postrema, and dorsal motor nucleus of the vagus. Neurochem Int 1985;7:191–211.
23. Gan TJ. Mechanisms underlying postoperative nausea and vomiting and neurotransmitter receptor antagonist-based pharmacotherapy. CNS Drugs 2007; 21(10):813–33.
24. Gan TJ, Meyer TA, Apfel CC, et al. Society for Ambulatory Anesthesia guidelines for the management of postoperative nausea and vomiting. Anesth Analg 2007; 105(6):1615–28.
25. Apfel CC, Kranke P, Eberhart LH, et al. Comparison of predictive models for postoperative nausea and vomiting. Br J Anaesth 2002;88(2):234–40.
26. Apfel CC, Kranke P, Eberhart LH. Comparison of surgical site and patient's history with a simplified risk score for the prediction of postoperative nausea and vomiting. Anaesthesia 2004;59(11):1078–82.
27. Apfel CC, Laara E, Koivuranta M, et al. A simplified risk score for predicting postoperative nausea and vomiting: conclusions from cross-validations between two centers. Anesthesiology 1999;91(3):693–700.
28. Pierre S, Corno G, Benais H, et al. A risk score-dependent antiemetic approach effectively reduces postoperative nausea and vomiting—a continuous quality improvement initiative. Can J Anaesth 2004;51(4):320–5.
29. Biedler A, Wermelt J, Kunitz O, et al. A risk adapted approach reduces the overall institutional incidence of postoperative nausea and vomiting. Can J Anaesth 2004;51(1):13–9.
30. Eberhart LH, Geldner G, Kranke P, et al. The development and validation of a risk score to predict the probability of postoperative vomiting in pediatric patients. Anesth Analg 2004;99(6):1630–7.
31. Kovac AL. Management of postoperative nausea and vomiting in children. Paediatr Drugs 2007;9(1):47–69.
32. Kranke P, Eberhart LH, Toker H, et al. A prospective evaluation of the POVOC score for the prediction of postoperative vomiting in children. Anesth Analg 2007;105(6):1592–7.
33. Sinclair DR, Chung F, Mezei G. Can postoperative nausea and vomiting be predicted? Anesthesiology 1999;91(1):109–18.
34. Apfel CC, Kranke P, Katz MH, et al. Volatile anaesthetics may be the main cause of early but not delayed postoperative vomiting: a randomized controlled trial of factorial design. Br J Anaesth 2002;88(5):659–68.
35. Roberts GW, Bekker TB, Carlsen HH, et al. Postoperative nausea and vomiting are strongly influenced by postoperative opioid use in a dose-related manner. Anesth Analg 2005;101(5):1343–8.
36. Leslie K, Myles PS, Chan MT, et al. Risk factors for severe postoperative nausea and vomiting in a randomized trial of nitrous oxide-based vs nitrous oxide-free anaesthesia. Br J Anaesth 2008;101(4):498–505.
37. Mraovic B, Simurina T, Sonicki Z, et al. The dose-response of nitrous oxide in postoperative nausea in patients undergoing gynecologic laparoscopic surgery: a preliminary study. Anesth Analg 2008;107(3):818–23.

38. White PF, Sacan O, Nuangchamnong N, et al. The relationship between patient risk factors and early versus late postoperative emetic symptoms. Anesth Analg 2008;107(2):459–63.
39. Kotiniemi LH, Ryhanen PT, Valanne J, et al. Postoperative symptoms at home following day-case surgery in children: a multicentre survey of 551 children. Anaesthesia 1997;52(10):963–9.
40. Villeret I, Laffon M, Duchalais A, et al. Incidence of postoperative nausea and vomiting in paediatric ambulatory surgery. Paediatr Anaesth 2002;12(8):712–7.
41. Hesketh PJ, Gandara DR. Serotonin antagonists: a new class of antiemetic agents. J Natl Cancer Inst 1991;83(9):613–20.
42. Scuderi PE. Pharmacology of antiemetics. Int Anesthesiol Clin 2003;41(4):41–66.
43. Barnes NM, Hales TG, Lummis SC, et al. The 5-HT3 receptor—the relationship between structure and function. Neuropharmacology 2009;56(1):273–84.
44. ZOFRAN (ondansetron hydrochloride) injection [prescribing information]. GlaxoSmithKline. Research Triangle Park (NC); 2009. Available at: http://us.gsk.com/products/assets/us_zofran.pdf. Accessed February 17, 2010.
45. KYTRIL (granisetron hydrochloride) injection [prescribing information]. Roche Laboratories. Nutley (NJ); 2009. Available at: http://www.gene.com/gene/products/information/kytril/pdf/pi_injection.pdf. Accessed February 17, 2010.
46. ANZEMET injection (dolasetron mesylate injection) [prescribing information]. Bridgewater (NJ): Sanofi-aventis; 2006. Available at: http://products.sanofi-aventis.us/Anzemet_Injection/anzemet_injection.html. Accessed February 17, 2010.
47. De Leon A. Palonosetron (Aloxi): a second-generation 5-HT(3) receptor antagonist for chemotherapy-induced nausea and vomiting. Proc (Bayl Univ Med Cent) 2006;19(4):413–6.
48. Sun R, Klein KW, White PF. The effect of timing of ondansetron administration in outpatients undergoing otolaryngologic surgery. Anesth Analg 1997;84(2):331–6.
49. Tang J, Wang B, White PF, et al. The effect of timing of ondansetron administration on its efficacy, cost-effectiveness, and cost-benefit as a prophylactic antiemetic in the ambulatory setting. Anesth Analg 1998;86(2):274–82.
50. Korttila KT, Jokinen JD. Timing of administration of dolasetron affects dose necessary to prevent postoperative nausea and vomiting. J Clin Anesth 2004;16(5):364–70.
51. Chen X, Tang J, White PF, et al. The effect of timing of dolasetron administration on its efficacy as a prophylactic antiemetic in the ambulatory setting. Anesth Analg 2001;93(4):906–11.
52. Kazemi-Kjellberg F, Henzi I, Tramèr MR. Treatment of established postoperative nausea and vomiting: a quantitative systematic review. BMC Anesthesiol 2001;1(1):2.
53. Tramèr MR, Reynolds DJ, Moore RA, et al. Efficacy, dose-response, and safety of ondansetron in prevention of postoperative nausea and vomiting: a quantitative systematic review of randomized placebo-controlled trials. Anesthesiology 1997;87(6):1277–89.
54. Jokela RM, Cakmakkaya OS, Danzeisen O, et al. Ondansetron has similar clinical efficacy against both nausea and vomiting. Anaesthesia 2009;64(2):147–51.
55. Carlisle JB, Stevenson CA. Drugs for preventing postoperative nausea and vomiting [Online]. Cochrane Database Syst Rev 2006;(3):CD004125.

56. Dershwitz M, Conant JA, Chang Y, et al. A randomized, double-blind, dose-response study of ondansetron in the prevention of postoperative nausea and vomiting. J Clin Anesth 1998;10(4):314–20.
57. Scuderi P, Wetchler B, Sung YF, et al. Treatment of postoperative nausea and vomiting after outpatient surgery with the 5-HT3 antagonist ondansetron. Anesthesiology 1993;78(1):15–20.
58. Claybon L. Single dose intravenous ondansetron for the 24-hour treatment of postoperative nausea and vomiting. Anaesthesia 1994;49(Suppl):24–9.
59. Tramèr MR, Moore RA, Reynolds DJ, et al. A quantitative systematic review of ondansetron in treatment of established postoperative nausea and vomiting. Clinical research ed. BMJ 1997;314(7087):1088–92.
60. Andrews PL, Bhandari P, Davey PT, et al. Are all 5-HT3 receptor antagonists the same? Eur J Cancer 1992;28A(Suppl 1):S2–6.
61. Gan TJ. Selective serotonin 5-HT3 receptor antagonists for postoperative nausea and vomiting: are they all the same? CNS Drugs 2005;19(3):225–38.
62. Mikawa K, Takao Y, Nishina K, et al. Optimal dose of granisetron for prophylaxis against postoperative emesis after gynecological surgery. Anesth Analg 1997; 85(3):652–6.
63. D'Angelo R, Philip B, Gan TJ, et al. A randomized, double-blind, close-ranging, pilot study of intravenous granisetron in the prevention of postoperative nausea and vomiting in patients abdominal hysterectomy. Eur J Anaesthesiol 2005;22(10):774–9.
64. Taylor AM, Rosen M, Diemunsch PA, et al. A double-blind, parallel-group, placebo-controlled, dose-ranging, multicenter study of intravenous granisetron in the treatment of postoperative nausea and vomiting in patients undergoing surgery with general anesthesia. J Clin Anesth 1997;9(8):658–63.
65. Graczyk SG, McKenzie R, Kallar S, et al. Intravenous dolasetron for the prevention of postoperative nausea and vomiting after outpatient laparoscopic gynecologic surgery. Anesth Analg 1997;84(2):325–30.
66. Rojas C, Stathis M, Thomas AG, et al. Palonosetron exhibits unique molecular interactions with the 5-HT3 receptor. Anesth Analg 2008;107(2):469–78.
67. Kloth DD. New pharmacologic findings for the treatment of PONV and PDNV. Am J Health Syst Pharm 2009;66(1 Suppl 1):S11–8.
68. Candiotti KA, Kovac AL, Melson TI, et al. A randomized, double-blind study to evaluate the efficacy and safety of three different doses of palonosetron versus placebo for preventing postoperative nausea and vomiting. Anesth Analg 2008; 107(2):445–51.
69. Kovac AL, Eberhart L, Kotarski J, et al. A randomized, double-blind study to evaluate the efficacy and safety of three different doses of palonosetron versus placebo in preventing postoperative nausea and vomiting over a 72-hour period. Anesth Analg 2008;107(2):439–44.
70. Grover VK, Mathew PJ, Hegde H. Efficacy of orally disintegrating ondansetron in preventing postoperative nausea and vomiting after laparoscopic cholecystectomy: a randomised, double-blind placebo controlled study. Anaesthesia 2009; 64(6):595–600.
71. Davis PJ, Fertal KM, Boretsky KR, et al. The effects of oral ondansetron disintegrating tablets for prevention of at-home emesis in pediatric patients after ear-nose-throat surgery. Anesth Analg 2008;106(4):1117–21.
72. Gan TJ, Franiak R, Reeves J. Ondansetron orally disintegrating tablet versus placebo for the prevention of postdischarge nausea and vomiting after ambulatory surgery. Anesth Analg 2002;94(5):1199–200.

73. Candiotti KA, Birnbach DJ, Lubarsky DA, et al. The impact of pharmacogenomics on postoperative nausea and vomiting: do CYP2D6 allele copy number and polymorphisms affect the success or failure of ondansetron prophylaxis? Anesthesiology 2005;102(3):543–9.
74. Rueffert H, Thieme V, Wallenborn J, et al. Do variations in the 5-HT3A and 5-HT3B serotonin receptor genes (HTR3A and HTR3B) influence the occurrence of postoperative vomiting? Anesth Analg 2009;109(5):1442–7.
75. Henzi I, Walder B, Tramèr MR. Dexamethasone for the prevention of postoperative nausea and vomiting: a quantitative systematic review. Anesth Analg 2000;90(1):186–94.
76. Wang JJ, Ho ST, Tzeng JI, et al. The effect of timing of dexamethasone administration on its efficacy as a prophylactic antiemetic for postoperative nausea and vomiting. Anesth Analg 2000;91(1):136–9.
77. Karanicolas PJ, Smith SE, Kanbur B, et al. The impact of prophylactic dexamethasone on nausea and vomiting after laparoscopic cholecystectomy: a systematic review and meta-analysis. Ann Surg 2008;248(5):751–62.
78. Elhakim M, Nafie M, Mahmoud K, et al. Dexamethasone 8 mg in combination with ondansetron 4 mg appears to be the optimal dose for the prevention of nausea and vomiting after laparoscopic cholecystectomy. Can J Anaesth 2002;49(9):922–6.
79. McCarthy BG, Peroutka SJ. Differentiation of muscarinic cholinergic receptor subtypes in human cortex and pons: implications for anti-motion sickness therapy. Aviat Space Environ Med 1988;59(1):63–6.
80. Kovac AL. Prevention and treatment of postoperative nausea and vomiting. Drugs 2000;59(2):213–43.
81. White PF, Tang J, Song D, et al. Transdermal scopolamine: an alternative to ondansetron and droperidol for the prevention of postoperative and postdischarge emetic symptoms. Anesth Analg 2007;104(1):92–6.
82. Kranke P, Morin AM, Roewer N, et al. The efficacy and safety of transdermal scopolamine for the prevention of postoperative nausea and vomiting: a quantitative systematic review. Anesth Analg 2002;95(1):133–43.
83. Sah N, Ramesh V, Kaul B, et al. Transdermal scopolamine patch in addition to ondansetron for postoperative nausea and vomiting prophylaxis in patients undergoing ambulatory cosmetic surgery. J Clin Anesth 2009;21(4):249–52.
84. Gan TJ, Sinha AC, Kovac AL, et al. A randomized, double-blind, multicenter trial comparing transdermal scopolamine plus ondansetron to ondansetron alone for the prevention of postoperative nausea and vomiting in the outpatient setting. Anesth Analg 2009;108(5):1498–504.
85. Henzi I, Sonderegger J, Tramèr MR. Efficacy, dose-response, and adverse effects of droperidol for prevention of postoperative nausea and vomiting. Can J Anaesth 2000;47(6):537–51.
86. McKeage K, Simpson D, Wagstaff AJ. Intravenous droperidol: a review of its use in the management of postoperative nausea and vomiting. Drugs 2006;66(16):2123–47.
87. Leslie JB, Gan TJ. Meta-analysis of the safety of 5-HT3 antagonists with dexamethasone or droperidol for prevention of PONV. Ann Pharmacother 2006;40(5):856–72.
88. White PF. Droperidol: a cost-effective antiemetic for over thirty years. Anesth Analg 2002;95(4):789–90.

89. Habib AS, Gan TJ. The use of droperidol before and after the Food and Drug Administration black box warning: a survey of the members of the Society of Ambulatory Anesthesia. J Clin Anesth 2008;20(1):35–9.
90. Dershwitz M. Droperidol: should the black box be light gray? [see comment]. J Clin Anesth 2002;14(8):598–603.
91. Granger B, Albu S. The haloperidol story. Ann Clin Psychiatry 2005;17(3): 137–40.
92. Buttner M, Walder B, von Elm E, et al. Is low-dose haloperidol a useful antiemetic? A meta-analysis of published and unpublished randomized trials. Anesthesiology 2004;101(6):1454–63.
93. Aouad MT, Siddik-Sayyid SM, Taha SK, et al. Haloperidol vs. ondansetron for the prevention of postoperative nausea and vomiting following gynaecological surgery. Eur J Anaesthesiol 2007;24(2):171–8.
94. Grecu L, Bittner EA, Kher J, et al. Haloperidol plus ondansetron versus ondansetron alone for prophylaxis of postoperative nausea and vomiting. Anesth Analg 2008;106(5):1410–3.
95. Rosow CE, Haspel KL, Smith SE, et al. Haloperidol versus ondansetron for prophylaxis of postoperative nausea and vomiting. Anesth Analg 2008;106(5): 1407–9, table of contents.
96. Khalil S, Philbrook L, Rabb M, et al. Ondansetron/promethazine combination or promethazine alone reduces nausea and vomiting after middle ear surgery. J Clin Anesth 1999;11(7):596–600.
97. Chen JJ, Frame DG, White TJ. Efficacy of ondansetron and prochlorperazine for the prevention of postoperative nausea and vomiting after total hip replacement or total knee replacement procedures: a randomized, double-blind, comparative trial. Arch Intern Med 1998;158(19):2124–8.
98. Habib AS, Reuveni J, Taguchi A, et al. A comparison of ondansetron with promethazine for treating postoperative nausea and vomiting in patients who received prophylaxis with ondansetron: a retrospective database analysis. Anesth Analg 2007;104(3):548–51.
99. Harrington RA, Hamilton CW, Brogden RN, et al. Metoclopramide. An updated review of its pharmacological properties and clinical use. Drugs 1983;25(5): 451–94.
100. Henzi I, Walder B, Tramèr MR. Metoclopramide in the prevention of postoperative nausea and vomiting: a quantitative systematic review of randomized, placebo-controlled studies. Br J Anaesth 1999;83(5):761–71.
101. Bolton CM, Myles PS, Carlin JB, et al. Randomized, double-blind study comparing the efficacy of moderate-dose metoclopramide and ondansetron for the prophylactic control of postoperative vomiting in children after tonsillectomy. Br J Anaesth 2007;99(5):699–703.
102. Kranke P, Morin AM, Roewer N, et al. Dimenhydrinate for prophylaxis of postoperative nausea and vomiting: a meta-analysis of randomized controlled trials. Acta Anaesthesiol Scand 2002;46(3):238–44.
103. Reeve BK, Cook DJ, Babineau D, et al. Prophylactic Diclectin reduces the incidence of postoperative vomiting. Can J Anaesth 2005;52(1):55–61.
104. DeBalli P. The use of propofol as an antiemetic. Int Anesthesiol Clin 2003;41(4): 67–77.
105. Gupta A, Stierer T, Zuckerman R, et al. Comparison of recovery profile after ambulatory anesthesia with propofol, isoflurane, sevoflurane and desflurane: a systematic review. Anesth Analg 2004;98(3):632–41.

106. Visser K, Hassink EA, Bonsel GJ, et al. Randomized controlled trial of total intravenous anesthesia with propofol versus inhalation anesthesia with isoflurane-nitrous oxide: postoperative nausea with vomiting and economic analysis. Anesthesiology 2001;95(3):616–26.
107. White H, Black RJ, Jones M, et al. Randomized comparison of two anti-emetic strategies in high-risk patients undergoing day-case gynaecological surgery. Br J Anaesth 2007;98(4):470–6.
108. Smith I, Thwaites AJ. Target-controlled propofol vs. sevoflurane: a double-blind, randomised comparison in day-case anaesthesia. Anaesthesia 1999;54(8): 745–52.
109. Ozkose Z, Ercan B, Unal Y, et al. Inhalation versus total intravenous anesthesia for lumbar disc herniation: comparison of hemodynamic effects, recovery characteristics, and cost. J Neurosurg Anesthesiol 2001;13(4):296–302.
110. Apfel CC, Malhotra A, Leslie JB. The role of neurokinin-1 receptor antagonists for the management of postoperative nausea and vomiting. Curr Opin Anaesthesiol 2008;21(4):427–32.
111. Saito R, Takano Y, Kamiya HO. Roles of substance P and NK(1) receptor in the brainstem in the development of emesis. J Pharmacol Sci 2003;91(2): 87–94.
112. Minami M, Endo T, Kikuchi K, et al. Antiemetic effects of sendide, a peptide tachykinin NK1 receptor antagonist, in the ferret. Eur J Pharmacol 1998; 363(1):49–55.
113. Diemunsch P, Joshi GP, Brichant JF. Neurokinin-1 receptor antagonists in the prevention of postoperative nausea and vomiting. Br J Anaesth 2009;103(1): 7–13.
114. Gan TJ, Apfel CC, Kovac A, et al. A randomized, double-blind comparison of the NK1 antagonist, aprepitant, versus ondansetron for the prevention of postoperative nausea and vomiting. Anesth Analg 2007;104(5):1082–9.
115. Diemunsch P, Gan TJ, Philip BK, et al. Single-dose aprepitant vs ondansetron for the prevention of postoperative nausea and vomiting: a randomized, double-blind phase III trial in patients undergoing open abdominal surgery. Br J Anaesth 2007;99(2):202–11.
116. Diemunsch P, Apfel C, Gan TJ, et al. Preventing postoperative nausea and vomiting: post hoc analysis of pooled data from two randomized active-controlled trials of aprepitant. Curr Med Res Opin 2007;23(10):2559–65.
117. Poli-Bigelli S, Rodrigues-Pereira J, Carides AD, et al. Addition of the neurokinin 1 receptor antagonist aprepitant to standard antiemetic therapy improves control of chemotherapy-induced nausea and vomiting. Results from a randomized, double-blind, placebo-controlled trial in Latin America. Cancer 2003;97(12): 3090–8.
118. Tsuchida D, Fukuda H, Koda K, et al. Central effect of mu-opioid agonists on antral motility in conscious rats. Brain Res 2004;1024(1–2):244–50.
119. Gan TJ, Ginsberg B, Glass PS, et al. Opioid-sparing effects of a low-dose infusion of naloxone in patient-administered morphine sulfate. Anesthesiology 1997; 87(5):1075–81.
120. Maxwell LG, Kaufmann SC, Bitzer S, et al. The effects of a small-dose naloxone infusion on opioid-induced side effects and analgesia in children and adolescents treated with intravenous patient-controlled analgesia: a double-blind, prospective, randomized, controlled study. Anesth Analg 2005;100(4):953–8.

121. Kim MK, Nam SB, Cho MJ, et al. Epidural naloxone reduces postoperative nausea and vomiting in patients receiving epidural sufentanil for postoperative analgesia. Br J Anaesth 2007;99(2):270–5.
122. Rowbotham DJ. Recent advances in the non-pharmacological management of postoperative nausea and vomiting. Br J Anaesth 2005;95(1):77–81.
123. Lee A, Fan LT. Stimulation of the wrist acupuncture point P6 for preventing postoperative nausea and vomiting. Cochrane Database Syst Rev 2009;(2): CD003281.
124. White A, Hayhoe S, Hart A, et al. Adverse events following acupuncture: prospective survey of 32 000 consultations with doctors and physiotherapists. Clinical research ed. BMJ 2001;323(7311):485–6.
125. Goll V, Akca O, Greif R, et al. Ondansetron is no more effective than supplemental intraoperative oxygen for prevention of postoperative nausea and vomiting. Anesth Analg 2001;92(1):112–7.
126. Greif R, Laciny S, Rapf B, et al. Supplemental oxygen reduces the incidence of postoperative nausea and vomiting. Anesthesiology 1999;91(5): 1246–52.
127. Orhan-Sungur M, Kranke P, Sessler D, et al. Does supplemental oxygen reduce postoperative nausea and vomiting? A meta-analysis of randomized controlled trials. Anesth Analg 2008;106(6):1733–8.
128. McKeen DM, Arellano R, O'Connell C. Supplemental oxygen does not prevent postoperative nausea and vomiting after gynecological laparoscopy. Can J Anaesth 2009;56(9):651–7.
129. Tramèr MR, Carroll D, Campbell FA, et al. Cannabinoids for control of chemotherapy induced nausea and vomiting: quantitative systematic review. Clinical research ed. BMJ 2001;323(7303):16–21.
130. Ernst E, Pittler MH. Efficacy of ginger for nausea and vomiting: a systematic review of randomized clinical trials. Br J Anaesth 2000;84(3):367–71.
131. Eberhart LH, Mayer R, Betz O, et al. Ginger does not prevent postoperative nausea and vomiting after laparoscopic surgery. Anesth Analg 2003;96(4): 995–8.
132. Tramèr M, Moore A, McQuay H. Meta-analytic comparison of prophylactic antiemetic efficacy for postoperative nausea and vomiting: propofol anaesthesia vs omitting nitrous oxide vs total i.v. anaesthesia with propofol. Br J Anaesth 1997; 78(3):256–9.
133. Tramèr M, Moore A, McQuay H. Omitting nitrous oxide in general anaesthesia: meta-analysis of intraoperative awareness and postoperative emesis in randomized controlled trials. Br J Anaesth 1996;76(2):186–93.
134. Tramèr MR, Fuchs-Buder T. Omitting antagonism of neuromuscular block: effect on postoperative nausea and vomiting and risk of residual paralysis. A systematic review. Br J Anaesth 1999;82(3):379–86.
135. Frighetto L, Loewen PS, Dolman J, et al. Cost-effectiveness of prophylactic dolasetron or droperidol vs rescue therapy in the prevention of PONV in ambulatory gynecologic surgery. Can J Anaesth 1999;46(6):536–43.
136. Tramèr MR, Phillips C, Reynolds DJ, et al. Cost-effectiveness of ondansetron for postoperative nausea and vomiting. Anaesthesia 1999;54(3):226–34.
137. Lachaine J. Therapeutic options for the prevention and treatment of postoperative nausea and vomiting: a pharmacoeconomic review. Pharmacoeconomics 2006;24(10):955–70.

138. Siegel JE, Weinstein MC, Russell LB, et al. Recommendations for reporting cost-effectiveness analyses. Panel on Cost-Effectiveness in Health and Medicine. JAMA 1996;276(16):1339–41.
139. Weinstein MC, Siegel JE, Gold MR, et al. Recommendations of the Panel on Cost-Effectiveness in Health and Medicine. JAMA 1996;276(15):1253–8.
140. Russell LB, Gold MR, Siegel JE, et al. The role of cost-effectiveness analysis in health and medicine. Panel on Cost-Effectiveness in Health and Medicine. JAMA 1996;276(14):1172–7.
141. Habib AS, El-Moalem HE, Gan TJ. The efficacy of the 5-HT3 receptor antagonists combined with droperidol for PONV prophylaxis is similar to their combination with dexamethasone. A meta-analysis of randomized controlled trials. Can J Anaesth 2004;51(4):311–9.
142. Pueyo FJ, Lopez-Olaondo L, Sanchez-Ledesma MJ, et al. Cost-effectiveness of three combinations of antiemetics in the prevention of postoperative nausea and vomiting. Br J Anaesth 2003;91(4):589–92.
143. Scuderi PE, James RL, Harris L, et al. Multimodal antiemetic management prevents early postoperative vomiting after outpatient laparoscopy. Anesth Analg 2000;91(6):1408–14.
144. Habib AS, White WD, Eubanks S, et al. A randomized comparison of a multimodal management strategy versus combination antiemetics for the prevention of postoperative nausea and vomiting. Anesth Analg 2004;99(1):77–81.
145. Kovac AL, O'Connor TA, Pearman MH, et al. Efficacy of repeat intravenous dosing of ondansetron in controlling postoperative nausea and vomiting: a randomized, double-blind, placebo-controlled multicenter trial. J Clin Anesth 1999;11(6):453–9.

Role of Regional Anesthesia in the Ambulatory Environment

Adam K. Jacob, MD, Michael T. Walsh, MD, John A. Dilger, MD*

KEYWORDS

• Regional anesthesia • Nerve block • Ambulatory • Outpatient

Ambulatory surgery has undergone tremendous growth in the past decade, from 20.8 million procedures in 1996 to 34.7 million in 2006.[1] Several factors have fueled this growth, including less-invasive surgical techniques, changes in practice patterns, and the use of anesthetic agents and techniques associated with fewer postoperative side effects. Postoperative pain management represents a particular challenge with ambulatory surgery because 40% of patients experience severe pain despite treatment.[2] Studies show that regional anesthesia (RA) improves pain scores, decreases narcotic use, and lowers the incidence of postoperative nausea and vomiting,[3,4] Thus, more patients can be discharged home in less time with high satisfaction.[5]

ORTHOPEDIC SURGERY

Perhaps more than any other specialty, orthopedic surgery lends itself to the practice of RA. Peripheral nerve or neuraxial blocks may be used as a primary anesthetic or as part of a combined technique to provide postoperative analgesia. For single-injection techniques, benefits generally last 8 to 12 hours, depending on the type of local anesthetic and adjuvants used. These short-term benefits include improved analgesia, fewer opioid-related side effects, and shorter length of stay in the ambulatory setting.[6–14] To further prolong postoperative analgesia, a continuous infusion of local anesthesia can be delivered through a perineural catheter. The use of continuous regional techniques for promise to broaden the scope of outpatient procedures that can be performed in an outpatient setting such as total shoulder and total hip arthroplasty.[15,16] These continuous techniques are discussed in detail, see the article by Swenson and colleagues elsewhere in this issue for further exploration of this topic.

This work was supported by Mayo Clinic Department of Anesthesiology.
Department of Anesthesiology, Mayo Clinic, 200 First Street Southwest, Rochester, MN 55905, USA
* Corresponding author.
E-mail address: dilger.john@mayo.edu

Anesthesiology Clin 28 (2010) 251–266
doi:10.1016/j.anclin.2010.02.009 **anesthesiology.theclinics.com**

Upper Extremity Surgery

Interscalene blockade (ISB) is a common technique for shoulder surgery. In a prospective study of 50 patients undergoing outpatient rotator cuff repair, patients randomized to receive single-injection ISB (vs general anesthesia [GA]) were more likely to bypass the postanesthesia care unit (PACU), report less pain, ambulate earlier, and meet home discharge criteria sooner.[8] Not unexpectedly, no difference was observed between groups in pain scores or opioid consumption at 24, 48, and 72 hours. These results support earlier retrospective findings comparing single-injection ISB with GA.[13,14] Because single-injection techniques can only provide 12 to 24 hours of relief when long-acting local anesthetics are used, patients may experience severe pain after the block resolves.[6] The addition of a perineural catheter and infusion may sustain analgesia for several days after surgery.[7,12,17,18] The benefits of catheter-based analgesia after shoulder surgery, however, remain controversial.[6,19]

Given the high incidence of phrenic nerve blockade during ISB, this technique may be contraindicated in patients who may not tolerate phrenic nerve blockade (eg, severe chronic obstructive pulmonary disease). Suprascapular nerve blockade (SSB) is an alternative technique that may provide analgesia after shoulder surgery. The suprascapular nerve innervates up to 70% of the posterior shoulder joint, the acromioclavicular joint, the subacromial bursa, and the coracoclavicular ligament. Furthermore, the location of blockade (in the supraspinatus fossa) eliminates the risk of inadvertent phrenic nerve blockade commonly encountered during ISB. In a study comparing single-injection ISB, SSB, intra-articular (IA) injection, and parenteral analgesia, SSB patients had lower pain verbal analog scale (VAS) scores with rest and movement up to 24 hours compared with parenteral or IA analgesia.[9] ISB patients consistently had the lowest pain scores overall, however.

For procedures below the shoulder, RA techniques also provide superior analgesia and shorter time to discharge compared with GA or systemic analgesics. Patients randomized to single-injection axillary brachial plexus block (vs GA) for ambulatory hand surgery were more likely to be fast-track eligible with a shorter duration of stay in the PACU and in the hospital after surgery.[10] In the RA group, pain scores up to 120 minutes after surgery were lower, but again there was no difference in pain, opioid consumption, adverse effects, Pain Disability Index, or satisfaction by postoperative day 1.

Infraclavicular brachial plexus blockade (INB), an alternative approach to upper extremity blockade for hand and wrist surgery, also provides short-term benefits in an ambulatory setting compared with GA. In a 2004 study by Hadzic and colleagues,[11] 52 patients undergoing outpatient hand or wrist surgery were randomized to INB or GA plus wound infiltration with local anesthetic. Compared with patients in the GA group, fewer patients in the INB group had pain (VAS >3) on arrival to the PACU and none requested treatment for pain when in the hospital (vs 48% of GA patients). Patients in the INB group reported less nausea, vomiting, and sore throat than GA patients and were, on average, discharged home approximately 100 minutes sooner than patients randomized to GA.

Lower Extremity Surgery

Hip arthroscopy is a surgical technique growing in popularity for treatment of a variety of painful hip conditions. Like many arthroscopic procedures, hip arthroscopy is commonly performed as outpatient surgery. Postoperative pain intensity may be a limiting factor for dismissing patients home postoperatively. IA bupivacaine injected at the conclusion of surgery lowers average pain scores at rest for 24 hours (18 vs 28 on 100-point scale) and with movement (23 vs 46 on 100-point scale) compared with 0.9% normal saline.[20] When 2-level paravertebral blockade (PVB) (L1 and L2) was added to IA bupivacaine, 2 patients experienced analgesia up to 36 and 48 hours, respectively.[21]

Total hip arthroplasty, a procedure that once required 2.5 to 3 weeks of inpatient recovery,[22] can now be performed on an ambulatory basis thanks to better pain control with continuous RA techniques. Investigators have described clinical pathways that include the use of 1 or more regional techniques, including lumbar plexus catheter and single-injection sciatic blockade, that enable patients undergoing minimally invasive total hip arthroplasty to be dismissed fewer than 23 hours after surgery.[16,23]

A variety of anesthetic and analgesic techniques are described for outpatient knee procedures. The most common methods of providing analgesia after knee arthroscopy, particularly with procedures involving ligament reconstruction, include femoral nerve blockade (with or without sciatic nerve blockade), lumbar plexus (ie, psoas) blockade, and IA injection. An ideal technique remains controversial.[24] Previous investigations have inconsistently compared the techniques, and variation in results may be due to differences in surgical and patient expectations as well as variations in postoperative nursing management.

Use of IA local anesthesia, often given in combination with an opioid, improves pain scores and early analgesic consumption after outpatient knee arthroscopy, regardless if the IA dose is administered pre- or post surgery.[25] Adding tramadol may potentiate the analgesic effects. In a recent study,[26] a combination of tramadol and 0.25% bupivacaine resulted in significantly lower pain VAS scores, decreased 24-hour analgesic consumption, prolonged time to first rescue analgesic, and shortened time to discharge compared with IA bupivacaine or tramadol alone. These benefits were seen without any detectable systemic effects. Recent evidence, however, suggests local anesthetics may be harmful to chondrocytes and may cause chondrolysis after IA infusion or even single injection.[27–30]

When used as a primary anesthetic agent, lumbar plexus blockade with or without sciatic nerve blockade provides short-term benefits compared with GA for outpatient knee surgery.[31,32] Patients who underwent peripheral blockade with 2-chloroprocaine 3% or mepivacaine 1.5% had lower immediate postoperative pain scores, shorter time to hospital dismissal, and higher satisfaction compared with patients who underwent GA.

In patients undergoing surgical procedures of the ankle or foot, several RA techniques exist that can provide anesthesia or analgesia of the operative extremity. Choice of technique largely depends on factors, such as surgical site (eg, hallux vs ankle), type of procedure (eg, hallux valgus correction vs ankle arthrodesis), use of a tourniquet, and the immediate weight-bearing status. A 2003 prospective, randomized study compared the analgesic benefits of a foot blockade (FB) (ie, ankle blockade) with 0.5% bupivacaine (20 mL) to sham blockade for outpatient bony midfoot surgery.[33] Patients who received an FB needed fewer intraoperative opioid supplements and, on average, had a significantly longer time to first perception of pain (12 vs 5.5 hours) compared with sham blockade. Again, the measured benefits were gone by postoperative day 1 with this single-injection technique.

The terminal branches of the sciatic and femoral nerves anesthetized during an FB can also be blocked more proximally in the popliteal fossa. In a prospective, randomized study comparing the efficacy of FB to popliteal blockade (PB) for outpatient forefoot surgery, Migues and colleagues[34] demonstrated equivalency of FBs and PBs. Specifically, both blocks were equally efficacious as primary anesthetic, and both blocks provided a similar duration of analgesia (FB, 11.0 hours, vs PB, 14.3 hours; $P = .13$) and patient satisfaction. By using a perineural catheter in the popliteal space, improved analgesia for ambulatory foot and ankle surgery can be extended up to 3 days compared with single-injection techniques.[35–37]

Neuraxial Techniques

A variety of neuraxial techniques have been studied for outpatient lower extremity procedures. With any approach, the anesthetic goals are the same: dense surgical anesthesia with rapid neurologic recovery and avoidance of neurotoxic effects (ie, transient neurologic syndrome). Although many combinations of local anesthetics, doses, additives, and approaches have been studied,[38–50] no single technique has emerged as the optimal choice. Each neuraxial anesthetic must be tailored to the patient and the procedure.

In the past 5 years, chloroprocaine has regained popularity for intrathecal use in ambulatory surgery. The rapid neurologic recovery (approximately 80–120 minutes) after intrathecal chloroprocaine makes it an attractive option for outpatient spinal anesthesia. At one time, chloroprocaine (or more specifically, the preservative sodium bisulfite) was thought to pose a significant risk of neurotoxicity. Recent animal evidence has disproved this,[51] and, thus far, no cases of neurotoxicity have been reported in several human volunteer and clinical studies.[43,52–58] Despite the growing body of clinical evidence illustrating the safety of spinal chloroprocaine, its use remains controversial.

An alternative to chloroprocaine for use in ambulatory surgery is low-dose bupivacaine. Many studies have examined a variety of drug doses, use of hyperbaric and isobaric drug preparations, with or without additives, and unilateral or bilateral spread of medication for a variety of surgical procedures.[39,42,44,55,59–71] Although low (<7.5 mg) and ultralow (2.5–4 mg) doses of spinal bupivacaine are used, these may come at the expense of additional sedation necessary for patient comfort during a procedure. In summary, each spinal anesthetic must be tailored to the patient, the procedure, and the practice style.

GENERAL SURGERY

Pain control after general surgery is challenging, and despite treatment, significant postoperative pain may result in unexpected hospital admission. Local anesthesia is used for subcutaneous injection providing anesthesia and analgesia, but the effects are limited by the short duration. An alternative method of providing prolonged unilateral (or bilateral) somatic and sympathetic nerve blockade is PVB. PVB involves the injection of local anesthetic at the nerve root just lateral to the neuraxial space and can be performed at 1 or more levels to increase the number of anesthetized dermatomes. PVB is commonly used to provide analgesia after procedures on the chest or abdominal wall, including breast surgery, hernia repair, and even laparoscopic procedures (eg, laparoscopic cholecystectomy).

Breast Surgery

PVB is used for major breast surgery. Analgesia for mastectomy, wide local excision, or lumpectomy should include nerve roots T1-T6, whereas procedures involving only sentinel node biopsy or axillary dissection involve nerve roots T1-T3. Injections typically require 3 to 5 mL of local anesthetic at each level (**Fig. 1**) or, alternatively, the entire dermatome coverage divided and a larger volume given at the midpoint. PVB may be used in conjunction with GA or as the primary anesthetic technique with sedation.

Demonstrated advantages of PVB over GA include decreased pain, lower narcotic usage, and earlier hospital discharge compared with patients having GA.[72] In addition to intraoperative anesthesia and analgesia, PVB using long-acting local anesthetics can prolong analgesia until the next day. This sustained analgesia results in significantly more same-day discharges, decreasing the costs associated with major breast surgery.[5] PVB also is associated with significantly less pain at 1, 6, and 12 months post procedure and a lower frequency of postmastectomy syndrome.[73] Additionally, PVB may inhibit the body's stress response to surgery, potentially limiting suppression of the immune system, including the action of natural killer cells, resulting in a lower recurrence of breast cancer up to 3 years after surgery.[74]

Although the benefits of thoracic PVB are well described, clear consideration must be given to the possibility of procedure-related complications, specifically pneumothorax. The risk of pneumothorax after a multiple injection technique is estimated to be 0.6%, and a postoperative chest radiograph is often ordered.[72] Although most pneumothoraces are small and asymptomatic, some may require chest tube placement and hospital admission. Ultrasound-guided PVB may be advantageous in that it allows for real-time visualization of the needle, costotransverse ligament, pleura, and spread of local anesthetic. In theory, the risk of complications, such as pneumothorax or intravascular injection, may be less when PVB is performed using ultrasonography, but these potential advantages are not yet proven.

Inguinal Hernia Repair

Analgesia after open inguinal herniorrhaphy is managed in many ways, although the use of local anesthesia is used increasingly due to superior outcomes. Simple wound infiltration is used commonly, and it is associated with an efficient recovery because side effects, such as urine retention, are uncommon (<0.5%).[75] The analgesic effects are limited by the brief duration of the local anesthetic used, but analgesia may be extended by placing a catheter in the wound. A continuous infusion for 2 days results in significantly lowered pain scores at 2 and 5 days postoperatively.[76]

PVB is an ideal perioperative technique for inguinal herniorrhaphy and lacks some of the risks (eg, pneumothorax) associated with thoracic-level paravertebral injections. For inguinal hernia surgery, blockade of T11-L2 nerve roots is required for adequate dermatomal analgesia. PVB for inguinal hernia repair is associated with less pain, less nausea, lower opioid requirements, and earlier home readiness compared with GA with local infiltration.[77] In addition, patients were able to urinate significantly sooner in the PVB group (128 vs 213 minutes).

An alternative technique that may be used to provide analgesia after hernia surgery is the transverse abdominus plane (TAP) block. Like PVB, TAP blocks may be unilateral or bilateral and involve injecting local anesthetic between the internal oblique and transverse abdominus muscle planes, resulting in blockade of T10-L3 segmental nerves and possibly the ilioinguinal and iliohypogastric nerves (**Fig. 2**).

Laparoscopic Surgery

Minimally invasive surgery using laparoscopy has dramatically expanded the number and type of cases that can be performed on an ambulatory basis. Cholecystectomy is a prime example. Although there is significantly less pain associated with the laparoscopic approach, pain is still the most common reason for admission to the hospital, with rates as high as 41%. The laparoscopic cholecystectomy pain state is unique even among other laparoscopic procedures with incisional somatic pain, abdominal visceral pain, and referred visceral pain to the shoulder. This complex pain state suggests

A
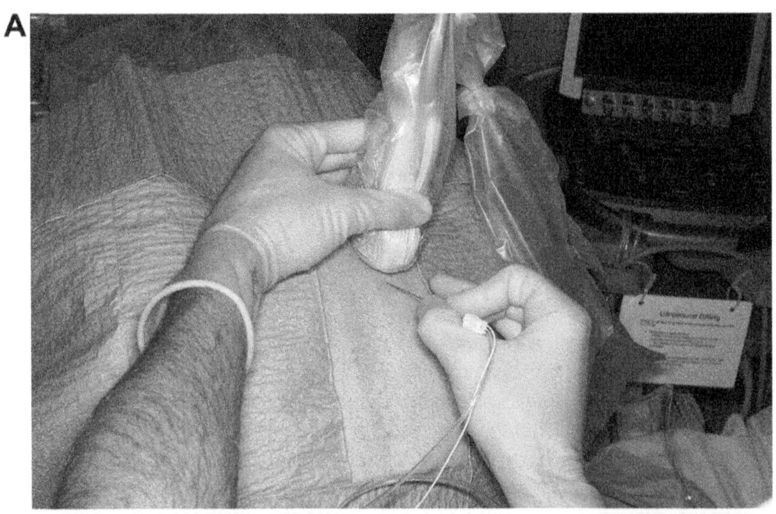

B
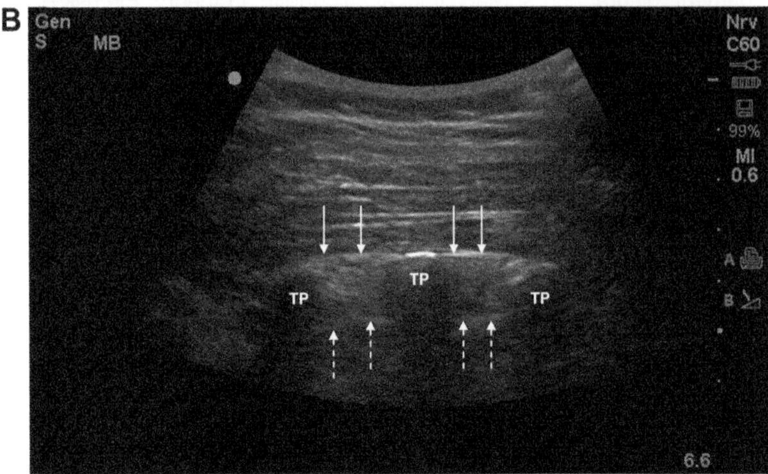
Gen
S MB
Nrv
C60
99%
MI
0.6
TP
TP
TP
A
B
6.6

C
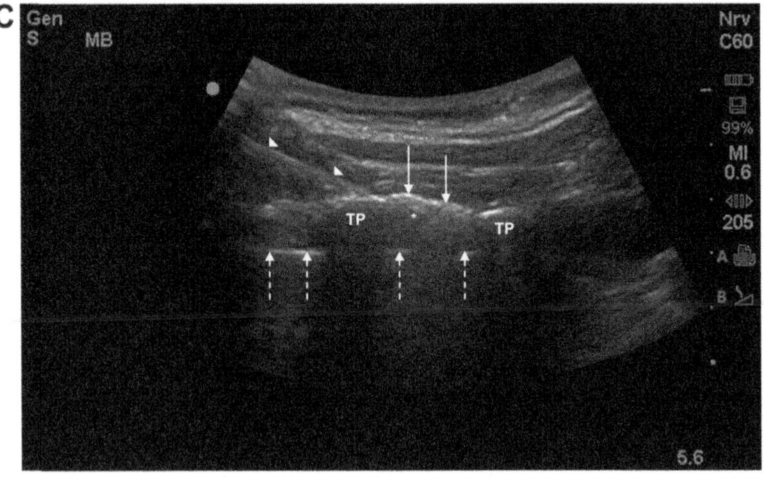
Gen
S MB
Nrv
C60
99%
MI
0.6
205
TP
TP
A
B
5.6

a role for multimodal analgesia. Acetaminophen and celecoxib are efficacious, and local anesthetic is applied in many ways to the postoperative pain with varying results.

Injecting the portholes with local anesthesia is efficacious although limited by the duration of local anesthesia. Ropivacaine injected to the portholes provides a median duration of analgesia of 2 to 3 hours, after which pain scores were similar to control patients.[78] Local anesthesia may also be applied to the intraperitoneal space for analgesia. The results have been excellent with an even greater efficacy resulting from injection of local anesthetic at the beginning of the procedure. Analgesia may last up to 4 hours.[79]

Bilateral PVB also seems efficacious after cholecystectomy, with the added benefit of longer duration. A combination of lidocaine and bupivacaine results in significantly less pain at 6, 12, and 24 hours postoperatively.[80]

TAP may be useful during cholecystectomy because it has an opioid-sparing effect perioperatively.[81] PVB and TAP blocks show some promise in managing pain after cholecystectomy, but incisional local combined with oral multimodal medications based on outcome data are the only regimen that demonstrate efficacy.

Many gynecologic procedures are done laparoscopically with GA, and local anesthesia is used to provide postoperative analgesia. When levobupivacaine is injected preoperatively in the port sites, laparoscopy patients experience significantly less pain, require fewer pain treatments, and ambulate earlier than patients not receiving local anesthesia.[82]

Postoperative pain control also is provided with local anesthetics applied to peritoneal surfaces intraoperatively. The efficacy of intraperitoneal local analgesia is conflicting in gynecologic surgery, and there is no compelling evidence to support its routine use as exists after laparoscopic cholecystectomy. The laparoscopic approach is similar in gynecologic and general surgery, but the procedures and pain states seem unique.

PLASTIC SURGERY

Local anesthesia has long been used in cosmetic surgery as much for its anesthetic potential as its vasoconstrictive properties when combined with epinephrine. Surgery may be conducted with the addition of light sedation, and this is preferred in rhytidectomy and blepharoplasty due to superior recovery compared with GA. In rhinoplasty, the local anesthetic cocaine is used for its anesthetic and vasoconstrictive properties, although there is concern for its arrhythmogenicity. Adrenalized lidocaine is also effective and combined with sedation or GA depending on the procedure. Liposuction uses the same lidocaine and epinephrine mixture in a different manner. Tumescent anesthesia, normal saline mixed with lidocaine 0.05% and epinephrine 1:1,000,000, is injected subdermally, so fluid distends adipocytes permitting thin cannula suctioning of the adipose tissue. Considerable amounts may be injected during liposuction raising concerns about hypervolemia and local anesthetic systemic toxicity. The maximum dose of adrenalized lidocaine is 7 mg/kg, but doses as high as 55 mg/kg have been used safely during liposuction, resulting in subtoxic serum lidocaine levels

Fig. 1. Ultrasound-guided thoracic PVB: (*A*) patient position, machine location, and hand position; (*B*) ultrasound anatomy: paraspinous tendon (*solid arrows*), parietal pleura (*dashed arrows*); TP, transverse process; and (*C*) ultrasound image showing needle approach and spread of local anesthetic in paravertebral space: paraspinous tendon (*solid arrows*); parietal pleura (*dashed arrows*); needle image with tip just below paraspinous tendon (*arrowheads*); final position of needle tip (*asterisk*); TP, transverse process.

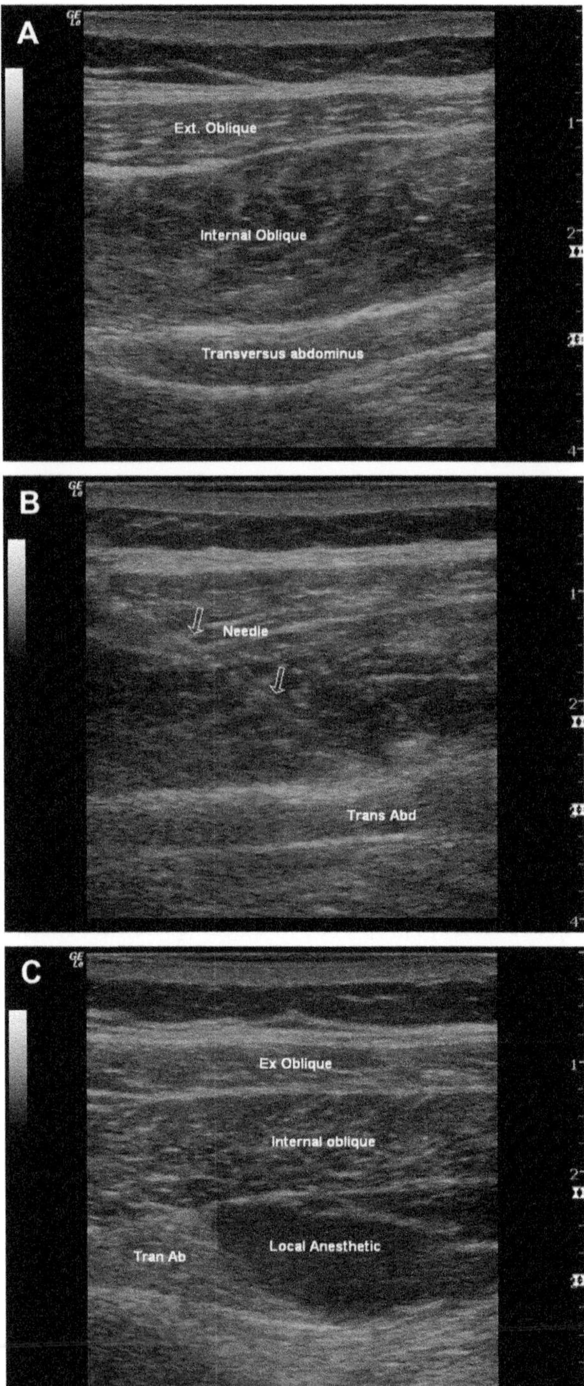

Fig. 2. Ultrasound-guided transversus abdominis plane blockade: (*A*) ultrasound anatomy, (*B*) ultrasound image showing needle (*arrows*) approach, and (*C*) ultrasound image showing injection of local anesthetic deep to fascial plane between transversus abdominis and internal oblique muscles.

(<5 μg/mL).[83] These doses of epinephrine do not cause tachycardia, arrhythmias, or hypertension. Cosmetic procedures use local anesthesia with epinephrine to provide anesthesia and limit bleeding, thus improving the surgical field conditions.

Breast surgery was discussed previously but bears mention because augmentation and reduction mammoplasty are unique. Paravertebral blocks also are used in the setting of plastic surgery. During submuscular breast augmentation, PVB provides intraoperative anesthesia and postoperative pain management, so patients may be discharged efficiently with minimal side effects.[84] Another analgesia technique in this setting involves a surgeon implanting catheters in the wound. Local anesthesia is infused providing prolonged analgesia.[85] Patients have significantly better analgesia, require less pain medication, and are more likely to be discharged on the same day compared with patients not receiving continuous wound infiltration.[86] This technique may have an advantage over PVB because analgesia is extended, no special training is required to place, and there is no risk of pneumothorax.

OFFICE-BASED SURGERY

Most of the growth in ambulatory surgery has taken place in offices or freestanding surgery centers. Although these smaller venues are usually associated with minor and less-invasive procedures, trends favor expansion of larger cases into smaller venues. All of the regional techniques (described previously) can (and eventually probably will) be done in offices as long as sufficient personnel and resources are available. Two examples of common office-based procedures are transrectal prostate biopsy and intrauterine surgery.

Transrectal prostate biopsy is a procedure commonly performed as an office-based procedure or in an ambulatory center. At one time, this procedure was thought well tolerated by most patients. Recent reviews have estimated, however, that 65% to 90% of patients experience discomfort and up to 30% may have significant pain. Many studies, including a recent meta-analysis, have compared the use of periprostatic nerve block to intrarectal local anesthesia or no local anesthesia during transrectal prostate biopsy. Periprostatic nerve block around the neurovascular bundles provided superior analgesia compared with intrarectal local anesthesia or no anesthesia with no increase in procedure-related complications.[87]

Intrauterine procedures, including dilation and curettage, diagnostic and operative hysteroscopy, oocyte retrieval, polypectomy, endometrial ablation, and sterilization, are often performed under GA or RA with sedation. Paracervical blockade, injection of local anesthetic around the cervix, is often used because anesthesia personnel are not present. The paracervical block seems of little value as a primary anesthetic or analgesic technique.[88] Patients anesthetized with paracervical block have equivalent intraoperative and postoperative pain compared with patients who receive no anesthesia at all. Therefore, intrauterine procedures should be done with deep sedation and there is no clear role for local analgesia.

Laparoscopy may be done in an office with only local anesthesia, and the laparoscopes are usually smaller with lower insufflation pressures in this setting. Laparoscopy is typically performed for diagnosis or treatment (eg, sterilization), and performing the procedure in this manner is associated with lower costs.[89] The gynecologic laparoscopic procedure may be done with local anesthesia or analgesia depending on the approach.

REGIONAL ANESTHESIA AND EFFICIENCY

Painful stimuli are initiated by tissue injury and transmitted by Aδ-fiber and C-fiber nociceptors to the spinal cord dorsal horn neurons. In response to this injury, a variety of neurotransmitters, such as prostaglandin, bradykinin, serotonin, and substance P, are released, which leads to increased activity of the dorsal horn neurons. If this input remains unmodulated, the result may be central sensitization. Preemptive analgesia is a pain control strategy implemented before a painful stimulus and in sufficient duration to limit or prevent sensitization of the central nervous system. This should result in less intense pain of shorter duration. Preemptive analgesia has been demonstrated in several animal models. In human studies by Moiniche and colleagues and Dahl and Moiniche and in the most recent meta-analysis by Ong and colleagues, preemptive analgesia could not be proved.[90–92] Their findings demonstrate it is unnecessary to provide analgesia before a painful stimulus, but it is critical to provide effective analgesia of sufficient duration. Local anesthesia inhibits the transmission of noxious afferent stimuli from the operative site to the spinal cord and brain, and it is desirable to maintain this effect well into the postoperative period. This sustained postoperative analgesia decreases the risks of hyperalgesia, allodynia, and increased pain.

The merits of local anesthetic-based analgesia are well established, and it is clear these techniques facilitate an earlier facility discharge with superior pain control. There is bias against RA because of the time commitment and possible delays associated with it. RA techniques may require additional time to perform, and this may have an impact on operating room efficiency and increase costs. Use of regional techniques result in an overall lower cost due to earlier discharge and fewer unplanned admissions.[93] More advanced techniques (eg, ultrasound-guided PVB) take time to administer and are best done in a time-neutral environment outside the operating room (eg, dedicated block room or PACU). Dedicated block rooms are time effective and contribute to an efficient outpatient practice while preserving analgesic outcomes.[94,95] This same level of efficiency and patient care has also been demonstrated in private practice settings.[96] These are barriers that must be overcome to use RA in any practice.[97,98]

SUMMARY

The use of local anesthetics in ambulatory surgery offers multiple benefits in line with the goals of modern-day outpatient surgery. A variety of regional techniques can be used for a wide spectrum of procedures; all are shown to reduce postprocedural pain; reduce the short-term need for opiate medications; reduce adverse effects, such as nausea and vomiting; and reduce the time to dismissal compared with patients who do not receive regional techniques. It is likely that the growth in ambulatory procedures will continue to rise with future advances in surgical techniques, changes in reimbursement, and the evolution of clinical pathways that include superior, sustained postoperative analgesia. Anticipating these changes in practice, the role of and demand for RA in outpatient surgery will continue to grow.

REFERENCES

1. Cullen KA, Hall MJ, Golosinskiy A. In: Ambulatory surgery in the United States, 2006, in reports NHS, vol. 11. Hyattsville (MD): United States Department of Health and Human Services; 2009. p. 1–28.
2. Chung F, Ritchie E, Su J. Postoperative pain in ambulatory surgery. Anesth Analg 1997;85(4):808–16.
3. Klein SM, Bergh A, Steele SM, et al. Thoracic paravertebral block for breast surgery. Anesth Analg 2000;90(6):1402–5.
4. Larsson S, Lundberg D. A prospective survey of postoperative nausea and vomiting with special regard to incidence and relations to patient characteristics,

anesthetic routines and surgical procedures. Acta Anaesthesiol Scand 1995; 39(4):539–45.

5. Boughey JC, Goravanchi F, Parris RN, et al. Improved postoperative pain control using thoracic paravertebral block for breast operations. Breast J 2009;15(5):483–8.
6. Trompeter A, Camilleri G, Narang K, et al. Analgesia requirements after interscalene block for shoulder arthroscopy: the 5 days following surgery. Arch Orthop Trauma Surg 2009;130(3):417–21.
7. Bryan NA, Swenson JD, Greis PE, et al. Indwelling interscalene catheter use in an outpatient setting for shoulder surgery: technique, efficacy, and complications. J Shoulder Elbow Surg 2007;16(4):388–95.
8. Hadzic A, Williams BA, Karaca PE, et al. For outpatient rotator cuff surgery, nerve block anesthesia provides superior same-day recovery over general anesthesia. Anesthesiology 2005;102(5):1001–7.
9. Singelyn FJ, Lhotel L, Fabre B. Pain relief after arthroscopic shoulder surgery: a comparison of intraarticular analgesia, suprascapular nerve block, and interscalene brachial plexus block. Anesth Analg 2004;99(2):589–92.
10. McCartney CJ, Brull R, Chan VW, et al. Early but no long-term benefit of regional compared with general anesthesia for ambulatory hand surgery. Anesthesiology 2004;101(2):461–7.
11. Hadzic A, Arliss J, Kerimoglu B, et al. A comparison of infraclavicular nerve block versus general anesthesia for hand and wrist day-case surgeries. Anesthesiology 2004;101(1):127–32.
12. Ilfeld BM, Morey TE, Wright TW, et al. Continuous interscalene brachial plexus block for postoperative pain control at home: a randomized, double-blinded, placebo-controlled study. Anesth Analg 2003;96(4):1089–95.
13. D'Alessio JG, Rosenblum M, Shea KP, et al. A retrospective comparison of interscalene block and general anesthesia for ambulatory surgery shoulder arthroscopy. Reg Anesth 1995;20(1):62–8.
14. Brown AR, Weiss R, Greenberg C, et al. Interscalene block for shoulder arthroscopy: comparison with general anesthesia. Arthroscopy 1993;9(3):295–300.
15. Ilfeld BM, Wright TW, Enneking FK, et al. Total shoulder arthroplasty as an outpatient procedure using ambulatory perineural local anesthetic infusion: a pilot feasibility study. Anesth Analg 2005;101(5):1319–22.
16. Mears DC, Mears SC, Chelly JE, et al. THA with a minimally invasive technique, multi-modal anesthesia, and home rehabilitation: factors associated with early discharge? Clin Orthop Relat Res 2009;467(6):1412–7.
17. Ilfeld BM, Morey TE, Wright TW, et al. Interscalene perineural ropivacaine infusion:a comparison of two dosing regimens for postoperative analgesia. Reg Anesth Pain Med 2004;29(1):9–16.
18. Nielsen KC, Greengrass RA, Pietrobon R, et al. Continuous interscalene brachial plexus blockade provides good analgesia at home after major shoulder surgery-report of four cases. Can J Anaesth 2003;50(1):57–61.
19. Klein SM, Steele SM, Nielsen KC, et al. The difficulties of ambulatory interscalene and intra-articular infusions for rotator cuff surgery: a preliminary report. Can J Anaesth 2003;50(3):265–9.
20. Morgenthaler K, Bauer C, Ziegeler S, et al. [Intra-articular bupivacaine following hip joint arthroscopy. Effect on postoperative pain]. Anaesthesist 2007;56(11): 1128–32 [in German].
21. Lee EM, Murphy KP, Ben-David B. Postoperative analgesia for hip arthroscopy: combined L1 and L2 paravertebral blocks. J Clin Anesth 2008;20(6): 462–5.

22. Charnley J. Present status of total hip replacement. Ann Rheum Dis 1971;30(6): 560–4.
23. Berger RA, Sanders SA, Thill ES, et al. Newer anesthesia and rehabilitation protocols enable outpatient hip replacement in selected patients. Clin Orthop Relat Res 2009;467(6):1424–30.
24. Horlocker TT, Hebl JR. Anesthesia for outpatient knee arthroscopy: is there an optimal technique? Reg Anesth Pain Med 2003;28(1):58–63.
25. Goodwin RC, Parker RD. Comparison of the analgesic effects of intra-articular injections administered preoperatively and postoperatively in knee arthroscopy. J Knee Surg 2005;18(1):17–24.
26. Zeidan A, Kassem R, Nahleh N, et al. Intraarticular tramadol-bupivacaine combination prolongs the duration of postoperative analgesia after outpatient arthroscopic knee surgery. Anesth Analg 2008;107(1):292–9.
27. McNaught AF, McCartney C. Bupivacaine chondrotoxicity. Br J Anaesth 2009; 103(1):133 [author reply: 33–4].
28. Dragoo JL, Korotkova T, Kanwar R, et al. The effect of local anesthetics administered via pain pump on chondrocyte viability. Am J Sports Med 2008;36(8): 1484–8.
29. Karpie JC, Chu CR. Lidocaine exhibits dose- and time-dependent cytotoxic effects on bovine articular chondrocytes in vitro. Am J Sports Med 2007; 35(10):1621–7.
30. Gomoll AH, Kang RW, Williams JM, et al. Chondrolysis after continuous intra-articular bupivacaine infusion: an experimental model investigating chondrotoxicity in the rabbit shoulder. Arthroscopy 2006;22(8):813–9.
31. Hadzic A, Karaca PE, Hobeika P, et al. Peripheral nerve blocks result in superior recovery profile compared with general anesthesia in outpatient knee arthroscopy. Anesth Analg 2005;100(4):976–81.
32. Jankowski CJ, Hebl JR, Stuart MJ, et al. A comparison of psoas compartment block and spinal and general anesthesia for outpatient knee arthroscopy. Anesth Analg 2003;97(4):1003–9.
33. Clough TM, Sandher D, Bale RS, et al. The use of a local anesthetic foot block in patients undergoing outpatient bony forefoot surgery: a prospective randomized controlled trial. J Foot Ankle Surg 2003;42(1):24–9.
34. Migues A, Slullitel G, Vescovo A, et al. Peripheral foot blockade versus popliteal fossa nerve block: a prospective randomized trial in 51 patients. J Foot Ankle Surg 2005;44(5):354–7.
35. Capdevila X, Dadure C, Bringuier S, et al. Effect of patient-controlled perineural analgesia on rehabilitation and pain after ambulatory orthopedic surgery: a multicenter randomized trial. Anesthesiology 2006;105(3):566–73.
36. Zaric D, Boysen K, Christiansen J, et al. Continuous popliteal sciatic nerve block for outpatient foot surgery–a randomized, controlled trial. Acta Anaesthesiol Scand 2004;48(3):337–41.
37. Ilfeld BM, Morey TE, Wang RD, et al. Continuous popliteal sciatic nerve block for postoperative pain control at home: a randomized, double-blinded, placebo-controlled study. Anesthesiology 2002;97(4):959–65.
38. O'Donnell D, Manickam B, Perlas A, et al. Spinal mepivacaine with fentanyl for outpatient knee arthroscopy surgery: a randomized controlled trial. Can J Anaesth 2009;57(1):32–8.
39. Merivirta R, Kuusniemi K, Jaakkola P, et al. Unilateral spinal anaesthesia for outpatient surgery: a comparison between hyperbaric bupivacaine and bupivacaine-clonidine combination. Acta Anaesthesiol Scand 2009;53(6):788–93.

40. Fanelli G, Danelli G, Zasa M, et al. Intrathecal ropivacaine 5 mg/ml for outpatient knee arthroscopy: a comparison with lidocaine 10 mg/ml. Acta Anaesthesiol Scand 2009;53(1):109–15.
41. Diallo T, Dufeu N, Marret E, et al. Walking in PACU after unilateral spinal anesthesia a criteria for hospital discharge: a 100 outpatient survey. Acta Anaesthesiol Belg 2009;60(1):3–6.
42. van Tuijl I, Giezeman MJ, Braithwaite SA, et al. Intrathecal low-dose hyperbaric bupivacaine-clonidine combination in outpatient knee arthroscopy: a randomized controlled trial. Acta Anaesthesiol Scand 2008;52(3):343–9.
43. Sell A, Tein T, Pitkanen M. Spinal 2-chloroprocaine: effective dose for ambulatory surgery. Acta Anaesthesiol Scand 2008;52(5):695–9.
44. Montes FR, Zarate E, Grueso R, et al. Comparison of spinal anesthesia with combined sciatic-femoral nerve block for outpatient knee arthroscopy. J Clin Anesth 2008;20(6):415–20.
45. Casati A, Fanelli G, Danelli G, et al. Spinal anesthesia with lidocaine or preservative-free 2-chlorprocaine for outpatient knee arthroscopy: a prospective, randomized, double-blind comparison. Anesth Analg 2007;104(4):959–64.
46. Boztug N, Bigat Z, Karsli B, et al. Comparison of ropivacaine and bupivacaine for intrathecal anesthesia during outpatient arthroscopic surgery. J Clin Anesth 2006; 18(7):521–5.
47. Cappelleri G, Aldegheri G, Danelli G, et al. Spinal anesthesia with hyperbaric levobupivacaine and ropivacaine for outpatient knee arthroscopy: a prospective, randomized, double-blind study. Anesth Analg 2005;101(1):77–82.
48. Korhonen AM, Valanne JV, Jokela RM, et al. A comparison of selective spinal anesthesia with hyperbaric bupivacaine and general anesthesia with desflurane for outpatient knee arthroscopy. Anesth Analg 2004;99(6): 1668–73.
49. Gurkan Y, Canatay H, Ozdamar D, et al. Spinal anesthesia for arthroscopic knee surgery. Acta Anaesthesiol Scand 2004;48(4):513–7.
50. Forssblad M, Jacobson E, Weidenhielm L. Knee arthroscopy with different anesthesia methods: a comparison of efficacy and cost. Knee Surg Sports Traumatol Arthrosc 2004;12(5):344–9.
51. Taniguchi M, Bollen AW, Drasner K. Sodium bisulfite: scapegoat for chloroprocaine neurotoxicity? Anesthesiology 2004;100(1):85–91.
52. Davis BR, Kopacz DJ. Spinal 2-chloroprocaine: the effect of added clonidine. Anesth Analg 2005;100(2):559–65.
53. Gonter AF, Kopacz DJ. Spinal 2-chloroprocaine: a comparison with procaine in volunteers. Anesth Analg 2005;100(2):573–9.
54. Kopacz DJ. Spinal 2-chloroprocaine: minimum effective dose. Reg Anesth Pain Med 2005;30(1):36–42.
55. Yoos JR, Kopacz DJ. Spinal 2-chloroprocaine: a comparison with small-dose bupivacaine in volunteers. Anesth Analg 2005;100(2):566–72.
56. Yoos JR, Kopacz DJ. Spinal 2-chloroprocaine for surgery: an initial 10-month experience. Anesth Analg 2005;100(2):553–8.
57. Kouri ME, Kopacz DJ. Spinal 2-chloroprocaine: a comparison with lidocaine in volunteers. Anesth Analg 2004;98(1):75–80.
58. Smith KN, Kopacz DJ, McDonald SB. Spinal 2-chloroprocaine: a dose-ranging study and the effect of added epinephrine. Anesth Analg 2004;98(1):81–8.
59. Kim SY, Cho JE, Hong JY, et al. Comparison of intrathecal fentanyl and sufentanil in low-dose dilute bupivacaine spinal anaesthesia for transurethral prostatectomy. Br J Anaesth 2009;103(5):750–4.

60. Gudaityte J, Marchertiene I, Karbonskiene A, et al. Low-dose spinal hyperbaric bupivacaine for adult anorectal surgery: a double-blinded, randomized, controlled study. J Clin Anesth 2009;21(7):474–81.
61. de Santiago J, Santos-Yglesias J, Giron J, et al. Low-dose 3 mg levobupivacaine plus 10 microg fentanyl selective spinal anesthesia for gynecological outpatient laparoscopy. Anesth Analg 2009;109(5):1456–61.
62. de Santiago J, Santos LJ, Giron J. Low-dose, low-concentration spinal anesthesia may help to detect surgery-related nerve injury. Acta Anaesthesiol Scand 2009; 53(9):1229–30.
63. Cuvas O, Gulec H, Karaaslan M, et al. The use of low dose plain solutions of local anaesthetic agents for spinal anaesthesia in the prone position: bupivacaine compared with levobupivacaine. Anaesthesia 2009;64(1):14–8.
64. Gurbet A, Turker G, Girgin NK, et al. Combination of ultra-low dose bupivacaine and fentanyl for spinal anaesthesia in out-patient anorectal surgery. J Int Med Res 2008;36(5):964–70.
65. Wassef MR, Michaels EI, Rangel JM, et al. Spinal perianal block: a prospective, randomized, double-blind comparison with spinal saddle block. Anesth Analg 2007;104(6):1594–6.
66. Korhonen AM. Use of spinal anaesthesia in day surgery. Curr Opin Anaesthesiol 2006;19(6):612–6.
67. Atallah MM, Shorrab AA, Abdel Mageed YM, et al. Low-dose bupivacaine spinal anaesthesia for percutaneous nephrolithotomy: the suitability and impact of adding intrathecal fentanyl. Acta Anaesthesiol Scand 2006;50(7):798–803.
68. Kaya M, Oguz S, Aslan K, et al. A low-dose bupivacaine: a comparison of hyperbaric and hypobaric solutions for unilateral spinal anesthesia. Reg Anesth Pain Med 2004;29(1):17–22.
69. Kararmaz A, Kaya S, Turhanoglu S, et al. Low-dose bupivacaine-fentanyl spinal anaesthesia for transurethral prostatectomy. Anaesthesia 2003;58(6):526–30.
70. Gupta A, Axelsson K, Thorn SE, et al. Low-dose bupivacaine plus fentanyl for spinal anesthesia during ambulatory inguinal herniorrhaphy: a comparison between 6 mg and 7. 5 mg of bupivacaine. Acta Anaesthesiol Scand 2003; 47(1):13–9.
71. Goel S, Bhardwaj N, Grover VK. Intrathecal fentanyl added to intrathecal bupivacaine for day case surgery: a randomized study. Eur J Anaesthesiol 2003;20(4): 294–7.
72. Coveney E, Weltz CR, Greengrass R, et al. Use of paravertebral block anesthesia in the surgical management of breast cancer: experience in 156 cases. Ann Surg 1998;227(4):496–501.
73. Kairaluoma PM, Bachmann MS, Rosenberg PH, et al. Preincisional paravertebral block reduces the prevalence of chronic pain after breast surgery. Anesth Analg 2006;103(3):703–8.
74. Exadaktylos AK, Buggy DJ, Moriarty DC, et al. Can anesthetic technique for primary breast cancer surgery affect recurrence or metastasis? Anesthesiology 2006;105(4):660–4.
75. Jensen P, Mikkelsen T, Kehlet H. Postherniorrhaphy urinary retention–effect of local, regional, and general anesthesia: a review. Reg Anesth Pain Med 2002; 27(6):612–7.
76. Sanchez B, Waxman K, Tatevossian R, et al. Local anesthetic infusion pumps improve postoperative pain after inguinal hernia repair: a randomized trial. Am Surg 2004;70(11):1002–6.

77. Hadzic A, Kerimoglu B, Loreio D, et al. Paravertebral blocks provide superior same-day recovery over general anesthesia for patients undergoing inguinal hernia repair. Anesth Analg 2006;102(4):1076–81.
78. Bisgaard T, Klarskov B, Kristiansen VB, et al. Multi-regional local anesthetic infiltration during laparoscopic cholecystectomy in patients receiving prophylactic multi-modal analgesia: a randomized, double-blinded, placebo-controlled study. Anesth Analg 1999;89(4):1017–24.
79. Boddy AP, Mehta S, Rhodes M. The effect of intraperitoneal local anesthesia in laparoscopic cholecystectomy: a systematic review and meta-analysis. Anesth Analg 2006;103(3):682–8.
80. Naja MZ, Ziade MF, Lonnqvist PA. General anaesthesia combined with bilateral paravertebral blockade (T5-6) vs. general anaesthesia for laparoscopic cholecystectomy: a prospective, randomized clinical trial. Eur J Anaesthesiol 2004;21(6):489–95.
81. El-Dawlatly AA, Turkistani A, Kettner SC, et al. Ultrasound-guided transversus abdominis plane block: description of a new technique and comparison with conventional systemic analgesia during laparoscopic cholecystectomy. Br J Anaesth 2009;102(6):763–7.
82. Alessandri F, Lijoi D, Mistrangelo E, et al. Effect of presurgical local infiltration of levobupivacaine in the surgical field on postsurgical wound pain in laparoscopic gynecological surgery. Acta Obstet Gynecol Scand 2006;85(7):844–9.
83. Ostad A, Kageyama N, Moy RL. Tumescent anesthesia with a lidocaine dose of 55 mg/kg is safe for liposuction. Dermatol Surg 1996;22(11):921–7.
84. Cooter RD, Rudkin GE, Gardiner SE. Day case breast augmentation under paravertebral blockade: a prospective study of 100 consecutive patients. Aesthetic Plast Surg 2007;31(6):666–73.
85. Pacik PT, Nelson CE, Werner C. Pain control in augmentation mammaplasty using indwelling catheters in 687 consecutive patients: data analysis. Aesthet Surg J 2008;28(6):631–41.
86. Lu L, Fine NA. The efficacy of continuous local anesthetic infiltration in breast surgery: reduction mammaplasty and reconstruction. Plast Reconstr Surg 2005;115(7):1927–34 [discussion: 35–6].
87. Tiong HY, Liew LC, Samuel M, et al. A meta-analysis of local anesthesia for transrectal ultrasound-guided biopsy of the prostate. Prostate Cancer Prostatic Dis 2007;10(2):127–36.
88. Tangsiriwatthana T, Sangkomkamhang US, Lumbiganon P, et al. Paracervical local anaesthesia for cervical dilatation and uterine intervention. Cochrane Database Syst Rev 2009;(1):CD005056.
89. DeQuattro N, Hibbert M, Buller J, et al. Microlaparoscopic tubal ligation under local anesthesia. J Am Assoc Gynecol Laparosc 1998;5(1):55–8.
90. Moiniche S, Kehlet H, Dahl JB. A qualitative and quantitative systematic review of preemptive analgesia for postoperative pain relief: the role of timing of analgesia. Anesthesiology 2002;96(3):725–41.
91. Dahl JB, Moiniche S. Pre-emptive analgesia. Br Med Bull 2004;71:13–27.
92. Ong CK, Lirk P, Seymour RA, et al. The efficacy of preemptive analgesia for acute postoperative pain management: a meta-analysis. Anesth Analg 2005;100(3):757–73.
93. Williams BA, Kentor ML, Vogt MT, et al. Femoral-sciatic nerve blocks for complex outpatient knee surgery are associated with less postoperative pain before

same-day discharge: a review of 1,200 consecutive cases from the period 1996-1999. Anesthesiology 2003;98(5):1206–13.

94. Armstrong KP, Cherry RA. Brachial plexus anesthesia compared to general anesthesia when a block room is available. Can J Anaesth 2004;51(1):41–4.
95. Mariano ER, Chu LF, Peinado CR, et al. Anesthesia-controlled time and turnover time for ambulatory upper extremity surgery performed with regional versus general anesthesia. J Clin Anesth 2009;21(4):253–7.
96. Fredrickson MJ, Ball CM, Dalgleish AJ. Successful continuous interscalene analgesia for ambulatory shoulder surgery in a private practice setting. Reg Anesth Pain Med 2008;33(2):122–8.
97. Mariano ER. Making it work: setting up a regional anesthesia program that provides value. Anesthesiol Clin 2008;26(4):681–92, vi.
98. Williams BA, Kentor ML. Making an ambulatory surgery centre suitable for regional anaesthesia. Best Pract Res Clin Anaesthesiol 2002;16(2):175–94.

Ambulatory Anesthesia and Regional Catheters: When and How

Jeffrey D. Swenson, MD*, Gloria S. Cheng, MD, Deborah A. Axelrod, MD, Jennifer J. Davis, MD

KEYWORDS

- Peripheral catheters • Ambulatory anesthesia
- Continuous peripheral nerve block

Several clinical trials have demonstrated the superiority of continuous peripheral nerve block (CPNB) compared with traditional opioid-based analgesia.[1–7] In addition to providing improved analgesia, CPNB is associated with less sedation, nausea, and pruritis.[8] Although single injection nerve blocks (SINB) can also provide excellent analgesia, CPNB allows added flexibility in both duration and density of local anesthetic effect. Recently there has been increased use of CPNB in the ambulatory surgery setting for both adults[9–11] and pediatric patients.[11–13] The ability to provide safe and effective CPNB at home is an attractive alternative to opioid-based analgesia with its related side effects. In some cases, CPNB shortens the duration[14] or eliminates the need[15] for hospitalization in patients who otherwise would require inpatient treatment for pain control.

In this article, several practical issues related to the use of CPNB in the ambulatory setting are discussed. Techniques for catheter placement, infusion regimens, patient education, and complications are reviewed. Recognizing that there are many institutional-based preferences for CPNB placement and management, special emphasis is placed on separating evidence-based techniques from institutional preferences.

WHY CHOOSE CPNB OVER SINGLE INJECTION?

Perhaps the most compelling reason to use CPNB is the increased flexibility in duration and block density that is possible compared with SINB. After orthopedic surgery, significant increases in visual analog scale scores may persist for 2 to 3 days.[16–18] Although SINB can provide up to 24 hours of analgesia, blocks of this duration require

Department of Anesthesiology, University of Utah Orthopaedics Hospital, University of Utah, 30 North 1900 East, 3C444, Salt Lake City, UT 84132, USA
* Corresponding author.
E-mail address: jeff.swenson@hsc.utah.edu

Anesthesiology Clin 28 (2010) 267–280
doi:10.1016/j.anclin.2010.02.010 **anesthesiology.theclinics.com**
1932-2275/10/$ – see front matter

concentrated local anesthetics that are associated with dense motor and sensory effect. By contrast, CPNB can be used to provide prolonged analgesia with low volumes of dilute local anesthetic.[1,2,5] Thus, flexibility in the duration and density of local anesthetic effect are provided while avoiding the need for initial injection of large volume, and potentially toxic doses, of local anesthetic.

Low-density nerve blocks are attractive for several reasons. Although most patients appreciate the excellent analgesia provided by nerve blocks, dense motor and sensory effect can be unpleasant and potentially dangerous. Patients may report decreased satisfaction when the extremity is "too numb" or "dead." Limb neglect caused by a dense motor and sensory block may also result in positioning injury and falls.[11,19] As more data emerge for infusions of dilute local anesthetic, improved patient satisfaction and safety are being documented. Already there are data showing that after shoulder surgery, lower concentration interscalene blocks (0.125% vs 0.25% bupivacaine) provide comparable analgesia but with improved diaphragm function and higher oxygen saturation.[20]

Finally, the cost savings from reduced need for hospitalization made possible with CPNB[14,15] have not been reported with SINB. Thus, the use of ambulatory catheters may represent an unprecedented example of improved patient care at a lower cost.

CPNB PLACEMENT TECHNIQUES

Techniques for CPNB placement have developed in large part from existing methods for SINB. Accurate needle placement has historically relied on eliciting a paresthesia or electrical stimulation (ES) of the nerve. Ultrasound (US) guidance has recently assumed a major, if not dominant, role in the performance of CPNB.

For several years, ES was the preferred technique for performing nerve blocks and enjoyed a "gold standard" status.[21] Although no data exist showing a consistent relationship between stimulating current and proximity to the nerve, this technique has remained popular due to the lack of a viable alternative.[22–24] Despite limitations, ES has been successfully used for many years with apparently few complications. Initial CPNB placement using ES techniques employed only stimulating needles. In the 1990s, ES catheters were introduced in hopes of improving the ease of placement and success rate for CPNB.[25] Unfortunately, when compared with conventional catheters, most studies have failed to show significant clinical benefit from these more costly catheters.[26–28]

The introduction of portable, high-resolution US has been an important development in regional anesthesia. Initially viewed as a novelty or a supplement to ES, US is now firmly recognized as a "stand-alone" technique.[29] In fact, a review of clinical trials comparing ES with US confirms that US-guided blocks are performed more quickly, with higher success rates, less procedure related pain, lower dose requirements, and fewer vascular punctures than those performed using ES.[21,30–34] In addition, the catheter tip position can be easily confirmed by injecting agitated local anesthetic or air through the catheter while imaging the nerve. These techniques, originally described anecdotally,[35,36] are now commonly reported as a method to verify catheter position.[33,34]

SKIN PREPARATION AND PATIENT DRAPING

Indwelling catheter placement requires strict adherence to sterile procedure. The American Society of Regional Anesthesia and Pain Medicine (ASRA) recommends sterile precautions, including antiseptic hand washing, sterile gloves, surgical hats and masks, and the use of alcohol-based chlorhexidine antiseptic solution.[37] These guidelines are extrapolations from data pertaining to neuraxial regional techniques and central venous access techniques. A sterile drape is applied to isolate the area of skin preparation. When using a US-guided technique, the transducer must either be covered with a sterile sleeve (**Fig. 1**) or be positioned outside of the sterile field (**Fig. 2**).

NEEDLE TYPE

The use of short beveled needles is a widely accepted practice in regional anesthesia. Many practitioners report an increased ability to recognize a "pop" or other tactile feedback when using a short beveled or Tuohy needle. The notion that nerve injury is less likely to occur with short beveled needles is controversial. A single animal study has suggested a relationship between bevel type and the incidence of nerve injury; however, this has never been validated clinically.[38] A subsequent study refuted the notion that short beveled needles are less prone to cause injury.[39] Recently there has been an increased interest in using US-guided techniques that do not require immediate proximity between the needle and the nerve. Since the transition to US-guided techniques, conventional thin-walled needles have also been used safely for CPNB placement.[11] If this trend continues, bevel type may play a less important role when choosing a needle. Nevertheless, the Tuohy needle remains a popular choice for many practitioners when transitioning from SINB to CPNB placement.

LOCAL ANESTHETIC INJECTION DURING CATHETER PLACEMENT

The timing, volume, and concentration of local anesthetic injected during the placement of CPNB may vary considerably between institutions. When using ES techniques, it is reported that local anesthetic injection through the stimulating needle may alter the threshold for nerve depolarization.[40] A theoretical disadvantage to injecting local anesthetic through the needle before catheter insertion is an inability to verify accurate placement by injection of local anesthetic through the catheter and

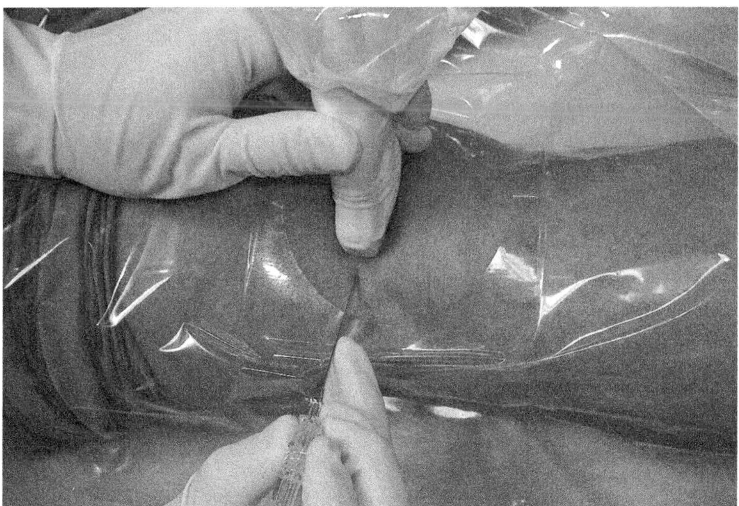

Fig. 1. An example in the left popliteal fossa of the US transducer covered with a sterile sleeve and positioned adjacent to the needle inside the sterile field.

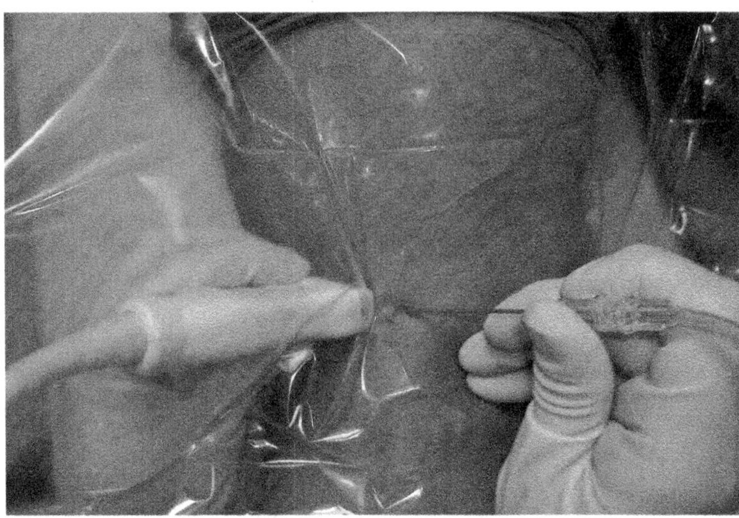

Fig. 2. An example in the left popliteal fossa of the US transducer positioned outside the sterile field. The needle is inserted through the skin within the sterile field and passes through the US beam, which is outside the field. A clear fenestrated drape with an adhesive border separates the needle and transducer.

observing subsequent sensory and motor effect.[41,42] The obvious concern for outpatients would be a scenario whereby initial bolus injection though the needle produced successful analgesia but subsequent infusion through the catheter failed. The ability to visualize catheter position relative to the nerve using US may eliminate this concern in the future.[36] **Figs. 3** and **4** demonstrate the appearance of agitated local anesthetic injected through existing interscalene and femoral catheters, respectively.

A significant advantage of CPNB placed for postoperative analgesia is that it does not require injection of a large, concentrated dose of local anesthetic. Interscalene catheters, for example, provide excellent analgesia after initial injection of only 20 mL of 0.125% bupivacaine.[20] This total dose of bupivacaine (25 mg) is considerably lower than doses typically used for SINB (100–150 mg).

SECURING THE CATHETER

As with many aspects of CPNB placement, there is variability among institutions regarding how to secure the catheter. Catheter dressing focuses on preventing leakage, dislodgment, and infection. Liquid adhesives are commonly applied to the skin before the dressing. Although they are very effective for securing tape and other coverings, a small percentage of patients may experience contact dermatitis from a common substance (styrax gum) found in both tincture of benzion and mastisol.[43] Sterile adhesive strips and other fixation devices can also be used at the catheter insertion site to prevent dislodgment.

Catheter tunneling is practiced at many institutions in hopes of minimizing infection and dislodgment. For CPNB, there are no prospective, randomized studies comparing infection rates for tunneled catheters versus catheters without tunneling. In fact, large infection-free series have been reported both with and without tunneling.[11,44] The risk of catheter dislodgment with and without tunneling has likewise not been assessed prospectively. Therefore, tunneling to prevent infection or dislodgment remains an

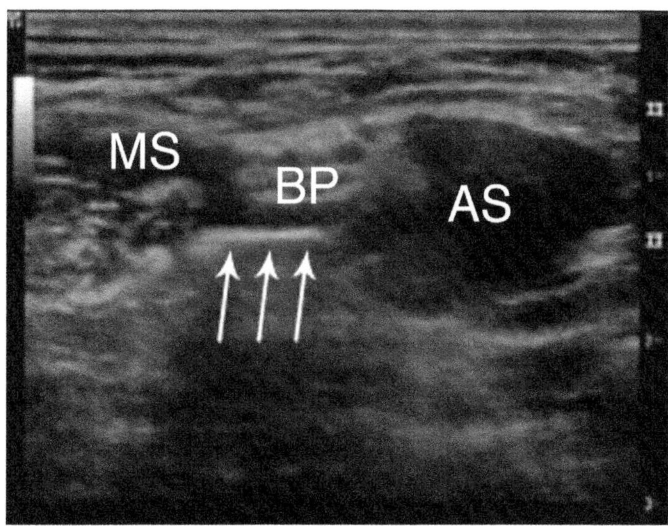

Fig. 3. Arrows highlight the position the catheter tip in the interscalene space (ISS). The injectate at the tip is hyperechoic due to local anesthetic containing microbubbles. The anterior scalene muscle (AS), middle scalene muscle (MS), and brachial plexus (BP) are displayed.

institutional preference rather than evidence-based practice. An important consideration for CPNB in the ambulatory setting is the ease with which the catheter can be withdrawn after the dressing has been removed. Patients should be instructed to seek consultation if any resistance is present during catheter removal. For this reason,

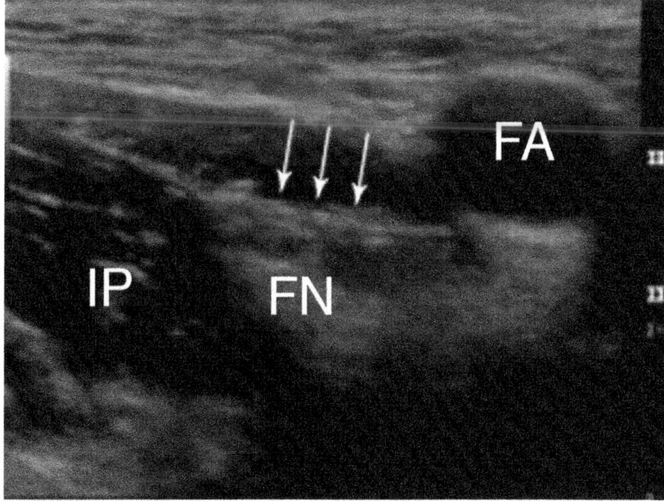

Fig. 4. Arrows highlight the position the catheter tip superficial to the femoral nerve (FN). The injectate at the tip is hyperechoic due to local anesthetic containing microbubbles. Also displayed are the femoral artery (FA) and the iliopsoas muscle (IP).

the ease with which a catheter can be withdrawn after removing the dressing is another consideration when deciding whether to tunnel the catheter.

PATIENT EDUCATION AND FOLLOW-UP

Successful ambulatory catheter programs provide focused education for patients and their caretakers. The goal of education should be to prepare patients to manage and remove their own catheters at home. With brief instruction, most questions and concerns about CPNB management can be answered for patients before discharge from the hospital. This education can be combined with written instructions and hospital contact information. Examples of these written instructions are included in Appendices 1 and 2.

At home, patients should have simple instructions to access hospital personnel. Although many anesthesiologists have concerns about the volume of patient calls, the actual need for intervention may be surprisingly low. In one large series, only 4% of patients required physician intervention after hospital discharge.[11] Only 1% of patients required intervention at night or on a weekend.[11] In this same series, only 1 of the 620 patients was unable to remove their catheter at home. Every effort should be made to simplify outpatient CPNB management. Patients may already be concerned with issues such as wound care and rehabilitation. Fixed-rate elastomeric pumps may be advantageous in this setting because they require little or no instruction for use, require no interaction by the patient, and can be discarded at home.

COST AND ECONOMIC EFFECT

The economic impact of CPNB on ambulatory surgery is increasingly evident. For selected orthopedic procedures, catheters may provide a significant reduction in hospital costs. In some cases, surgeries that have historically required hospitalization for pain control can be performed as outpatients.[15] Patients with obstructive sleep apnea represent another potential application for CPNB. Current guidelines recommend hospital admission and monitoring for some patients with obstructive sleep apnea who require postoperative treatment with opioid analgesics.[45] By using CPNB as the primary mode of analgesia, postoperative opioids may be minimized or avoided altogether. Thus, catheter use may provide improved safety as well as decreased cost of hospitalization for these patients.

Equipment costs are an important consideration when establishing a CPNB program. At present, ES and US are the 2 dominant modalities used to guide catheter placement. Although US is a viable stand-alone method, initial equipment costs can be considerable. Each institution must balance the initial investment in imaging equipment with the ongoing needle and catheter costs associated with ES methods.

Infusion pumps are probably the area of greatest cost disparity in CPNB practice. Prices for disposable pumps vary from $55 for fixed rate elastomeric pumps to more than $300 for bolus/basal capable pumps.[46] Although there is ample evidence demonstrating improved analgesia and decreased side effects with CPNB infused at a basal rate, the data supporting the addition of a bolus capability are less consistent.[16,17] Hence, the significant increase in cost and complexity for bolus/basal pumps should be balanced against any individual benefit.

LOCAL ANESTHETICS, INFUSION RATES, AND DELIVERY SYSTEMS

After CPNB placement, there are a variety of local anesthetics, dosing regimens, and delivery systems that have been successfully used. The number of existing techniques suggests there is still no established best practice. Usually a low concentration of long-acting local anesthetic is administered through the catheter. The delivery of short-acting local anesthetics such as lidocaine and mepivacaine seems reasonable, but studies on their use are limited.[47] The most commonly reported drugs, bupivacaine and ropivacaine, both seem to provide adequate analgesia without toxicity. However, innate property differences between the two may lead to differences in motor blockade. Ropivacaine has been described as being more "motor sparing" in comparison with bupivacaine.[48] Although ropivacaine is also reportedly less cardiotoxic than bupivacaine, this difference may only be clinically relevant when large doses are anticipated. Extensive experience with prolonged infusions of bupivacaine (up to 25 mg/h) has not revealed clinically detectable toxicity.[49] Instead, toxicity with both bupivacaine and ropivacaine is associated almost exclusively with a single large injection such as an SINB or catheter bolus. Although the addition of clonidine has been shown to increase the duration of analgesia associated with SINB,[50] its benefits as an adjuvant to CPNB remain unproven. In studies thus far, the addition of clonidine to ropivacaine for CPNB has not resulted in improved analgesia or decreased local anesthetic use.[51,52]

The optimal combination of local anesthetic concentration and volume to be infused through a perineural catheter also remains to be determined. One trend that seems to be consistent is that analgesia can be achieved at most locations using low concentrations of long-acting local anesthetics (ropivacaine 0.2%, bupivacaine 0.125%) infused at rates from 5 to 12 mL per hour.[11,16–18]

Catheter infusion regimens (ie, basal, basal-bolus, bolus only) have also been the subject of many studies. An important finding of these reports is the significant pain relief and reduction in opioid requirements provided by a simple basal infusion.[1,3,11,13] Bolus-only regimens may be associated with higher pain scores, oral analgesic use, and number of sleep disturbances compared with techniques with a basal infusion.[16,17] In comparing basal-bolus and basal-only techniques, however, pain scores and patient satisfaction are mixed.[16–18]

Many types of pumps exist for the outpatient setting,[46] including reusable and disposable, electronic and nonelectronic, basal-only and basal-bolus capable. Nonelectronic disposable infusion pumps include elastomeric, positive-pressure (spring-powered and gas-pressure–powered), and negative-pressure (vacuum) pumps.[53] In choosing an appropriate model, several factors should be considered including cost, ease of use, flow-rate accuracy, programmability, and bolus capability. Electronic pumps offer more accuracy in hourly volume delivery than the elastomeric pumps.[54] Such pumps also allow infusion rates and bolus doses to be readily programmed and changed depending on the individual patient's needs. However, they are associated with more technical problems and are considerably more expensive than more simple devices.[55] In clinical trials comparing electronic-programmable pumps with the simple elastomeric variety, elastomeric pumps provided similar postoperative analgesia, fewer technical problems, and decreased cost.[55] Furthermore, the lack of programming ability eliminates any risk of programming error by the practitioner or the patient. Reusable electronic pumps may be cost effective over time but require a mechanism for their return by patients, making them less convenient. In summary, if cost is a major consideration, elastomeric pumps offer adequate functionality at a price significantly less than their electronic counterparts. Though they are less accurate, the variability in dose delivery has not been shown to be clinically significant, nor reported to be the cause of adverse events.[56] By contrast, if programmability and the ability to deliver patient-controlled boluses are important, then consideration should be given to electronic infusion pumps.

In summary, no particular combination of drug, rate, regimen, or pump has been established as best practice. In most CPNB studies, accurately positioned catheters at reasonable range of basal infusions (5–10 mL/h) will provide analgesia that is superior to opioid-based techniques. When considering the cost of outpatient catheter programs, the measurable differences between various pumps and local anesthetics should be carefully considered.

COMPLICATIONS

Complications associated with the outpatient use of CPNB are largely similar to those associated with their use in the hospital setting.[57] In recent years, a large body of literature has been assembled to identify the most notable adverse events associated with continuous catheter techniques. A working knowledge of these complications is important when discussing these treatment options with patients. Such complications include infection, neurologic complications, and local anesthetic toxicity.

Infection

Most studies reporting infection associated with CPNB are from hospitalized patients; however, data for large outpatient series are accumulating as well. For inpatients, incidence of catheter infection ranges from 0% to 3.2%,[44,57,58] while outpatient rates are less than 1%.[11,59] The American Society of Regional Anesthesia and Pain Medicine (ASRA) recommends sterile precautions, including antiseptic hand washing, sterile gloves, surgical hats and masks, and the use of alcohol-based chlorhexidine antiseptic solution. These guidelines are extrapolations from data pertaining to neuraxial and central venous access techniques. Added to these recommendations should be a provision for sterile precautions while filling infusion pumps. At least one report of severe, deep cellulitis has been attributed to contaminated infusate from a pump that was not filled under sterile conditions.[60]

Several specific risk factors associated with infection have been identified. Those applicable to the outpatient setting include duration of catheter use longer than 48 hours, lack of antibiotic prophylaxis, and axillary or femoral location.[59] Although tunneling has been recommended to reduce of bacterial colonization, this practice has never been confirmed as a factor in reducing infection.

Neurologic Complications

Although neurologic injury associated with CPNB is usually transient and ranges from 0.3% to 2.0%,[11,57] it remains one of the anesthesiologist's primary concerns. Injury may occur during performance of the block as well as during the postoperative period. Because placement techniques are similar between hospitalized and ambulatory patients, this discussion focuses on unique aspects of patients treated at home with catheters.

There are few reports of nerve injury in patients who go home with CPNB; however, pressure injury has been implicated as a likely cause.[11] For patients with an extremity in which there is little or no sensation, special precautions must be taken during application of casts, splints, and other dressings. Likewise, the patient must position the extremity carefully at all times. When determining the rate and concentration of local anesthetic infusions, the desire to achieve complete analgesia with the nerve block should be balanced against the risks of "limb neglect." Multimodal approaches to analgesia have recently been explored, which may prove beneficial in preserving more motor function and proprioception while providing excellent analgesia.[61]

A somewhat more novel neurologic concern associated with outpatient CPNB is the risk of falls. In a recent report, 4 of 233 patients (1.7%) treated with continuous femoral nerve block after knee surgery fell as outpatients.[19] These falls occurred despite patients receiving instruction not to bear weight on the affected extremity. This complication, although uncommon, is another example of the potential benefit in providing low-concentration blocks that preserve more motor function and proprioception.

Local Anesthetic Toxicity

As previously mentioned, one advantage of CPNB over SINB is the ability to provide prolonged analgesia without initial large-volume injections of concentrated local anesthetics. Indeed, recent data suggest that US-guided interscalene injection of bupivacaine, 25 mg (20 mL, 0.125%) provides excellent postoperative analgesia after shoulder surgery.[20] Most investigators report subsequent basal hourly infusion rates of 5 to 10 mL per hour using dilute solutions of either ropivacaine or bupivicaine.[11,16–18] With these low rates of infusion, it is not surprising that local anesthetic toxicity is not listed as a complication in any large published series of CPNB to date. However, even with these favorable results, it should be noted that although continuous infusion is unlikely to result in sudden onset of toxicity, patients with a pump allowing bolus capability could theoretically be at risk if intravascular migration should occur.

SUMMARY

The use of CPNB provides improved analgesia with fewer side effects than traditional opioid-based techniques. These benefits are increasingly relevant in the ambulatory surgery setting where more complex procedures are being performed as outpatients. Safe and effective use of these catheters at home has been demonstrated in large trials whose patients manage and remove their own catheters. Although variations exist between institutions with respect to placement and management strategies, several trends are becoming apparent. First, US is rapidly emerging as a dominant technique for placing CPNB. Second, patients are able to successfully manage and remove catheters at home with minimal supervision and low complication rates. Finally, by containing catheter-related expenses and reducing the need for hospitalization, the elusive goal of improved care at lower cost could be achieved.

APPENDIX 1
INTERSCALENE CATHETER: PATIENT INSTRUCTIONS (EXAMPLE)

You have received a nerve catheter to help control pain control after surgery. We have provided the information below to answer questions you may have.

1. In addition to the catheter, you may take pain medication prescribed by your surgeon as needed.
2. Keep the dressing clean and dry until it is time to remove the catheter. A small amount of blood and/or clear fluid under the dressing is normal.
3. If you detect any increased pain, swelling, or redness at the site of the catheter, notify the Doctor named below immediately.
4. The pump attached to this catheter will work in any position and is not affected by gravity. You may attach it anywhere that is convenient for you. The "balloon" inside empties very slowly and may not appear to be changing in size.
5. Some normal side effects that may be present with this catheter include:
   Drooping eyelid
   Slight redness in the eye

A smaller pupil
Hoarseness of the voice
Slight shortness of breath (diaphragm weakness).

6. Be aware that without normal sensation in your arm and hand, you must keep it well-padded and protected from injury.
7. Your catheter should be removed on_______, when the bottle is empty. Simply remove the tape and adhesive and pull the catheter out. The catheter should come out very easily.
8. For any questions or concerns you may reach Dr_______ directly at phone # _______.

APPENDIX 2
FEMORAL NERVE CATHETER: PATIENT INSTRUCTIONS (EXAMPLE)

You have received a nerve catheter to help control pain control after surgery. We have provided the information below to answer questions you may have.

1. In addition to the catheter, you may take pain medication prescribed by your surgeon as needed.
2. Keep the dressing clean and dry until it is time to remove the catheter. A small amount of blood and/or clear fluid under the dressing is normal.
3. If you detect any increased pain, swelling, or redness at the site of the catheter, notify the Doctor named below immediately.
4. You should not bear weight or walk without assistance or crutches until the sensation has completely returned to your leg.
5. The pump attached to this catheter will work in any position and is not affected by gravity. You may attach it anywhere that is convenient for you. The "balloon" inside empties very slowly and may not appear to be changing in size.
6. Be aware that without normal sensation in your leg, you must keep it well-padded and protected from injury.
7. Your catheter should be removed on_______, when the bottle is empty. Simply remove the tape and adhesive and pull the catheter out. The catheter should come out very easily.
8. For any questions or concerns you may reach Dr_______ directly at phone #_______.

REFERENCES

1. Edwards ND, Wright EM. Continuous low-dose 3-in-1 nerve blockade for postoperative pain relief after total knee replacement. Anesth Analg 1992;75(2):265–7.
2. Ilfeld BM, Morey TE, Wang RD, et al. Continuous popliteal sciatic nerve block for postoperative pain control at home: a randomized, double-blinded, placebo-controlled study. Anesthesiology 2002;97(4):959–65.
3. White PF, Issioui T, Skrivanek GD, et al. The use of a continuous popliteal sciatic nerve block after surgery involving the foot and ankle: does it improve the quality of recovery? Anesth Analg 2003;97(5):1303–9.
4. Borgeat A, Tewes E, Biasca N, et al. Patient-controlled interscalene analgesia with ropivacaine after major shoulder surgery: PCIA vs PCA. Br J Anaesth 1998;81(4):603–5.
5. Borgeat A, Schappi B, Biasca N, et al. Patient-controlled analgesia after major shoulder surgery: patient-controlled interscalene analgesia versus patient-controlled analgesia. Anesthesiology 1997;87(6):1343–7.

6. Borgeat A, Perschak H, Bird P, et al. Patient-controlled interscalene analgesia with ropivacaine 0.2% versus patient-controlled intravenous analgesia after major shoulder surgery: effects on diaphragmatic and respiratory function. Anesthesiology 2000;92(1):102–8.
7. Ilfeld BM, Morey TE, Wright TW, et al. Continuous interscalene brachial plexus block for postoperative pain control at home: a randomized, double-blinded, placebo-controlled study. Anesth Analg 2003;96(4):1089–95.
8. Richman JM, Liu SS, Courpas G, et al. Does continuous peripheral nerve block provide superior pain control to opioids? A meta-analysis. Anesth Analg 2006; 102(1):248–57.
9. Mariano ER, Afra R, Loland VJ, et al. Continuous interscalene brachial plexus block via an ultrasound-guided posterior approach: a randomized, triple-masked, placebo-controlled study. Anesth Analg 2009;108(5):1688–94.
10. Fredrickson MJ, Ball CM, Dalgleish AJ. Successful continuous interscalene analgesia for ambulatory shoulder surgery in a private practice setting. Reg Anesth Pain Med 2008;33(2):122–8.
11. Swenson JD, Bay N, Loose E, et al. Outpatient management of continuous peripheral nerve catheters placed using ultrasound guidance: an experience in 620 patients. Anesth Analg 2006;103(6):1436–43.
12. Ganesh A, Cucchiaro G. Multiple simultaneous perineural infusions for postoperative analgesia in adolescents in an outpatient setting. Br J Anaesth 2007;98(5): 687–9.
13. Ganesh A, Rose JB, Wells L, et al. Continuous peripheral nerve blockade for inpatient and outpatient postoperative analgesia in children. Anesth Analg 2007;105(5):1234–42.
14. Ilfeld BM, Mariano ER, Williams BA, et al. Hospitalization costs of total knee arthroplasty with a continuous femoral nerve block provided only in the hospital versus on an ambulatory basis: a retrospective, case-control, cost-minimization analysis. Reg Anesth Pain Med 2007;32(1):46–54.
15. Hunt KJ, Higgins TF, Carlston CV, et al. Continuous peripheral nerve blockade a spost-operative analgesia for open treatment of calcaneal fractures. J Orthop Trauma 2010;24(3):148–55.
16. Capdevila X, Dadure C, Bringuier S, et al. Effect of patient-controlled perineural analgesia on rehabilitation and pain after ambulatory orthopedic surgery: a multicenter randomized trial. Anesthesiology 2006;105(3):566–73.
17. Ilfeld BM, Thannikary LJ, Morey TE, et al. Popliteal sciatic perineural local anesthetic infusion: a comparison of three dosing regimens for postoperative analgesia. Anesthesiology 2004;101(4):970–7.
18. Ilfeld BM, Morey TE, Enneking FK. Infraclavicular perineural local anesthetic infusion: a comparison of three dosing regimens for postoperative analgesia. Anesthesiology 2004;100(2):395–402.
19. Williams BA, Kentor ML, Bottegal MT. The incidence of falls at home in patients with perineural femoral catheters: a retrospective summary of a randomized clinical trial. Anesth Analg 2007;104(4):1002.
20. Thackery E, Swenson J, Greis PE, et al. Diaphragm function and room air oxygen saturation are affected less with 0.125% bupivacaine interscalene blocks [abstract #P291]. Am Acad Orthop Surg 2010. [Epub ahead of print].
21. Abrahams MS, Aziz MF, Fu RF, et al. Ultrasound guidance compared with electrical neurostimulation for peripheral nerve block: a systematic review and meta-analysis of randomized controlled trials. Br J Anaesth 2009;102(3): 408–17.

22. Rigaud M, Filip P, Lirk P, et al. Guidance of block needle insertion by electrical nerve stimulation: a pilot study of the resulting distribution of injected solution in dogs. Anesthesiology 2008;109(3):473–8.
23. Urmey WF, Stanton J. Inability to consistently elicit a motor response following sensory paresthesia during interscalene block administration. Anesthesiology 2002;96(3):552–4.
24. Bollini CA, Urmey WF, Vascello L, et al. Relationship between evoked motor response and sensory paresthesia in interscalene brachial plexus block. Reg Anesth Pain Med 2003;28(5):384–8.
25. Boezaart AP, de Beer JF, du Toit C, et al. A new technique of continuous interscalene nerve block. Can J Anaesth 1999;46(3):275–81.
26. Tran de QH, Munoz L, Russo G, et al. Ultrasonography and stimulating perineural catheters for nerve blocks: a review of the evidence. Can J Anaesth 2008;55(7):447–57.
27. Barrington MJ, Olive DJ, McCutcheon CA, et al. Stimulating catheters for continuous femoral nerve blockade after total knee arthroplasty: a randomized, controlled, double-blinded trial. Anesth Analg 2008;106(4):1316–21.
28. Hayek SM, Ritchey RM, Sessler D, et al. Continuous femoral nerve analgesia after unilateral total knee arthroplasty: stimulating versus nonstimulating catheters. Anesth Analg 2006;103(6):1565–70.
29. Sites BD, Neal JM, Chan V. Ultrasound in regional anesthesia: where should the "focus" be set? Reg Anesth Pain Med 2009;34(6):531–3.
30. Oberndorfer U, Marhofer P, Bosenberg A, et al. Ultrasonographic guidance for sciatic and femoral nerve blocks in children. Br J Anaesth 2007;98(6):797–801.
31. Kapral S, Greher M, Huber G, et al. Ultrasonographic guidance improves the success rate of interscalene brachial plexus blockade. Reg Anesth Pain Med 2008;33(3):253–8.
32. Perlas A, Brull R, Chan VW, et al. Ultrasound guidance improves the success of sciatic nerve block at the popliteal fossa. Reg Anesth Pain Med 2008;33(3):259–65.
33. Mariano ER, Loland VJ, Sandhu NS, et al. Ultrasound guidance versus electrical stimulation for femoral perineural catheter insertion. J Ultrasound Med 2009;28(11):1453–60.
34. Mariano ER, Loland VJ, Bellars RH, et al. Ultrasound guidance versus electrical stimulation for infraclavicular brachial plexus perineural catheter insertion. J Ultrasound Med 2009;28(9):1211–8.
35. Sandhu NS, Capan LM. Ultrasound-guided infraclavicular brachial plexus block. Br J Anaesth 2002;89(2):254–9.
36. Swenson JD, Davis JJ, DeCou JA. A novel approach for assessing catheter position after ultrasound-guided placement of continuous interscalene block. Anesth Analg 2008;106(3):1015–6.
37. Hebl JR. The importance and implications of aseptic techniques during regional anesthesia. Reg Anesth Pain Med 2006;31(4):311–23.
38. Selander D, Dhuner KG, Lundborg G. Peripheral nerve injury due to injection needles used for regional anesthesia. An experimental study of the acute effects of needle point trauma. Acta Anaesthesiol Scand 1977;21(3):182–8.
39. Rice AS, McMahon SB. Peripheral nerve injury caused by injection needles used in regional anaesthesia: influence of bevel configuration, studied in a rat model. Br J Anaesth 1992;69(5):433–8.
40. Tsui BC, Wagner A, Finucane B. Electrophysiologic effect of injectates on peripheral nerve stimulation. Reg Anesth Pain Med 2004;29(3):189–93.

41. Zaric D, Boysen K, Christiansen J, et al. Continuous popliteal sciatic nerve block for outpatient foot surgery—a randomized, controlled trial. Acta Anaesthesiol Scand 2004;48(3):337–41.
42. Ekatodramis G, Nadig M, Blumenthal S, et al. Continuous popliteal sciatic nerve block. How to be sure the catheter works? Acta Anaesthesiol Scand 2004;48(10): 1342–3 [author reply: 1343].
43. James WD, White SW, Yanklowitz B. Allergic contact dermatitis to compound tincture of benzoin. J Am Acad Dermatol 1984;11(5 Pt 1):847–50.
44. Compere V, Legrand JF, Guitard PG, et al. Bacterial colonization after tunneling in 402 perineural catheters: a prospective study. Anesth Analg 2009;108(4):1326–30.
45. Gross JB, Bachenberg KL, Benumof JL, et al. Practice guidelines for the perioperative management of patients with obstructive sleep apnea: a report by the American Society of Anesthesiologists Task Force on Perioperative Management of patients with obstructive sleep apnea. Anesthesiology 2006;104(5):1081–93 [quiz: 1117–88].
46. Ilfeld BM, Enneking FK. Continuous peripheral nerve blocks at home: a review. Anesth Analg 2005;100(6):1822–33.
47. Buettner J, Klose R, Hoppe U, et al. Serum levels of mepivacaine-HCl during continuous axillary brachial plexus block. Reg Anesth 1989;14(3):124–7.
48. Borgeat A, Kalberer F, Jacob H, et al. Patient-controlled interscalene analgesia with ropivacaine 0.2% versus bupivacaine 0.15% after major open shoulder surgery: the effects on hand motor function. Anesth Analg 2001;92(1):218–23.
49. Emanuelsson BM, Zaric D, Nydahl PA, et al. Pharmacokinetics of ropivacaine and bupivacaine during 21 hours of continuous epidural infusion in healthy male volunteers. Anesth Analg 1995;81(6):1163–8.
50. Popping DM, Elia N, Marret E, et al. Clonidine as an adjuvant to local anesthetics for peripheral nerve and plexus blocks: a meta-analysis of randomized trials. Anesthesiology 2009;111(2):406–15.
51. Ilfeld BM, Morey TE, Thannikary LJ, et al. Clonidine added to a continuous interscalene ropivacaine perineural infusion to improve postoperative analgesia: a randomized, double-blind, controlled study. Anesth Analg 2005;100(4):1172–8.
52. Ilfeld BM, Morey TE, Enneking FK. Continuous infraclavicular perineural infusion with clonidine and ropivacaine compared with ropivacaine alone: a randomized, double-blinded, controlled study. Anesth Analg 2003;97(3):706–12.
53. Skryabina EA, Dunn TS. Disposable infusion pumps. Am J Health Syst Pharm 2006;63(13):1260–8.
54. Remerand F, Vuitton AS, Palud M, et al. Elastomeric pump reliability in postoperative regional anesthesia: a survey of 430 consecutive devices. Anesth Analg 2008;107(6):2079–84.
55. Capdevila X, Macaire P, Aknin P, et al. Patient-controlled perineural analgesia after ambulatory orthopedic surgery: a comparison of electronic versus elastomeric pumps. Anesth Analg 2003;96(2):414–7.
56. Dadure C, Pirat P, Raux O, et al. Perioperative continuous peripheral nerve blocks with disposable infusion pumps in children: a prospective descriptive study. Anesth Analg 2003;97(3):687–90.
57. Capdevila X, Pirat P, Bringuier S, et al. Continuous peripheral nerve blocks in hospital wards after orthopedic surgery: a multicenter prospective analysis of the quality of postoperative analgesia and complications in 1416 patients. Anesthesiology 2005;103(5):1035–45.
58. Neuburger M, Buttner J, Blumenthal S, et al. Inflammation and infection complications of 2285 perineural catheters: a prospective study. Acta Anaesthesiol Scand 2007;51(1):108–14.

59. Capdevila X, Bringuier S, Borgeat A. Infectious risk of continuous peripheral nerve blocks. Anesthesiology 2009;110(1):182–8.
60. Capdevila X, Jaber S, Pesonen P, et al. Acute neck cellulitis and mediastinitis complicating a continuous interscalene block. Anesth Analg 2008;107(4):1419–21.
61. Hebl JR, Dilger JA, Byer DE, et al. A pre-emptive multimodal pathway featuring peripheral nerve block improves perioperative outcomes after major orthopedic surgery. Reg Anesth Pain Med 2008;33(6):510–7.

Sedation: Not Quite That Simple

Peter M. Hession, MD, Girish P. Joshi, MBBS, MD, FFARCSI*

KEYWORDS

- Sedation • Analgesia • Diagnostic & surgical procedures
- Complications

In recent years, the number of diagnostic and surgical procedures performed with sedation has increased exponentially, with the majority of the growth occurring in ambulatory surgical centers, physicians' offices, and hospital locations outside the operating room (also referred to as remote locations).[1] Sedation and analgesia minimize patient anxiety and discomfort, and allow patients to remain immobile for the procedure. Other benefits include the avoidance of airway interventions, as well as general anesthesia and its associated complications. Furthermore, sedation/analgesia facilitates and expedites procedures and allows early recovery and discharge.[2] Sedation provides for a superior patient experience that may improve overall patient satisfaction.[3] However, sedation/analgesia techniques can be associated with significant adverse events that might increase morbidity and mortality.[4,5]

This article reviews the complications associated with sedation/analgesia techniques and provides an approach for their safe administration, and discusses the newer drugs and devices used for provision of sedation/analgesia.

COMPLICATIONS ASSOCIATED WITH SEDATION/ANALGESIA TECHNIQUES

The overall complication rate associated with sedation/analgesia techniques remains unknown because the literature is sparse and of limited quality. Nevertheless, it is well accepted that although the mortality of sedation is low, the associated morbidity can be significant. Complications of sedation/analgesia include respiratory complications such as loss of airway patency, airway obstruction, and respiratory depression. That may lead to life-threatening hypoxia and hypercarbia as well as cardiovascular complications such as hypotension and cardiac arrhythmias.[4,5] In addition, depression of protective airway reflexes during excessive sedation can lead to an unprotected airway and thereby increase the risk regurgitation and aspiration of gastric contents. The risks inherent in the procedures as well as risk of patient movement that may

Department of Anesthesiology and Pain Management, University of Texas Southwestern Medical Center, 5323 Harry Hines Boulevard, Dallas, TX 75390-9068, USA
* Corresponding author.
E-mail address: girish.joshi@utsouthwestern.edu

Anesthesiology Clin 28 (2010) 281–294
doi:10.1016/j.anclin.2010.02.007 anesthesiology.theclinics.com
1932-2275/10/$ – see front matter

be detrimental to the patient should also be taken into consideration. Another concern, although rare, is the potential for drug interactions or adverse reactions, including anaphylaxis. Of note, residual sedative effects have the potential to cause delayed complications (eg, hypoxia after discharge) that can be hazardous to unsupervised patients.

Analysis of the American Society of Anesthesiologists (ASA) closed claim database of monitored anesthesia care (MAC) cases found that more than 40% of claims associated with MAC involved death or permanent brain damage, and the incidence was similar to claims associated with general anesthesia.[5] Respiratory depression with hypoventilation after absolute or relative overdose of sedative-hypnotics and/or opioids was the most common mechanism of injury. The investigators reviewing these claims concluded that nearly 50% of complications were preventable.

Another analysis by Metzner and colleagues[6] of the ASA closed claims database, comparing liability in the operating room with that in remote locations (eg, gastrointestinal suite, interventional cardiology suite, interventional radiology suite, and magnetic resonance imaging suite), found that 50% of remote location liability claims involved MAC. The proportion of claims of death was higher in remote locations than in the operating room. Inadequate oxygenation/ventilation secondary to oversedation accounted for more than a third of the claims. In addition, sedation in the prone position, for example, during endoscopic retrograde cholangiopancreatography (ERCP), may further increase the complication rate due to difficulty in securing the airway and resuming adequate ventilation.[6] Similar to the previous report,[5] this study also determined that better monitoring could have prevented the substandard care that led to complications. These investigators emphasize that monitoring standards and guidelines used for general anesthesia should be used for sedation care outside the operating room.[5,6]

A recent study evaluated the safety and efficacy of propofol/opioid sedation, administered by anesthesia providers, for advanced endoscopic procedures that require deep sedation (eg, ERCP and endoscopic ultrasound).[7] In this study of 799 patients, airway manipulations were required in 14.4% of cases. The incidence of hypoxemia was 12.8%, hypotension occurred in 0.5%, and premature termination of the procedure was required in 0.6% of patients. No patient required bag-mask ventilation or tracheal intubation. Predictors of airway manipulation included male gender, higher body mass index (weight in kilograms divided by height in meters squared), and ASA physical status of 3 or higher. The dose of propofol used in this study was similar to that required for provision of general anesthesia. The propofol dose to induce sedation was 2.41 $\pm$ 1.13 mg/kg when used alone and 1.37 $\pm$ 0.75 mg/kg when used in combination with opioids, while the propofol dose used for maintenance of sedation was 0.23 $\pm$ 0.1 mg/kg/min when used alone and 0.17 $\pm$ 0.11 mg/kg/min when used in combination with opioids. In addition, 87.2% of patients had no response to insertion of the endoscope, which also suggests that the patients experienced deep sedation or general anesthesia. Thus, the procedures were essentially performed under general anesthesia (ie, total intravenous anesthesia) without tracheal intubation. Therefore, this study questions the routine use of general anesthesia with tracheal intubation for patients undergoing advanced gastrointestinal endoscopic procedures, which is in contrast to the recommendation by Metzner and colleagues.[6,7]

An analysis of patients developing apnea and cardiopulmonary arrest during and after endoscopy found that the majority of complications occurred around the time of drug administration or after the procedure had ended, usually around 30 minutes after the last dose of sedative-hypnotic and/or opioid administration.[8] The investigators also reported that although pulse oximetry did not reduce the complication rate, it allowed early recognition of apnea and cardiopulmonary arrest. This study emphasizes that postsedation observation is critical, particularly in the elderly and patients with comorbidities.

In recent years, there has been an increasing trend toward propofol use by nonanesthesia practitioners, including registered nurses, which has become a subject of major controversy.[9] The safety of nonanesthesia practitioner administered propofol (NAAP) was observed in 646,080 patients undergoing gastrointestinal endoscopic procedures. These observational studies reported a low complication rate, which included the need for tracheal intubation in 11 patients and death in 4 patients, but no patient who survived had any permanent neurologic injury.[9] Mask ventilation was required in 0.1% cases. Overall, the safety of NAAP for upper endoscopy and colonoscopy is the same as that of a benzodiazepine/opioid technique.[10] Of note, the reported mortality with a conventional benzodiazepine and opioid combination is 11 deaths per 100,000 cases.[9] A recent study reported that deep sedation frequently occurred with midazolam/meperidine sedation during endoscopic sedation.[11]

A position statement by the American Association for the Study of Liver Diseases, the American College of Gastroenterology, the American Gastroenterological Association Institute, and the American Society for Gastrointestinal Endoscopy claims that the safety profile of NAAP is equivalent to that of standard benzodiazepine/opioid sedation. It must be noted, however, that the majority of the observational trials included in the evaluation of the safety of NAAP sedation are from a select few endoscopic units with extensive experience. Also, the sedation for endoscopy was provided by the sole use of propofol. It is likely that the complication rate may increase if propofol is used in combination with benzodiazepines and/or opioids, which is usually necessary for more painful procedures. Furthermore, there is a paucity of data on the safety of propofol administered by nonanesthesia practitioners for procedures other than gastrointestinal endoscopies. Therefore, widespread indiscriminate use of propofol by non-anesthesia practitioner may compromise patient safety.

In an interesting editorial endorsing the use of propofol in the emergency unit, Green and Krauss[12] identified risk of aspiration as the most serious risk rather than airway obstruction and respiratory depression. Green and Krauss recommended clinicians to "avoid assisting ventilations" and to "simply 'wait out' an occurrence of propofol-associated respiratory depression" so as to minimize the risk of aspiration. Such statements obviously confirm that these investigators, who are supposed to be experts on sedation in the emergency unit, lack the understanding of risks associated with propofol use. Similarly, a recent article on nurse-administered propofol sedation for gastrointestinal endoscopic procedures[13] states that "when using a multidrug protocol with propofol, the clinician may be able to exploit the therapeutic actions of the individual agents while reducing the possibility of sedation dose-related complications." This standpoint is contrary to the established principles of polypharmacy emphasizing that the risk of hypoxia, hypercarbia, and airway compromise are actually worsened when propofol is combined with benzodiazepines and/or opioids. A lack of appreciation for the risks associated with sedation and inappropriate management of complications will lead to increased morbidity and mortality.

FACTORS INFLUENCING SEDATION-RELATED COMPLICATIONS

Some of the factors that influence sedation/analgesia complications include patient characteristics, type of procedure, drug selection and dosing, monitoring, and training. Patient characteristics that influence sedation-related complications include extremes of age,[14] significant airway abnormalities, obstructive sleep apnea (OSA), morbid obesity,[15] and ASA physical status of 3 or greater. The increased risk of developing complications in this patient population is due to increased sensitivity to sedative-hypnotics and opioids and/or altered pharmacokinetics and drug clearance.[4,16] Similarly, certain types of procedures (eg, those requiring deeper levels of sedation to prevent patient movement) may not be suitable for sedation/analgesia, and it may be safer to perform them using general anesthesia. Also, the frequency of complications may be influenced by expectations of deeper levels of sedation by patients and proceduralists.[17]

Achieving an appropriate level of sedation remains a clinical challenge, as sedation represents a continuum of progressive impairment of consciousness that extends from wakefulness to general anesthesia.[18] As the patient transitions between stages, they clearly become subject to respiratory and cardiovascular complications.[19,20] Because of wide variability in patient response to sedative regimens, the appropriate dosage needed to achieve a specific level of sedation cannot always be predicted. Another factor that might influence the complication rate is the synergistic effects of combinations of sedative-hypnotics and opioids[21–25] as well as the accumulation of active metabolites (eg, midazolam).[26] Lysakowski and colleagues[27] administered opioids to achieve a specific effect-site concentration (fentanyl, 1.5 ng/mL; alfentanil, 100 ng/mL; remifentanil, 6 ng/mL; and sufentanil, 0.2 ng/mL; or placebo) to a group of patients who then received propofol infusions. At the time of loss of consciousness (LOC), the effect-site concentration of propofol was recorded. The investigators found that, compared with placebo, patients who had received any of the 4 opioids achieved LOC at lower propofol concentrations. Training and skills, patient selection, including identification of patients and procedures that may be more safely performed by using a general anesthetic, and monitoring and vigilance also influence the sedation-related complication rate.

SAFE USE OF SEDATION AND ANALGESIA TECHNIQUES

The goals of a sedation/analgesia technique require a balance between patient comfort and safety (ie, avoidance of respiratory and cardiovascular adverse effects and delayed recovery and discharge home). It is important that the patient is prepared appropriately and is not promised total amnesia, sleep, and oblivion, or complete absence of pain.[17] The level of sedation must be coupled with the invasiveness of the procedure as well as the anxiety and cooperation of the patient. Sedative-hypnotics and opioids should be administered prior to the noxious stimuli, rather than at the time of the stimulus, as they have slow blood-brain equilibrium times. In fact, drug administration at the time of the noxious stimuli may result in inadvertent overdosing. Similarly, drug boluses should be adequately spaced, based on the time to peak effect, to avoid overdosing. Furthermore, it is important to avoid using deeper levels of sedation to compensate for inadequate analgesia.

Many professional associations have recently published sedation guidelines to ensure high standards of patient care.[28–31] The guidelines include recommendations for preprocedure evaluation and selection, sedation techniques, monitoring, recovery, and discharge protocols as well as the availability of appropriate facilities, equipment, staffing, and training.

SEDATIVE-HYPNOTIC MEDICATIONS

Although several medication options exist, sedation in adults is typically achieved by a combination of benzodiazepines (eg, midazolam) and opioids (eg, meperidine or fentanyl). Midazolam provides reliable anxiolysis, sedation, and amnesia as well as centrally mediated muscle relaxation. In addition, it has a wide margin of safety and can be quickly reversed by administration of the benzodiazepine antagonist flumazenil. However, midazolam produces a dose-dependent cardiorespiratory depression, which might be further exaggerated due to a synergistic effect when combined with other sedatives and opioids. Another major limitation of midazolam is that it has a slow onset and a prolonged duration that might delay recovery, discharge home, and the return to daily living.[32]

Propofol

Propofol, an intravenous hypnotic drug with rapid onset and short duration of action, can be used to provide moderate to deep sedation. The rapid onset of action allows early achievement of the desired level of sedation. Because of its short duration of action and lack of accumulation, propofol allows a more rapid recovery of cognitive function. Other benefits of propofol include antiemetic and euphoric effects. Propofol sedation has been associated with improved patient satisfaction compared with benzodiazepine/opioid combinations. Furthermore, propofol reduces recovery room stay (and improves throughput) and allows an early return to daily living. Because of these numerous exceptionally desirable characteristics, propofol has become an attractive option for sedation.

Propofol is, however, associated with hemodynamic effects (eg, hypotension) as well as respiratory depression and airway obstruction. Propofol has no analgesic effects and therefore it may have to be combined with opioids for painful procedures. Concomitant use of propofol and opioids or benzodiazepines can cause significant cardiorespiratory depression. Propofol has a narrow therapeutic range, which may result in a deeper than expected depth of sedation, and it lacks a reversal agent.

Fospropofol

Fospropofol is a water-soluble prodrug of propofol that was recently approved for sedation/analgesia. Fospropofol is metabolized by endothelial alkaline phosphatases to propofol, phosphate, and formaldehyde.[33–36] Formaldehyde is readily converted to formate, which is metabolized in the liver to water and carbon dioxide. Although formate toxicity can cause lactate acidosis, this has not been reported even with long-term fospropofol infusion. Fospropofol is formulated in an aqueous solution with some potential benefits over propofol (eg, pain on injection and safety issues related to lipid-containing formulation such as hyperlipidemia and risk of infection). Although fospropofol does not cause pain on injection, a side effect commonly seen with propofol, it has been associated with paresthesias (burning sensations and tingling) in the perianal and perineal area. The mechanism of this is still unknown. However, the paresthesias are usually described as mild in intensity, transient, and self-limited, typically lasting for 1 to 2 minutes. Also, similar to its metabolite, propofol, fospropofol can cause dose-dependent hypotension, respiratory depression, and apnea.[33,36]

The sedative properties of fospropofol are similar to those of propofol, but with a slower onset and offset.[35,36] The slower offset of fospropofol may allow a short procedure (approximately 20–25 minutes) to be performed without repeated dosing. However, clinical experience with fospropofol, particularly in nongastrointestinal procedures, is limited. Also, currently recommended fospropofol dosing is complex and based on its use by nonanesthesia practitioners. Similar to propofol, the US Food and Drug Administration (FDA) approval information and product label state that when used to induce and maintain anesthesia, fospropofol "should be administered only by persons trained in the administration of general anesthesia."

MANAGEMENT OF PROCEDURAL PAIN

Pain during interventional and invasive procedures can be managed with opioids and/or nonopioid analgesics. The sole use of sedative-hypnotics, which do not have analgesic effects, during painful procedures will require deep sedation and increase the risk of cardiopulmonary complications. Therefore, sedative-hypnotics should not be used to compensate for inadequate analgesia (eg, an inadequate local anesthetic technique). The use of analgesics as adjuncts to hypnotic-sedatives may provide adequate pain relief and reduce the total dose of hypnotic-sedative, but may also increase the incidence of cardiopulmonary complications due to the synergistic effects of combining multiple drug classes.

Opioids

Opioids (eg, fentanyl, sufentanil, and remifentanil) are commonly used as adjuncts to sedatives to provide analgesia and reduce the autonomic effects of noxious stimuli. Remifentanil has a short duration of action that does not increase with longer duration of administration because of rapid clearance (elimination half-life of 20–30 minutes context-sensitive half-time is 3–5 minutes) and lack of accumulation. Therefore, remifentanil (0.05–0.5 μg/kg/min) is useful for conscious sedation and allows titratable balance between analgesic and respiratory depressant effects.[37] Although the combination of opioids with hypnotic-sedatives in appropriate doses may be beneficial with respect to recovery and side effect profile, inappropriate doses and combinations may significantly increase the incidence of undesirable side effects such as respiratory depression, hypoxemia, and nausea and vomiting, as well as delay of recovery.[25,38] It is important that opioids should be avoided or the dose limited in at-risk patient groups such as the elderly, morbidly obese, and those with OSA.

Ketamine

Ketamine is a dissociative anesthetic with analgesic properties. Ketamine has cardiovascular-stimulating effects (ie, increased heart rate and blood pressure) but no respiratory-depressive effects. Therefore, combining ketamine (0.25–1 mg/kg) with propofol should reduce propofol requirements and mitigate the respiratory and hemodynamic side effects of propofol. The analgesic effects of ketamine should improve the quality of procedural sedation. Furthermore, ketamine produces positive mood effects with perceptual changes, provides prolonged analgesia that extends into the postprocedure period, and allows earlier recovery of cognitive function.

Despite the potential benefits of a propofol/ketamine combination it is not commonly used, likely due to lack of knowledge about the optimal ketamine dose as well as concerns about ketamine's side effects.[39] A systematic review of the combination of low-dose ketamine with propofol for procedural sedation/analgesia in the emergency department concluded that a ketamine/propofol combination reduced the incidence of significant hemodynamic and respiratory compromise. The need for active interventions, however, including fluid/vasopressor administration, need for supplemental analgesia, or assisted ventilation, was similar. The time to discharge was also similar. Patients who received higher doses of ketamine had a higher incidence of nausea, vomiting, and emergence reactions after the procedure. Because the total number of patients included in the 11 trials who were evaluated in the systematic review was small, the investigators concluded that insufficient evidence exists to recommend the routine use of a ketamine/propofol combination for sedation in the emergency department setting.

Ketamine can cause copious secretions that might lead to laryngospasm. In addition, it produces skeletal muscle hypertonus and involuntary purposeful movements. Larger ketamine doses can result in deep sedation or general anesthesia, and associated complications including reduced gag reflex and airway obstruction. Another major concern with ketamine is the potential for emergence reactions manifested by vivid dreams and hallucinations. These complications may be avoided if the dose of ketamine is limited to 0.25 to 0.5 mg/kg boluses with a maximum of 2 mg/kg over a 30-minute period.

Glucocorticoids

Glucocorticoids have anti-inflammatory properties and therefore have the potential to reduce the inflammatory response to surgical stress and improve postoperative outcome.[40,41] Dexamethasone (4–8 mg) causes analgesia and euphoria. Dexamethasone has also been shown to reduce postoperative nausea and vomiting. Thus, the combination of dexamethasone with the sedation/analgesia technique has the potential for improving the quality of procedural sedation. Although no side effects have been observed with a single dose of dexamethasone in large studies,[42] there is a potential for increased gastrointestinal side effects as well as delayed wound healing.[43]

Dexmedetomidine

Dexmedetomidine is a centrally acting α_2 agonist with hypnotic, analgesic, and sympatholytic properties. Dexmedetomidine is gaining popularity for procedural sedation because it has sedative as well as analgesic effects. In addition, it has minimal effects on ventilation. Although it causes a decrease in minute ventilation, similar to that seen during natural sleep, it maintains the normal ventilatory response to hypercarbia. Therefore, dexmedetomidine may be beneficial in select patient populations sensitive to sedative-hypnotics, resulting in life-threatening respiratory depression and airway obstruction (eg, morbidly obese and OSA). A recent study reported that compared with a midazolam/fentanyl sedation technique, a dexmedetomidine bolus of 1 μg/kg over 10 minutes followed by an infusion of 0.2 to 1 μg/kg/h provided superior patient satisfaction, with lower opioid requirements and a lower incidence of respiratory depression. Another study found that dexmedetomidine was less effective than propofol/fentanyl for sedation during ERCP.[44] However, dexmedetomidine can cause bradycardia and hypotension.[45,46] Hypertension has also been observed with increasing plasma levels. Other limitations of dexmedetomidine include a slow onset and longer duration of action, and a duration of action based on the duration of infusion as well as the infusion rate.[47] In a recent study, 49 patients undergoing outpatient extracorporeal shock wave lithotripsy were randomized to receive dexmedetomidine or midazolam/fentanyl sedation. The investigators found prolonged recovery time (116 vs 51 minutes; $P<.001$) and a greater requirement of rescue midazolam (96% vs 58%; $P = .002$) in the dexmedetomidine group.[48] Avoidance of a bolus dose may reduce the hemodynamic adverse effects. Therefore, an initial infusion rate of 1 μg/kg/h, which is then titrated to a sedation level and/or hemodynamics, is recommended. A combination of ketamine with dexmedetomidine may reduce dexmedetomidine requirements and associated side effects as well as improve procedural sedation.

MONITORING DURING SEDATION AND ANALGESIA

Early detection of upper airway obstruction, respiratory depression, and apnea, which are the most common sedation-related complications, should prevent hypoxia and hypercarbia and associated complications such as permanent brain damage and death. Many critical events could be detected early or avoided entirely by appropriate monitoring, particularly respiratory monitoring.[5,6,49]

Because the procedures performed under sedation/analgesia are minimally invasive (or relatively noninvasive), one may be lulled into complacency. An inappropriate assumption may be made that the degree of care and vigilance required during sedation could be less intense or less thorough. Signs of airway obstruction include snoring, retraction of the suprasternal notch, and paradoxic pattern of breathing. Monitoring of oxygen saturation has become the standard of care; however, there is a considerable delay between the onset of hypoxemia and the detection of desaturation by a pulse oximeter. This is particularly true in patients receiving supplemental oxygen, which has also become the standard of care during sedation. An analysis of deaths during upper gastrointestinal endoscopy ($n = 153$) revealed that 88% occurred during sedation while only 56% were monitored with pulse oximetry and none had expired carbon dioxide (CO_2) monitoring.[50]

Monitoring of ventilation during sedation can be accomplished by auscultation of breath sounds using a precordial stethoscope, electrical impedance, or capnography monitoring. Precordial auscultation and electrical impedance monitoring detect respiratory efforts but not upper airway obstruction. In contrast, capnography (ie, monitoring of the exhaled CO_2 waveform rather than just the value of end-tidal CO_2 concentration) allows early detection of airway obstruction and apnea, and reliably predicts impending hypoxemia.[51,52] In a study by Soto and colleagues,[51] apnea for more than 20 seconds was detected by capnography but not by clinical signs of obstruction and pulse oximetry. Thus, exhaled CO_2 monitoring should be routinely used during moderate to deep sedation.

SUPPLEMENTAL OXYGEN

Supplemental oxygenation prolongs the time to desaturation.[53] Supplemental oxygen increases oxygen reserves and decreases the likelihood of hypoxemia, thus providing an additional margin of safety. However, this may provide a false sense of security, and delay the diagnosis of airway obstruction and respiratory depression. Therefore, the need for vigilance cannot be overemphasized.

STAFFING

Adequate staffing is critical in maintaining patient safety. There must be a minimum of 3 appropriately trained staff members present, which could include the proceduralist, the practitioner administering sedation (with the sole responsibility of monitoring the patient), and at least 1 additional staff member to provide assistance to the proceduralist and/or the practitioner providing sedation.

TRAINING FOR SEDATION BY NONANESTHESIA PRACTITIONERS

Training and responsibilities of health care workers providing procedural sedation is critical in maintaining patient safety. It is clear that the skills and abilities that must be acquired to safely provide deep sedation (eg, propofol sedation) are distinct from those required for minimal to moderate sedation (eg, conventional benzodiazepine/opioid sedation).

Important elements of a training program include the understanding of the pharmacology of the drugs used to provide sedation/analgesia and the ability to recognize the various levels of sedation. In addition, students should become proficient in the identification and management of potential complications, including advanced airway management techniques and cardiopulmonary resuscitation. Training should include both didactic and hands-on practical learning experience using life-size manikins and/or human simulators. In addition, proficiency should be acquired through preceptorship supervised by an anesthesiologist or a qualified clinician with privileges to administer deep sedation and/or general anesthesia. Certification in advanced cardiac life support alone clearly is not adequate. There should be regular retraining with emphasis on cardiovascular resuscitation, airway management, and exposure to new and updated clinical information.

The American Association for the Study of Liver Diseases, the American College of Gastroenterology, the American Gastroenterological Association Institute, and the American Society for Gastrointestinal Endoscopy collaborated recently to provide recommendations for NAAP for gastrointestinal endoscopy.[29] The position statement states that nonanesthesiologists can safely administer propofol for gastrointestinal endoscopy provided they are properly trained and select patients wisely. This standpoint is in contradiction to the ASA statement that propofol should be used by practitioners trained in the administration of general anesthesia because of propofol's narrow therapeutic range and lack of a reversal agent. The ASA recommends that the practitioners of moderate sedation should be able to rescue a patient transiting into deep sedation, while those practicing deep sedation should be able to rescue patients who inadvertently move into general anesthesia.[28]

DEVICES FOR SEDATION/ANALGESIA ADMINISTRATION

One of the factors that might influence procedural sedation/analgesia in the future is the introduction of automated drug administration systems. Numerous sedation administration devices designed to achieve optimal procedural sedation/analgesia with improved patient safety have been investigated. These devices include patient-controlled sedation (PCS), target-controlled sedation, and computer-assisted personalized sedation (CAPS) systems.

PCS is a concept based on patient-controlled analgesia (PCA), which has become a standard of care for pain management. PCS attempts to address some of the limitations of current sedation/analgesia practices including variations in patients' response to sedative-hypnotics, variations in patients' expectations of the degree of sedation, and variations in requirements of sedation based on the level of stimulus.[54] During PCS, patients can self-administer a sedative-hypnotic (eg, propofol) to their desired needs. Patient satisfaction with PCS can be greater because of greater participation in the sedation process. Similar to PCA, there is an inherent safety in the PCS system, as patient feedback is necessary to administer a sedative-hypnotic. A PCS system would administer a predetermined dose of a sedative/hypnotic with a lockout period during which no drug will be administered. A recent study in patients undergoing colonoscopy reported that compared with PCS with midazolam and fentanyl, PCS with propofol and remifentanil provided rapid induction of sedation and early recovery.[55]

Target-controlled infusion devices (TCI) are designed to achieve steady-state drug concentration based on pharmacokinetic-guided models.[56] However, the TCI devices have some inherent limitations such as variations in pharmacokinetics. In contrast to these closed-loop systems, the newer automated anesthesia systems using pharmacodynamic-guided models (eg, bispectral index-guided propofol administration) show promise. These devices appear to be superior to manual control devices, allow more rapid recovery, and improve quality of patient care.[57] Of course, before such devices become the "standard of care," the limitations of the pharmacodynamic variables (eg, bispectral index) used to guide drug administration will have to be addressed. In addition, the safety of these devices must be proven under varying clinical conditions. Further studies are needed to determine the optimal delivery system that would enhance patient safety.

A CAPS system (Sedasys; Ethicon Endo-Surgery, Inc, Cincinnati, OH, USA), comprising an automated propofol delivery device designed to provide minimal to moderate sedation, is currently seeking the approval of the FDA. This device integrates monitoring with pulse oximetry, capnography, electrocardiography, noninvasive blood pressure, and patient feedback to determine the dose of propofol.[58] The Sedasys system responds to hypoxia and low respiratory rate or apneic episodes by encouraging the patient to breathe and/or stopping or slowing the propofol infusion, as well as increasing the flow rate of supplemental oxygen.

A recent study reported that compared with the midazolam/fentanyl technique, the Sedasys device precisely controlled propofol administration to achieve minimal to moderate sedation in patients undergoing gastrointestinal endoscopic procedures, and allowed early postprocedure recovery.[59] However, this study can be criticized for several reasons. First, the dose of midazolam and fentanyl was higher than that used in routine practice. In addition, patients in the midazolam/fentanyl group received lower oxygen flow rate (2 L/min) compared with higher variable oxygen flow rate with the Sedasys device, which may have masked the incidence of hypoxia. Propofol boluses were required in 77% of procedures, suggesting a need for intervention as well as indicating the limitations of the alert system, as it can be overridden. The higher doses of midazolam/fentanyl in the "standard of care" group and the extra propofol boluses suggest the use of deeper levels of sedation in these patient groups.

The device is designed to provide a propofol infusion rate of less than 75 μg/kg/min with a 3-minute lockout between increases in maintenance dose, assuming that the-patient responds appropriately to the periodic requests by the device. The health care provider using the device can administer additional propofol boluses of 25 μg/kg with a lockout interval of 90 seconds. This protocol allows for a maximum propofol dose of 200 μg/kg/min. Because the propofol dose for the maintenance of general anesthesia is 100 to 200 μg/kg/min, the Sedasys system may allow administration of general anesthesia by nonanesthesia practitioners, which may compromise patient safety. The device is equipped with red and yellow alerts, which indicate different levels of hypoxia and apnea. The device does not allow administration of propofol boluses during these alerts, which are specifically designed to prevent further propofol dosing.

In addition, in response to hypoventilation, the device increases the flow of fresh oxygen. As described earlier, supplemental oxygen in the setting of hypopnea or apnea can allow hypercarbia to go unnoticed for extended periods of time and delay intervention. The device will also encourage the subject to increase ventilation when inadequate ventilation is assessed either by respiratory rate or end-tidal CO_2. As mentioned previously, capnography allows for an accurate assessment of ventilation quality and can detect impending hypoxemia earlier than pulse oximetry.

It is recommended that this device be used only in patients younger than 70 years, in the presence of a 3-person clinical team whereby one person will have the sole responsibility of monitoring the patient, the device, and managing the patient's airway.

This dedicated person must have advanced training and at least the skills of a nurse. Physicians using the device must complete a stringent educational program as well as demonstrate continuing competency (see earlier discussion). Finally, there is a need for further research to assess the appropriate use and safety of this device in older and sicker patients with comorbidities.

SUMMARY

The advantages conferred by the sedation and analgesia techniques have increased their popularity. The goal of sedation must be to minimize risk while maintaining an acceptable level of patient and practitioner satisfaction. In achieving adequate patient comfort, it is important to avoid compromising patient safety. Because the differences between the levels of sedation may be subtle and patients frequently move to a deeper level than originally intended (which can result in significant morbidity and mortality), the degree of care provided should be the same for all patients receiving sedation. Of importance is that the risks of deep sedation may even exceed those of general anesthesia in which the airway is already secured. Therefore, it is necessary to develop protocols for instituting training programs, patient selection and preparation, monitoring, sedation/analgesia techniques, and postprocedure recovery and discharge, as well as diagnosis and treatment of potential complications. Finally, anesthesiologists can play an important role in development of protocols, training programs, and quality assurance programs.

REFERENCES

1. National Center for Health Statistics, Centers for Disease Control and Prevention. Results from the National Survey of Ambulatory Surgery (preliminary data). Available at: http://www.cdc.gov/nchs/nsas/about_nsas.htm. Accessed March 29, 2010.
2. Joshi GP. Efficiency in ambulatory surgery center. Curr Opin Anaesthesiol 2008; 21:695–8.
3. Fung D, Cohen MM, Stewart S, et al. What determines patient satisfaction with cataract care under topical local anesthesia and monitored sedation in a community hospital setting? Anesth Analg 2005;100:1644–50.
4. Hug CC. MAC should stand for maximum anesthesia caution, not minimal anesthesiology care. Anesthesiology 2006;104:221–3.
5. Bhananker SM, Posner KL, Cheney FW, et al. Injury and liability associated with monitored anesthesia care: a closed claims analysis. Anesthesiology 2006;104: 228–34.
6. Metzner J, Posner KL, Domino KB. The risk and safety of anesthesia at remote locations: the US closed claims analysis. Curr Opin Anaesthesiol 2009;22:502–8.
7. Coté GA, Hovis RM, Ansstas MA, et al. Incidence of sedation-related complications with propofol use during advanced endoscopic procedures. Clin Gastroenterol Hepatol 2009;8:137–42.
8. Iber FL, Livak A, Kruss DM. Apnea and cardiopulmonary arrest during and after endoscopy. J Clin Gastroenterol 1992;14:109–13.
9. Rex DK, Deenadayalu VP, Eid E, et al. Endoscopist directed administration of propofol: a world-wide safety experience. Gastroenterology 2009;137:1229–37.
10. American Society for Gastrointestinal Endoscopy. Sedation and anesthesia in GI endoscopy. Gastrointest Endosc 2008;68:815–26.

11. Patel S, Vargo JJ, Khandwala F, et al. Deep sedation occurs frequently during elective endoscopy with meperidine and midazolam. Am J Gastroenterol 2005; 100:2689–95.
12. Green SM, Krauss B. Propofol in emergency medicine: pushing the sedation frontier. Ann Emerg Med 2003;42:792–7.
13. Sipe BW, Scheidler M, Baluyut A, et al. A prospective safety study of a low-dose propofol sedation protocol for colonoscopy. Clin Gastroenterol Hepatol 2007;5(5): 563–6.
14. Ekstein M, Gavish D, Ezri T, et al. Monitored anaesthesia care in the elderly: guidelines and recommendations. Drugs Aging 2008;25:477–500.
15. Vargo JJ. Procedural sedation and obesity: waters left uncharted. Gastrointest Endosc 2009;70:980–4.
16. Qadeer MA, Rocio Lopez A, Dumot JA, et al. Risk factors for hypoxemia during ambulatory gastrointestinal endoscopy in ASA I-II patients. Dig Dis Sci 2009; 54(5):1035–40.
17. Esaki RK, Mashour GA. Levels of consciousness during regional anesthesia and monitored anesthesia care: patient expectations and experiences. Anesth Analg 2009;108:1560–3.
18. American Society of Anesthesiology. Position on monitored anesthesia care. Available at: http://www.asahq.org/publicationsAndServices/standards/23.pdf. Accessed December 23, 2009.
19. Win NN, Fukayama H, Kohase H, et al. The different effects of intravenous propofol and midazolam sedation on hemodynamic and heart rate variability. Anesth Analg 2005;101:97–102.
20. Ebert TJ. Sympathetic and hemodynamic effects of moderate and deep sedation with propofol in humans. Anesthesiology 2005;103(1):20–4.
21. Vuyk J, Lim T, Engbers FH, et al. The pharmacodynamic interaction of propofol and alfentanil during lower abdominal surgery in women. Anesthesiology 1995; 83(1):8–22.
22. Smith C, McEwan AI, Jhaveri R, et al. The interaction of fentanyl on the Cp50 of propofol for loss of consciousness and skin incision. Anesthesiology 1994;81(4): 820–8.
23. Short TG, Plummer JL, Chui PT. Hypnotic and anaesthetic interactions between midazolam, propofol and alfentanil. Br J Anaesth 1992;69:162–7.
24. Miner JR, Gray RO, Stephens D, et al. Randomized clinical trial of propofol with and without alfentanil for deep procedural sedation in the emergency department. Acad Emerg Med 2009;16:825–34.
25. Moerman AT, Struys M, Vereecke HE, et al. Remifentanil used to supplement propofol does not improve quality of sedation during spontaneous respiration. J Clin Anesth 2004;16:237–43.
26. Bauer TM, Ritz R, Haberthur C, et al. Prolonged sedation due to accumulation of conjugated metabolites of midazolam. Lancet 1995;346:145–7.
27. Lysakowski C, Dumont L, Pellégrini M, et al. Effects of fentanyl, alfentanil, remifentanil and sufentanil on loss of consciousness and bispectral index during propofol induction of anaesthesia. Br J Anaesth 2001;86(4):523–7.
28. American Society of Anesthesiologists. Practice guidelines for sedation and analgesia by non-anesthesiologists. An updated report by the American Society of Anesthesiologists Task Force on Sedation and Analgesia by Non-Anesthesiologists. Anesthesiology 2002;96:1004–17.

29. Vargo JJ, Cohen LB, Rex DK, et al. Position statement: nonanesthesiologist administration of propofol for GI endoscopy. Gastroenterology 2009;137: 2161–7.
30. American College of Cardiology/Society for Cardiac Angiography and Interventions Clinical Expert Consensus Document on Cardiac Catheterization Laboratory Standards. Available at: http://www.acc.org/qualityandscience/clinical/consensus/angiography/angiography_X.htm. Accessed January 4, 2009.
31. ACR practice guideline for adult sedation/analgesia. Available at: http://www.acr.org/SecondaryMainMenuCategories/quality_safety/guidelines/iv/adult_sedation.asas. Accessed January 4, 2009.
32. Dunn T, Mossop D, Newton A, et al. Propofol for procedural sedation in the emergency department. Emerg Med J 2007;24(7):459–61.
33. Moore GD, Walker AM, MacLaren R. Fospropofol: a new sedative-hypnotic agent for monitored anesthesia care. Ann Pharmacother 2009;43:1802–8.
34. Cohen LB. Clinical trial: a dose-response study of fospropofol disodium for moderate sedation during colonoscopy. Aliment Pharmacol Ther 2008;27: 597–608.
35. Cohen LB, Cattau E, Goetsch A, et al. A randomized, double-blind, phase 3 study of fospropofol disodium for sedation during colonoscopy. J Clin Gastroenterol 2009. [Epub ahead of print].
36. Silvestri GA, Vincent BD, Wahidi MM, et al. A phase 3, randomized, double-blind study to assess the efficacy and safety of fospropofol disodium injection for moderate sedation in patients undergoing flexible bronchoscopy. Chest 2009; 135:41–7.
37. Akcaboy ZN, Akcaboy EY, Albayrak D, et al. Can remifentanil be a better choice than propofol for colonoscopy during monitored anesthesia care? Acta Anaesthesiol Scand 2006;50:736–41.
38. Sinclair RCF, Faleiro RJ. Delayed recovery of consciousness after anaesthesia. Cont Educ Anaesth Crit Care Pain 2006;6(3):114–8.
39. Loh G, Dalen D. Low-dose ketamine in addition to propofol for procedural sedation and analgesia in the emergency department. Ann Pharmacother 2007;41: 485–92.
40. Aasboe V, Raeder JC, Groegaard B. Betamethasone reduces postoperative pain and nausea after ambulatory surgery. Anesth Analg 1998;87:319–23.
41. Kehlet H. Glucocorticoids for peri-operative analgesia: how far are we from general recommendations? Acta Anaesthesiol Scand 2007;51:1133–5.
42. Holte K, Kehlet H. Perioperative single-dose glucocorticoid administration—pathophysiological effects in clinical implications. J Am Coll Surg 2002;195:694–711.
43. Joshi GP. Multimodal analgesia techniques and postoperative rehabilitation. Anesthesiol Clin North America 2005;23:185–202.
44. Muller S, Borowics SM, Fortis EA, et al. Clinical efficacy of dexmedetomidine alone is less than propofol for conscious sedation during ERCP. Gastrointest Endosc 2008;67:651–9.
45. Candiotti KA, Bergese SD, Bokesch PM, et al. MAC Study Group. Monitored anesthesia care with dexmedetomidine: a prospective, randomized, double-blind, multicenter trial. Anesth Analg 2010;110(1):47–56.
46. Jalowiecki P, Rudner R, Gonciarz M, et al. Sole use of dexmedetomidine has limited use for conscious sedation during outpatient colonoscopy. Anesthesiology 2005;103:268–73.

47. Bloor BC, Ward DS, Belleville JP, et al. Effects of intravenous dexmedetomidine in humans. II. Hemodynamic changes. Anesthesiology 1992;77(6):1134–42.
48. Zeyneloglu P, Pirat A, Candan S, et al. Dexmedetomidine causes prolonged recovery when compared with midazolam/fentanyl combination in outpatient shock wave lithotripsy. Eur J Anaesthesiol 2008;25(12):961–7.
49. Qadeer M, Vargo JJ, Dumot JA, et al. Capnographic monitoring of respiratory activity improves safety of sedation for endoscopic cholangiopancreatography and ultrasonography. Gastroenterology 2009;136:1568–76.
50. Thompson AM, Wright DJ, Murray W, et al. Analysis of 153 deaths after upper gastrointestinal endoscopy: room for improvement? Surg Endosc 2004;18:22–5.
51. Soto RG, Fu ES, Vila H Jr, et al. Capnography accurately detects apnea during monitored anesthesia care. Anesth Analg 2004;99:379–82.
52. Srinivasa V, Kodali BS. Capnometry in the spontaneously breathing patient. Curr Opin Anaesthesiol 2004;17:517–20.
53. Fu ES, Downs JB, Schweiger JW, et al. Supplemental oxygen impairs detection of hypoventilation by pulse oximetry. Chest 2004;126(5):1552–8.
54. Stonell CA, Leslie K, Absalom AR. Effect-site targeted patient-controlled sedation with propofol: comparison with anesthesiologist administration for colonoscopy. Anaesthesia 2006;61:240–7.
55. Mandel JE, Tanner JW, Lichtenstein GR, et al. A randomized, controlled, double-blind trial of patient-controlled sedation with propofol/remifentanil versus midazolam/fentanyl for colonoscopy. Anesth Analg 2008;106:434–9.
56. Fields AM, Fields KM, Cannon JW. Closed-loop systems for drug delivery. Curr Opin Anaesthesiol 2008;21:446–51.
57. Leslie K, Absalom A, Kenny GN. Closed loop control of sedation for colonoscopy using the bispectral index. Anaesthesia 2002;57:693–7.
58. Pambianco DJ, Whitten CJ, Moerman A, et al. An assessment of computer-assisted personalized sedation: a sedation delivery system to administer propofol for gastrointestinal endoscopy. Gastrointest Endosc 2008;68:542–7.
59. Pambianco DJ, Pruitt RE, Hardi R, et al. A computer-assisted personalized sedation system to administer propofol versus standard-of-care sedation for colonoscopy and esophagogastroduodenoscopy: a 1000-subject randomized, controlled, multicenter pivotal trial [abstract]. Gastroenterology 2008;135:294.

Supraglottic Airway Devices in the Ambulatory Setting

Katarzyna Luba, MD, MS*, Thomas W. Cutter, MD, MAEd

KEYWORDS

• Supraglottic device • Airway • Ambulatory setting
• Outpatient surgery

Modern anesthesia practice was made possible by the invention of the endotracheal tube (ET), which made lengthy and complex surgical procedures feasible without the disastrous complications of airway obstruction, aspiration of gastric contents, or asphyxia. For decades, endotracheal intubation or bag-and-mask ventilation were the mainstays of airway management. In 1983 this changed with the invention of the laryngeal mask airway (LMA), the first supraglottic airway device (SGA) that blended features of the facemask with those of the ET,[1] providing ease of placement and hands-free maintenance, along with a relatively secure airway.

In the United States, more than 75% of all surgical procedures are performed on an outpatient basis.[2] This situation has created an ever-increasing demand for anesthetic agents and techniques that improve the efficiency and safety of anesthesia, aiming for faster induction, emergence and recovery, fewer and milder side effects, and earlier discharge of the patient. SGAs lend themselves particularly well to outpatient anesthesia, offering several advantages over the ET.

Insertion of an SGA may be less stimulating to the sympathetic nervous system than direct laryngoscopy and placement of a semirigid ET into the trachea, thereby decreasing the risk of adverse cardiovascular events in patients with coronary artery disease. The laryngeal mask airway (LMA) is also tolerated at lighter levels of anesthesia than an ET,[3] potentially decreasing side effects and length of stay. While one study showed no differences between an LMA and an ET in average time to placement of the two airway devices or time from end of surgery to removal of the airway device, length of stay in the postanesthesia care unit and time to ambulation were significantly shorter in the LMA group, although there were no differences in the times to "home readiness."[4] Another study did demonstrate that LMAs reduce induction time when

Department of Anesthesia and Critical Care, Pritzker School of Medicine, University of Chicago Medical Center, University of Chicago, 5841 South Maryland Avenue, MC 4028, Chicago, IL, 60637, USA
* Corresponding author.
E-mail address: kluba@dacc.uchicago.edu

Anesthesiology Clin 28 (2010) 295–314
doi:10.1016/j.anclin.2010.02.004 anesthesiology.theclinics.com
1932-2275/10/$ – see front matter

compared with endotracheal intubation, although emergence times were again similar.[5] For outpatients undergoing dentoalveolar procedures under general anesthesia, the LMA group did have a shorter procedure time than the ET group and had a significantly shorter recovery time.[6] The incidence of postoperative sore throat is also significantly less in patients receiving the LMA[4,7] Another advantage is that an SGA typically does not require neuromuscular blockade, thereby avoiding any associated morbidity and side effects of the medication or its antagonists.

Following the success of the LMA, the last two decades have seen a proliferation of SGAs. To be suitable for clinical use, an SGA must bridge the oropharyngeal space efficiently, seal the upper airway during spontaneous and positive pressure ventilation, have low resistance to respiratory gas flow, provide some degree of protection of the subglottic airway from upper airway secretions and gastric contents, and have a low incidence of airway morbidity and adverse events. The success of any SGA in clinical practice depends on its accept/reject profile, which describes the potential for acceptance or rejection of a foreign body by the oropharynx.[8,9] This profile depends on the device's shape, material, cuff volume, and cuff position in the oropharynx.

The use of SGAs is limited to certain patient populations and surgical procedures. Compared with ETs, SGAs only partially protect against aspiration of gastric contents. This limitation precludes their use in patients with a full stomach or other risk factors for aspiration. Delivery of positive pressure ventilation is limited by the SGA's airway leak pressure, which for many lies between 20 and 25 cm H_2O.[10,11] Airway pressure above this range may result in gastric insufflation and increased risk for regurgitation and aspiration of gastric contents. Delivery of positive pressure ventilation may be inadequate in the presence of decreased lung and chest compliance. Thus, the utility of SGAs is limited in morbidly obese patients, in patients with restrictive and obstructive lung disease, or for laparoscopic surgery, especially when performed on a patient in steep Trendelenburg position. Newer SGA designs aspire to address these limitations and to expand the use of supraglottic ventilating techniques.

SUPRAGLOTTIC AIRWAY DEVICES IN CLINICAL USE

LMA Classic (LMA North America, Inc)

The LMA Classic may be the most important development in airway management in the last 25 years. This device became commercially available in Europe in 1988 and was approved by the Food and Drug Administration (FDA) for clinical use in the United States in 1992.

The LMA Classic (**Fig. 1**) consists of a "bowl-shaped" mask surrounded by an oval, inflatable, silicone cuff designed to seal around the laryngeal inlet. Two elastic bars across the bowl aperture prevent obstruction by the epiglottis. The bowl and aperture of the mask are continuous with a curved, wide-bore tube that can be connected to a self-inflating (eg, Ambu) bag or a ventilatory circuit. The LMA Classic, available in sizes 1 to 6, is designed to fit most airways, from neonates through large adults; it is reusable up to 40 times with steam autoclaving.

After placement in the oropharynx, the cuff of the LMA is inflated with enough air to yield an airway leak pressure between 20 and 25 cm H_2O. If the LMA is misplaced, it may result in a low airway leak pressure, but merely inflating the cuff with more air will not necessarily contain the leak, and may cause pressure ischemia of the pharyngeal mucosa and sore throat postoperatively. A low-pressure airway leak should be corrected by adjusting the LMA position (with gentle pushing or pulling or with jaw thrust) or by withdrawing and reinserting (**Table 1**).

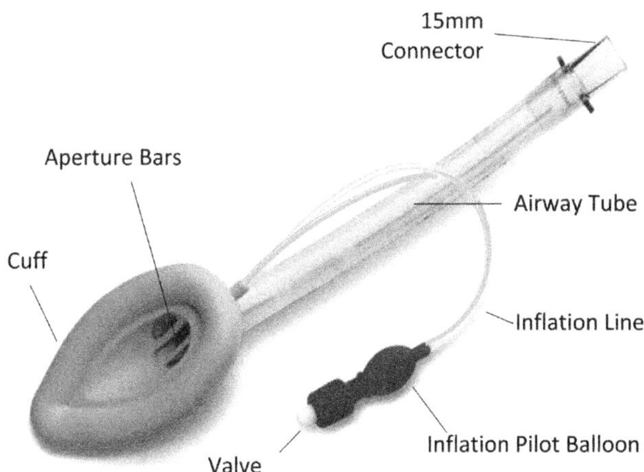

Fig. 1. Laryngeal mask airway LMA Classic. (*Courtesy of* LMA North America, Inc; with permission.)

The LMA Classic was originally developed for use during routine general anesthesia with spontaneous ventilation. The device can also be used with positive pressure ventilation at peak airway pressures not exceeding 20 to 25 cm H_2O or with pressure support ventilation. Although designed for elective airway management, it has been used successfully as an airway rescue device in emergencies, including resuscitation. The LMA Classic is now listed in the American Society of Anesthesiologists (ASA) Difficult Airway Algorithm[12] and the American Heart Association 2000 Guidelines for Cardiopulmonary Resuscitation and Emergency Cardiovascular Care[13] as a primary ventilatory device or as a conduit for the ET in pediatric and adult patients in whom ventilation with a facemask or intubation is difficult or impossible. The success rate for blind intubation through the LMA Classic varies, but the use of a fiberoptic scope for intubation through the LMA increases the success rate.[14]

The LMA Classic remains the most widely used SGA. At present, about 30% to 60% of all general anesthetics are performed with an LMA, and it has been used in more than 200 million patients worldwide.[8] The incidence of major complications and airway morbidity has been consistently low, and no apparent deaths have been attributed to its use.[8,15] The LMA primarily substitutes for a facemask, making airway management "hands-free" during general anesthesia. The LMA is contraindicated for patients with decreased lung or chest compliance and increased airway resistance, glottic or subglottic airway obstruction, oropharyngeal anatomic abnormalities, or who are at high risk for aspiration.

The LMA Classic has been successfully used as a primary ventilatory device for laparoscopic cholecystectomy and laparoscopic gynecologic surgery.[16–18] However, clinical studies of the use of the LMA for laparoscopic surgery have excluded patients at risk for failure or complications of the use of the LMA, including patients with a full stomach, those with a body mass index (BMI) of 30 kg/m^2 or more, those of ASA physical status III and above, or with a Mallampati score III or IV.[16–18]

LMA Unique (LMA North America, Inc)

The LMA Unique (**Fig. 2**) was among the first single-use equivalents of the original, reusable SGAs. The development of this device was motivated by concerns about the transmission of infectious agents, especially prions, by residual proteinaceous

Table 1
Tips for troubleshooting problems after LMA ProSeal insertion

Problems After Insertion	Possible Cause(s)	Possible Solution(s)
Poor airway seal/Air leak (audible air leak, poor ventilation)	Mask seated too high in pharynx	Advance mask in further and resecure airway tubes with tape
	Inadequate anesthesia	Deepen anesthesia
	Poor fixation	Ensure palatal pressure and proper fixation
	Overinflation of cuff	Check cuff pressure at start and periodically during case, especially if using nitrous oxide to ensure not >60 cm H_2O (adjust if necessary)
	Herniation of cuff	Confirm cuff integrity before use; deflate entirely before autoclaving
Gas leakage up the drain tube with or without PPV	Mask seated too high in pharynx	Advance mask in further and resecure airway tubes with tape
	Incorrect placement in laryngeal vestibule	Remove and reinsert
	Open upper esophageal sphincter	Monitor
Airway obstruction (difficult ventilation, phonation, stridor)	Incorrect placement in laryngeal vestibule	Remove and reinsert
	Distal tip of mask pressing on glottic inlet with mechanical closure of vocal cords	Ensure adequate anesthesia and correct cuff inflation pressures Place patient's head/neck in sniffing position Try PPV or add PEEP
	Folding of cuff walls medially	Consider insertion of 1 size smaller LMA ProSeal Ensure correct cuff inflation pressures

Gastric insufflation	Distal tip of mask folded backward	Remove and reinsert of digitally sweep behind the tip
	Mask seated to high in pharynx	Advance mask in further and resecure airway tubes with tape
Migration/Rotation/Mask popping out of mouth	Overinflation of cuff	Check cuff pressure at start and periodically during case, especially if using nitrous oxide to ensure not >60 cm H_2O
	Herniation of cuff	Confirm cuff integrity before use
	Accidental displacement	Ensure proper fixation
	Distal tip of mask folding backward	Remove and reinsert or digitally sweep behind the tip
	Poor fixation	Ensure palatal pressure and proper fixation
Resistance to OG tube insertion	Insufficient lubrication	Add lubricant and re-attempt passing OG tube
	Distal tip of mask folded backward	Remove and insert or digitally sweep behind the tip
	Mask seated to high in pharynx	Advance mask in further and resecure airway tubes with tape
	Incorrect placement in laryngeal vestibule	Remove and reinsert
	Gross overinflation of cuff	Check cuff pressure at start and periodically during case, especially if using nitrous oxide to ensure not >60 cm H_2O

Abbreviations: OG, orogastric; PEEP, positive end-expiratory pressure; PPV, positive pressure ventilation.
Courtesy of LMA North America, Inc; with permission.

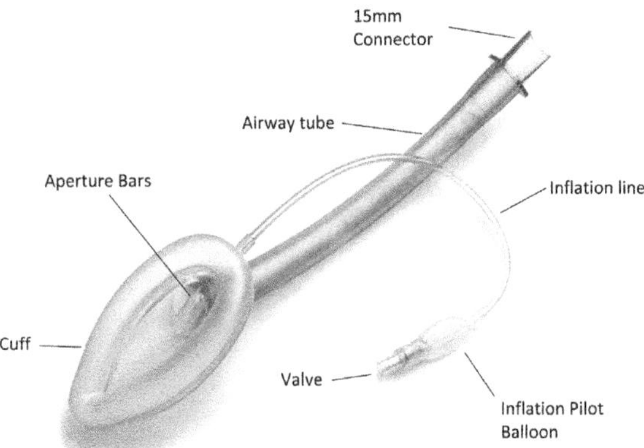

Fig. 2. Laryngeal mask airway LMA Unique. (*Courtesy of* LMA North America, Inc; with permission.)

material found on autoclaved airway management equipment.[15,19,20] The LMA Unique is a disposable, sterile version of the LMA Classic, is available in 5 sizes, and has clinical applications and performance similar to those of the LMA Classic.

LMA Classic Excel (LMA North America, Inc)

The LMA Classic Excel (**Fig. 3**) improves on the LMA Classic with the addition of an epiglottic elevating bar and removable connector to facilitate introduction of an ET through the LMA after placement. The LMA Classic Excel is available in sizes 3 to 5 and accommodates ETs up to size 7.5; it is reusable up to 60 times.

LMA Flexible (LMA North America, Inc)

The LMA Flexible (**Fig. 4**) combines the original LMA cuff design with a narrower, longer, wire-reinforced flexible airway tube. Intubation through this device is impossible because of its longer and narrower airway tube, but because of its flexibility and extra length, it can be positioned away from the surgical field without cuff displacement. This feature makes it particularly useful for those procedures in which the surgeon and the anesthesiologist work in the same area, such as during

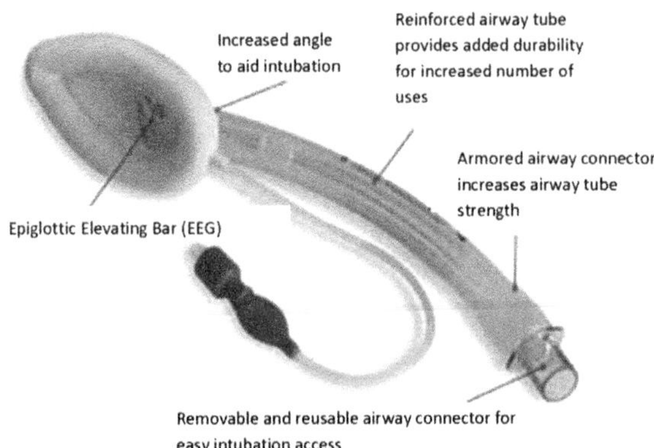

Fig. 3. Laryngeal mask airway LMA Classic Excel. (*Courtesy of* LMA North America, Inc; with permission.)

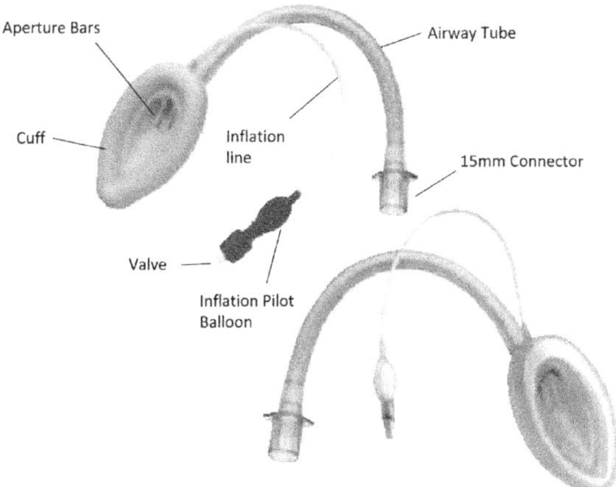

Fig. 4. Laryngeal mask airway LMA Flexible. Reusable version (*top*) and single-use version (*bottom*). (*Courtesy of* LMA North America, Inc; with permission.)

ear/nose/throat, maxillofacial, or dental procedures. The LMA Flexible is available in sizes 2 to 6 in both reusable and disposable versions.

LMA ProSeal (LMA North America, Inc)

The LMA ProSeal (**Fig. 5**) modifies the LMA Classic with a better airway seal and separate access to the gastrointestinal and respiratory tracts. These features improve the safety and efficacy of positive pressure ventilation, provide a means of gastric suctioning, reduce the risk of regurgitation and aspiration of gastric contents, and help confirm correct mask position (**Fig. 6**). The cuff of the LMA ProSeal has an additional chamber to form a tighter pharyngeal seal when the perilaryngeal cuff is pushed

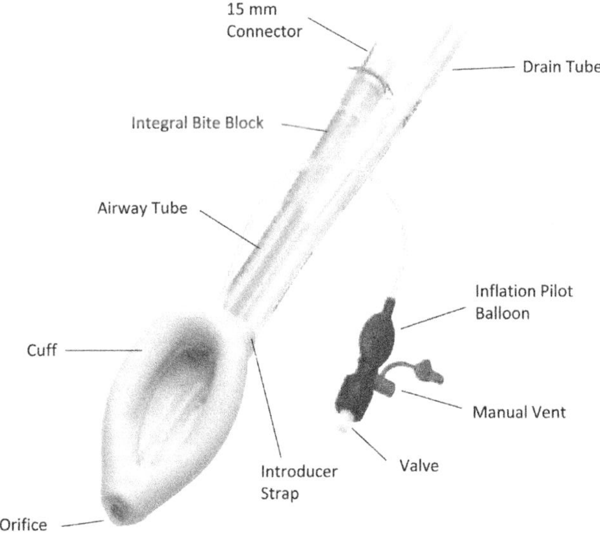

Fig. 5. Laryngeal mask airway LMA ProSeal. (*Courtesy of* LMA North America, Inc; with permission.)

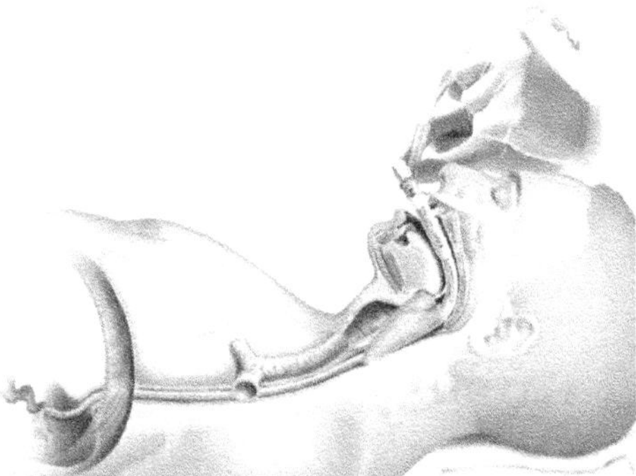

Fig. 6. Correct placement of the LMA ProSeal. Gastric tube placed in the esophageal lumen enables gastric emptying and assessment of the position of the distal end of the LMA ProSeal at the upper esophageal sphincter. (*Courtesy of* LMA North America, Inc; with permission.)

against the laryngeal inlet, permitting positive pressure ventilation up to 30 cm H_2O. A built-in esophageal drain opens at the esophageal tip of the mask and can accommodate a 14-F gastric tube (see **Fig. 6**). Because it is impossible to pass the gastric tube through an obstructed distal opening of the esophageal drain, a misplaced LMA (eg, folding the tip of the mask over backward) can be discovered quickly (see **Table 1**). The LMA ProSeal is available in sizes 1.5 to 5 and is reusable. The airway tube is wire-reinforced and fused with the esophageal drain at the incisor level by a built-in, silicone bite block.

In 2005, 59 controlled randomized trials or other clinical studies and 79 other publications from January 1998 to March 2005 were reviewed.[21] Compared with the LMA Classic, the LMA ProSeal had an equal insertion success rate and 50% improvement in the airway seal. Because of the esophageal port, diagnosis of misplacement was prompt, gastric drainage was possible, gastric inflation was reduced, and regurgitated stomach contents could be vented. Evidence suggested, but did not prove, that a properly placed LMA ProSeal reduces aspiration risk compared with the LMA Classic. The LMA ProSeal also caused less coughing and sympathetic stimulation than an ET. Comparative trials of the LMA ProSeal and other SGAs demonstrated the superior performance of the LMA ProSeal during positive pressure ventilation, under conditions of both normal and elevated (ie, during laparoscopic surgery) intra-abdominal pressure.[22–24] The ProSeal was also associated with less analgesic requirement in patients undergoing laparoscopic gynecologic surgery in the first six hours after surgery in comparison with intubated patients.[25] Postoperative nausea and vomiting, analgesic requirements, and airway morbidity were also less in a similar study looking at both laparoscopic and breast surgery.[7]

LMA Supreme (LMA North America, Inc)

Like the LMA ProSeal, the LMA Supreme (**Fig. 7**) has a modified cuff that achieves a 50% higher airway seal pressure than the Classic or the Unique, and a gastric drain to suction the stomach, vent regurgitated stomach contents, and confirm placement of the tip of the mask at the upper esophageal sphincter. A reinforced tip and molded distal cuff prevent folding. The curve and shape of the airway tube make insertion easier and placement more stable. The LMA Supreme is a single-use device, available in adult sizes 3 to 5; its clinical utility is similar to that of the LMA ProSeal.

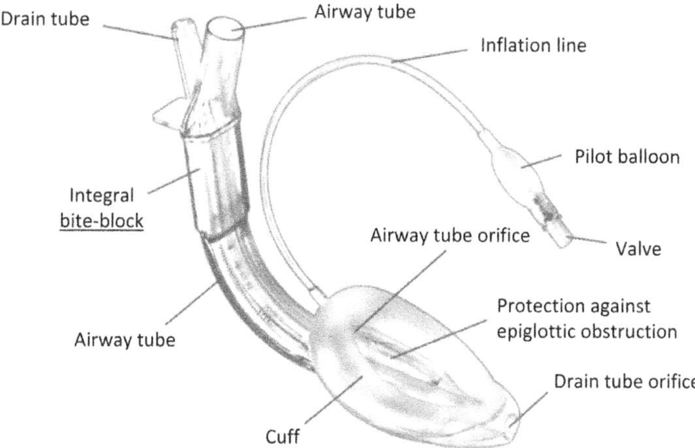

Fig. 7. Laryngeal mask airway LMA Supreme. (*Courtesy of* LMA North America, Inc; with permission.)

LMA Fastrach (LMA North America, Inc)

Although the LMA Fastrach (**Fig. 8**) may function as a ventilating supraglottic airway, it is primarily an intubating tool and was designed as a conduit for placement of an ET in cases of anticipated or actual difficult direct laryngoscopy. Its rigid, anatomically shaped airway tube is wide enough to accommodate a size 8 ET and short enough for placement of the ET cuff below the vocal cords. The LMA Fastrach was intended for blind endotracheal intubation but also can be used with a fiberoptic bronchoscope, lighted stylets, or the Flexible Airway Scope; it is available in sizes 3 to 5 and comes with a specially designed, reusable, wire-reinforced LMA Fastrach ET (**Fig. 9**).

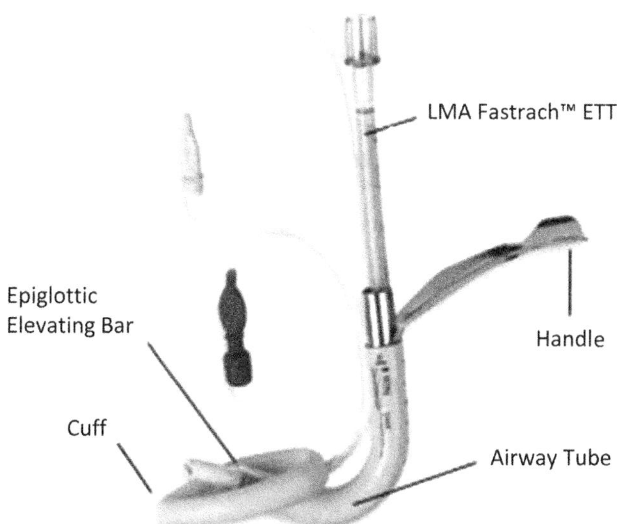

Fig. 8. Laryngeal mask airway LMA FasTrach. LMA ET Tube is placed in the airway tube. The tip of the ET tube protrudes under the epiglottic elevating bar. (*Courtesy of* LMA North America, Inc; with permission.)

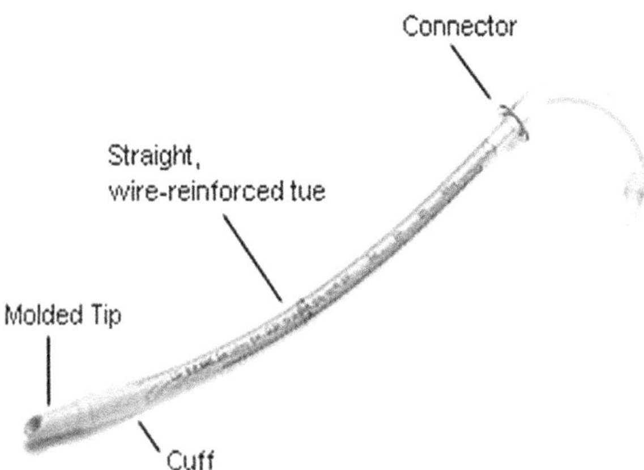

Fig. 9. Endotracheal tube LMA ET Tube, for use with the LMA FasTrach. (*Courtesy of* LMA North America, Inc; with permission.)

LMA CTrach (LMA North America, Inc)

The LMA CTrach (**Fig. 10**) is an LMA Fastrach with built-in fiberoptics for real-time visualization during intubation of the trachea. Ventilation is possible during intubation attempts through the mask portion of the LMA CTrach.

Other SGAs Similar To LMA Laryngeal Masks

There are several laryngeal masks available for clinical use in the United States. Their design generally follows that of the LMA Classic and its later variants, with minor modifications depending on the manufacturer. Most of them are single-use devices. The list of the laryngeal masklike devices includes Sheridan Laryngeal Mask (Teleflex Medical), Portex Soft Seal Laryngeal Mask (Smiths Medical), Aura40 Reusable Laryngeal Mask, AuraStraight Disposable Laryngeal Mask, AuraFlex Disposable Laryngeal

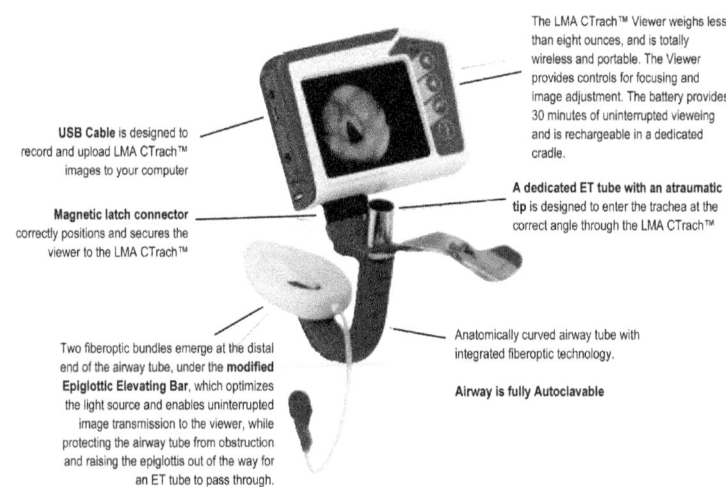

Fig. 10. Intubating laryngeal mask airway LMA CTrach. (*Courtesy of* LMA North America, Inc; with permission.)

Mask, and AuraOnce Disposable Laryngeal Mask (Ambu, Inc), as well as Ultra CPV and UltraFlex CPV (AES, Inc).

OTHER SGA DESIGNS

Combitube (Covidien)

The Combitube (**Fig. 11**) is a disposable, double-lumen tube that combines the features of a conventional ET with those of an esophageal obturator airway. The Combitube has a large proximal oropharyngeal balloon and a distal esophageal (or tracheal), low-pressure small cuff, with eight ventilatory holes between the cuffs, and a single ventilatory port at the distal tip (**Fig. 12**). There is ventilation with the Combitube regardless of whether the distal tip is in the esophagus (common) (**Fig. 13**) or in the trachea (rare).[26] In the latter case, the device functions like a conventional ET when the distal cuff is inflated. When the distal tip is in the esophagus, the distal cuff seals the esophagus against regurgitation of gastric contents, and a gastric tube can be placed through the esophageal lumen.

The Combitube has been used worldwide for more than 20 years as an emergency airway,[27] chiefly in the prehospital setting. The Combitube is an easy-to-use device in a "cannot-ventilate-cannot- intubate" scenario that has been used in challenging

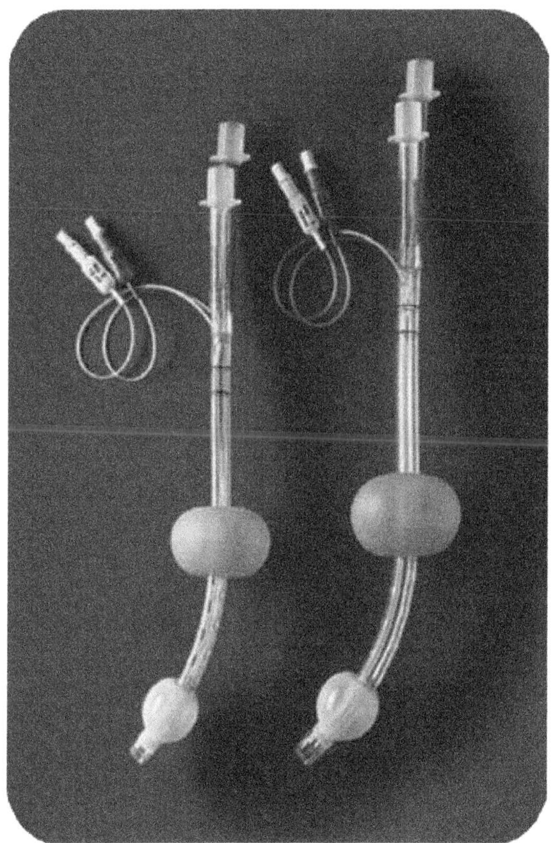

Fig. 11. Combitube esophageal/tracheal double-lumen airway: 2 different sizes. (*Courtesy of* Covidien-Nellcor and Puritan Bennett, Boulder, CO; with permission.)

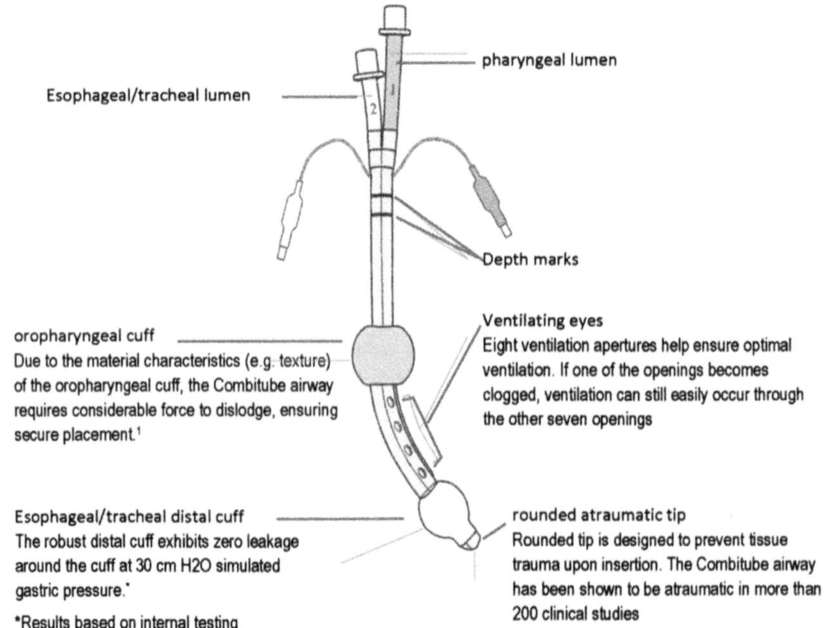

Fig. 12. Combitube esophageal/tracheal double-lumen airway. (*Courtesy of* Covidien-Nellcor and Puritan Bennett, Boulder, CO; with permission.)

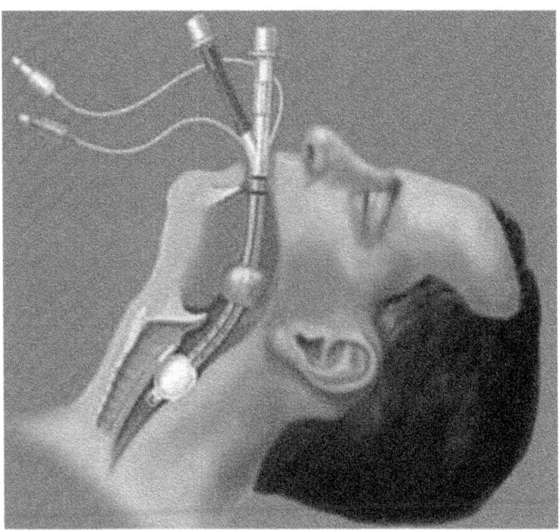

Fig. 13. Combitube placement in esophagus. The tube is advanced until the 2 black depth marks are at the level of the teeth. The distal esophageal cuff is inflated with 10 mL of air to seal the esophagus. The proximal pharyngeal cuff is inflated with 80 mL of air, securing the tube in place and sealing off the oral and nasal cavity. The patient's lungs are ventilated through lumen 1 (pharyngeal lumen). (*Courtesy of* Covidien-Nellcor and Puritan Bennett, Boulder, CO; with permission.)

situations at accident sites, such as for individuals trapped in an automobile wreck where access to the airway is severely limited.

One study compared the Combitube, the LMA ProSeal, and the Laryngeal Tube S (LTS) in 90 patients who underwent general anesthesia for minor gynecologic procedures. All patients were ASA physical status class I, II, or III, and had a BMI less than 35 kg/m^2. The Combitube was inferior for the technical aspects of ventilation (time to successful placement and ventilation, failure rate), produced the highest cuff pressures, and resulted in the highest incidence of airway morbidity.[28] Increased airway morbidity with the Combitube compared with the LMA during routine surgery has also been demonstrated by another study,[29] and airway management with the Combitube during routine general anesthesia is not recommended.[28,29]

King LT and King LTS (King Systems/VBM Medizintechnik, GmbH)

The Laryngeal Tube (LT) (**Fig. 14**) is a single-lumen, silicone tube with a large oropharyngeal and smaller esophageal, low-pressure cuff, two ventilation outlets between the cuffs, insertion marks, and a blind esophageal tip. Superficially it resembles a shorter Combitube. The LT is easy to insert and may offer some protection against aspiration. The reusable version may be used up to 50 times and is available in sizes 2 to 5. A disposable version is also available.

The Laryngeal Tube S (LTS) has a second lumen for placement of a gastric tube for drainage of stomach contents (**Fig. 15**). The LTS is available in reusable and disposable versions in sizes 3 to 5.

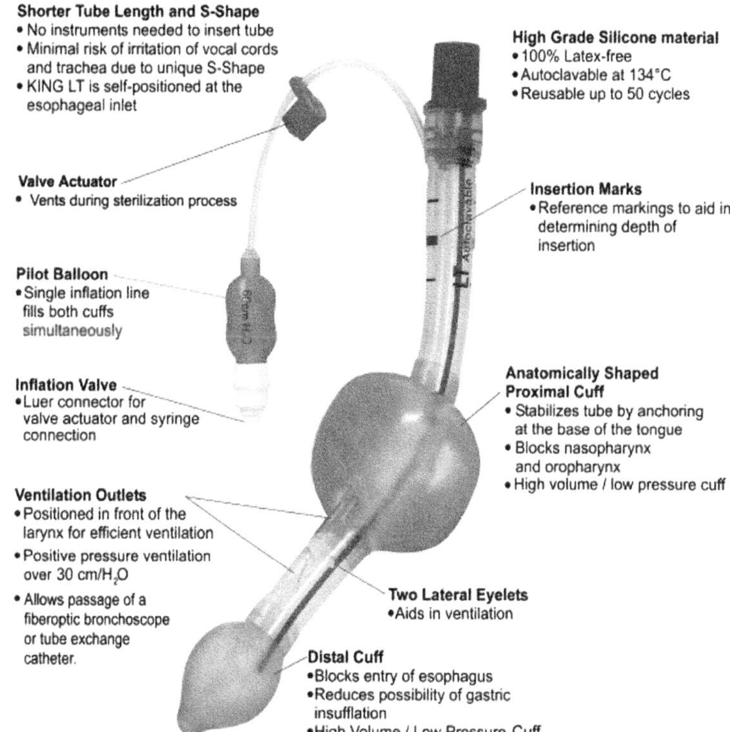

Fig. 14. Supraglottic airway device King LT. (*Courtesy of* King Systems Corporation, Noblesville, IN; with permission.)

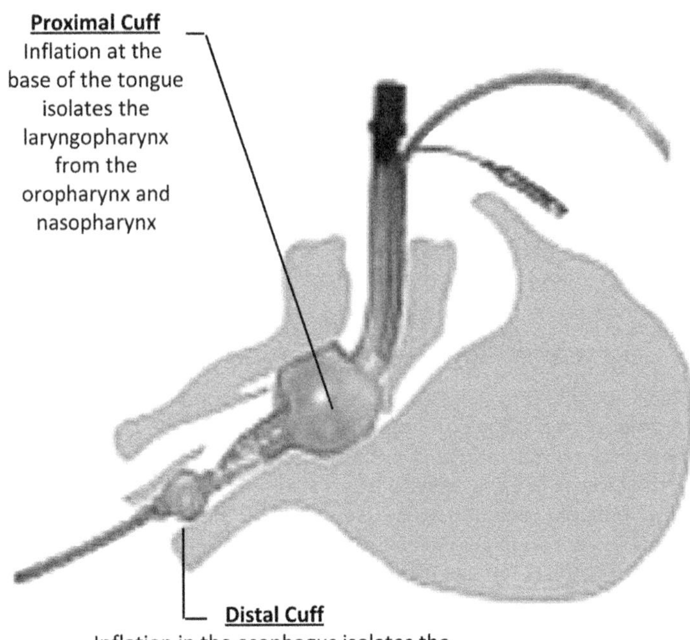

Fig. 15. Supraglottic airway device King LTS: a correct placement with distal tip at the upper esophageal sphincter. A gastric tube is placed in the esophageal channel. (*Courtesy of* King Systems Corporation, Noblesville, IN; with permission.)

The LT and LTS can be used with a spontaneously breathing patient or with positive pressure ventilation. Their ventilatory seal characteristics are comparable with those of the LMA ProSeal. Since its introduction into clinical practice in 2002, several studies have compared the LTS with the LMA ProSeal.[22,23,28,30] In three studies, the airway seal of the LTS was adequate during positive pressure ventilation, even under conditions of elevated intra-abdominal pressure during laparoscopy, but excluded from the studies were patients whose ASA physical status class was III or higher, whose BMI was greater than 35 kg/m^2, or who were at a risk for aspiration. During laparoscopy, intra-abdominal pressure was limited to 18 cm H_2O, and Trendelenburg position did not exceed 15°. In a fourth study, the LTS was inferior to the LMA ProSeal with regard to insertion time and success, airway leak pressure, peak and plateau airway pressure, and ease of passage of a gastric tube.[23] The incidence of throat soreness and dysphagia appeared to be lower with the use of the LMA ProSeal.[22,28]

Overall, the data suggest that the LTS is a safe and effective airway device in adult patients whose lungs are mechanically ventilated.[8]

Cobra PLA (Engineered Medical Systems)

The Cobra Perilaryngeal Airway (PLA) (**Fig. 16**) is a cuffed, disposable SGA. The Cobra PLA has a tapered, striated head, a large, circumferential pharyngeal cuff, and a breathing tube; it is available in eight sizes for use from neonates through large adults. The ventilatory opening at the junction of the tube and the head is protected from obstruction by the epiglottis by a soft "grill" on the anterior (laryngeal) aspect of the head. A size 8 ET can be advanced through Cobra sizes 4 to 6. Several

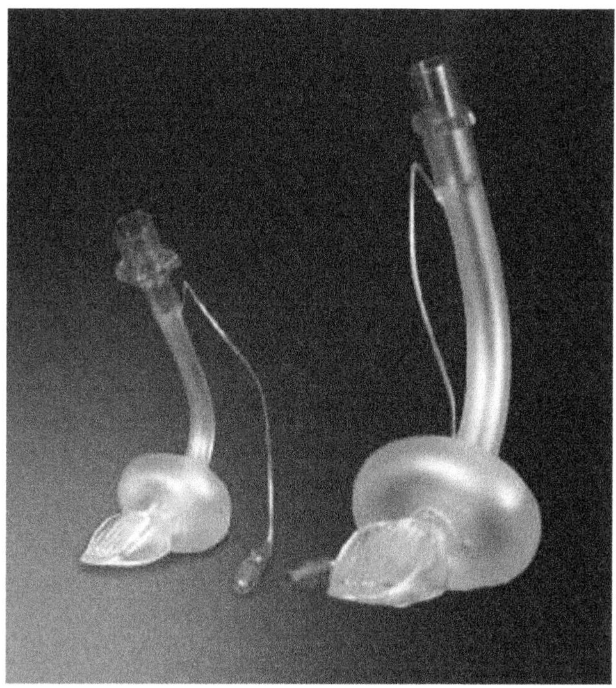

Fig. 16. Cobra supraglottic airway device. (*Courtesy of* Focus Medical Hellas S.A., Attiki, Greece; with permission.)

studies[16,31–33] evaluated the Cobra during spontaneous and positive pressure ventilation in adults and children. Patients were ASA physical status class I or II, had a Mallampati score of I or II, BMI less than 30 kg/m^2, and no history of gastroesophageal reflux disease (GERD). In all studies, the Cobra was a suitable primary ventilatory device that provided a higher airway seal pressure than the LMA Unique. However, another study comparing the Cobra and the LMA Classic during anesthesia for elective surgery was terminated after pulmonary aspiration occurred in two patients with the Cobra PLA.[34] This study excluded patients with a history of GERD, a difficult airway, or morbid obesity.

SLIPA (SLIPA Medical Ltd)

The Streamlined Liner of the Pharynx Airway (SLIPA) (**Fig. 17**) is a noncuffed, single-use SGA, made of soft plastic in the shape of a pressurized pharynx. The SLIPA has a hollow, boot-shaped chamber, with a toe bridge that seals at the base of the tongue and a heel that anchors the device in place between the esophagus and the nasopharynx (**Fig. 18**). The hollow chamber can store up to 50 mL of regurgitant gastric liquid. The SLIPA is available in six adult sizes, 47 to 57, that match the width of the thyroid cartilage and are equivalent to LMA sizes 3 to 5.5.

The SLIPA is intended as a primary airway device during general anesthesia of short duration. Its efficacy and complication rate are comparable to those of the LMA Classic.[31,35,36] The SLIPA is not recommended for patients placed in positions other than supine or when the risk of aspiration is increased. Even though the SLIPA includes a chamber to capture regurgitant gastric contents, more clinical evidence is needed to demonstrate that it confers protection against aspiration.

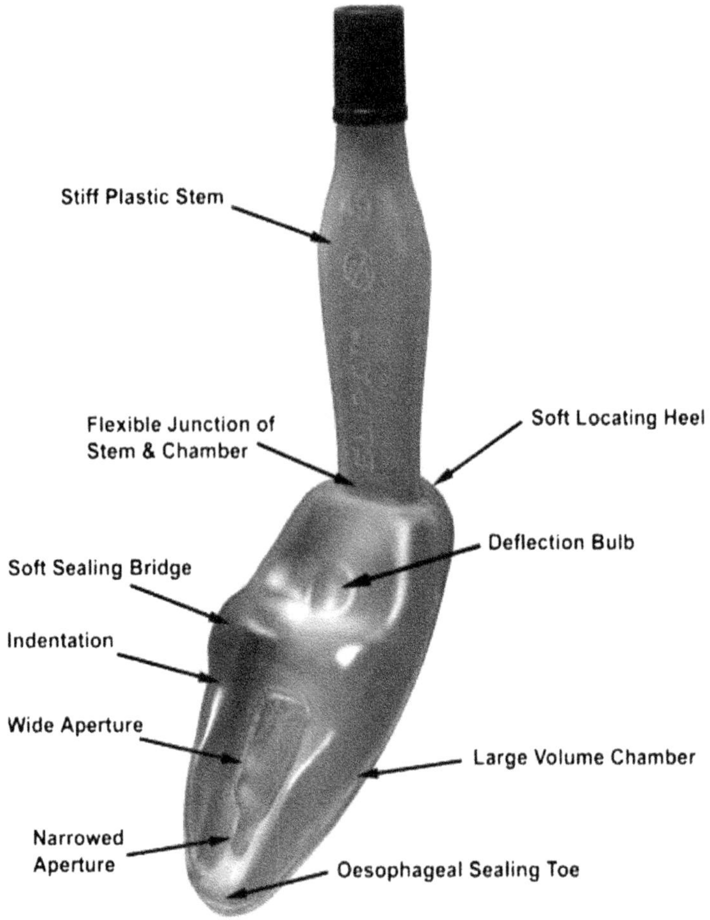

Stiff Plastic Stem
Flexible Junction of Stem & Chamber
Soft Locating Heel
Deflection Bulb
Soft Sealing Bridge
Indentation
Wide Aperture
Large Volume Chamber
Narrowed Aperture
Oesophageal Sealing Toe

Fig. 17. SLIPA supraglottic airway device. (*Courtesy of* ARC Medical, Inc, Tucker, GA; with permission.)

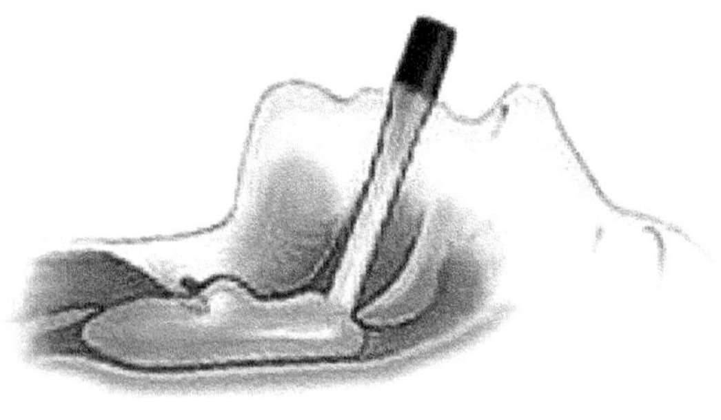

Fig. 18. SLIPA supraglottic airway device placement in the oropharynx. (*Courtesy of* ARC Medical, Inc, Tucker, GA; with permission.)

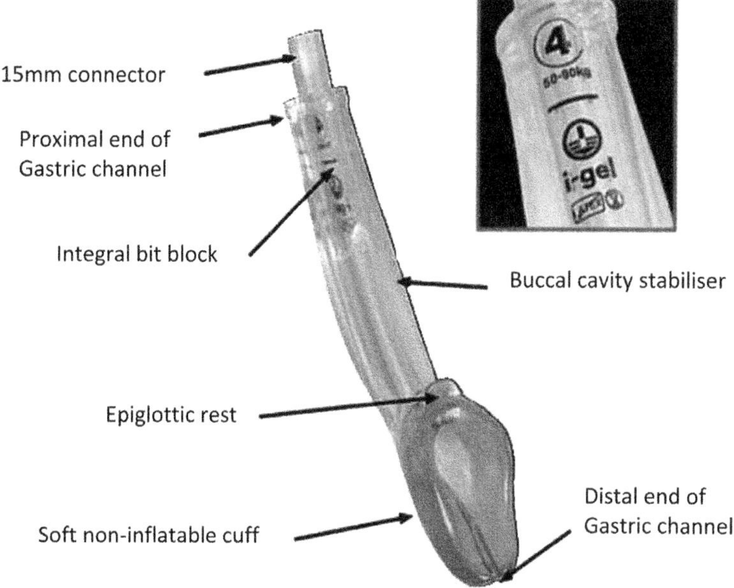

Fig. 19. i-gel supraglottic airway device. (*Courtesy of* i-gel Intersurgical Ltd, Wokingham, Berkshire, UK; with permission.)

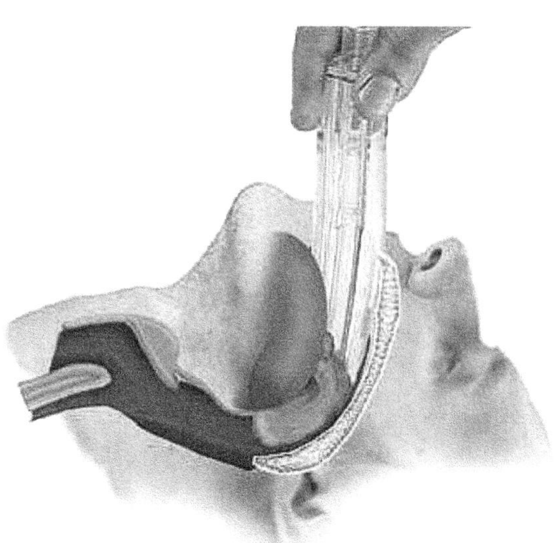

Fig. 20. Placement of the i-gel supraglottic airway device in the oropharynx. (*Courtesy of* i-gel Intersurgical Ltd, Wokingham, Berkshire, UK; with permission.)

Intersurgical i-gel (Intersurgical Inc)

The i-gel (**Fig. 19**) is the latest addition to the SGA arsenal. The i-gel is a single-use device that has an integral bite block, a gastric tube channel, and a soft, noninflatable cuff that adapts to the hypopharyngeal anatomy after blind placement (**Fig. 20**). The i-gel was found to be safe and effective during positive pressure ventilation in adults with a BMI less than 35 kg/m^2,[37,38] and in nonobese children,[39] but another study looking at 280 uses of the i-gel yielded three cases of regurgitation, with one resulting in nonfatal aspiration.[40]

SUMMARY

Supraglottic airway devices have become prevalent in the ambulatory setting because they typically are more user-friendly than a face mask and avoid many of the problems associated with endotracheal intubation. The LMA Classic and the LMA ProSeal have an established record of safety and efficacy for routine cases in healthy adult and pediatric patients with no significant comorbidities such as morbid obesity, pulmonary disease, or aspiration risk. While this reputation has resulted in a tendency to expand the use of supraglottic airway devices to laparoscopic surgery and to procedures in morbidly obese or pregnant patients, these practices remain controversial. The LMA ProSeal may provide a better airway seal and protection against aspiration than the LMA Classic, although the latter claim has not been definitively demonstrated. Often, disposable LMAs match the performance of the reusable devices.

Over the last two decades, the enormous success of the LMA has been followed by the proliferation of other supraglottic airway devices, each claiming advantages over devices already in use. The Laryngeal Tube and the Laryngeal Tube S are somewhat inferior to the LMA and the LMA ProSeal, respectively, in terms of airway morbidity and delivery of positive pressure ventilation, but they are suitable for routine use. The Combitube should not be used for routine airway management during anesthesia because its incidence of airway morbidity is higher than that of other supraglottic airway devices. Recently developed noninflatable devices, the SLIPA and the i-gel, await more clinical trials to establish their suitability in either the outpatient or the inpatient setting. While more research and development are indicated, SGAs are already proven to be indispensable in the ambulatory setting.

ACKNOWLEDGMENTS

The authors wish to thank Sally Kozlik for editorial help, and Susan Yager and Sandra Nunnally for technical assistance in preparing this article.

REFERENCES

1. Brain AI. The laryngeal mask—a new concept in airway management. Br J Anaesth 1983;55(8):801–5.
2. Twersky RS. Ambulatory surgery update. Can J Anaesth 1998;45(5 Pt 2):R76–90.
3. Wilkins CJ, Cramp PG, Staples J, et al. Comparison of the anesthetic requirement for tolerance of laryngeal mask airway and endotracheal tube. Anesth Analg 1992;75(5):794–7.
4. Joshi GP, Inagaki Y, White PF, et al. Use of the laryngeal mask airway as an alternative to the tracheal tube during ambulatory anesthesia. Anesth Analg 1997; 85(5):573–7.

5. Hartmann B, Banzhaf A, Junger A, et al. Laryngeal mask airway versus endotracheal tube for outpatient surgery: analysis of anesthesia-controlled time. J Clin Anesth 2004;16(3):195–9.
6. Todd DW. A comparison of endotracheal intubation and use of the laryngeal mask airway for oral surgery patients. J Oral Maxillofac Surg 2002;60(1):2–4.
7. Hohlrieder M, Brimacombe J, von Goedecke A, et al. Postoperative nausea, vomiting, airway morbidity, and analgesic requirements are lower for the ProSeal laryngeal mask airway than the tracheal tube in females undergoing breast and gynaecological surgery. Br J Anaesth 2007;99(4):576–80.
8. Bein B, Scholz J. Supraglottic airway devices. Best Pract Res Clin Anaesthesiol 2005;19(4):581–93.
9. Brain AI. The development of the Laryngeal Mask—a brief history of the invention, early clinical studies and experimental work from which the Laryngeal Mask evolved. Eur J Anaesthesiol Suppl 1991;4:5–17.
10. Brimacombe J, Keller C, Fullerkrug B, et al. A multicenter study comparing the ProSeal and Classic laryngeal mask airway in anesthetized, nonoparalyzed patients. Anesthesiology 2002;96(2):289–95.
11. Asai T, Kawashima A, Hidaka I, et al. The laryngeal tube compared with the laryngeal mask: insertion, gas leak pressure and gastric insufflations. Br J Anaesth 2002;89(5):729–32.
12. American Society of Anesthesiologists Task Force on Management of the Difficult Airway. Practice guidelines for management of the difficult airway: an updated report by the American Society of Anesthesiologists Task Force on Management of the Difficult Airway. Anesthesiology 2003;98(5):1269–77.
13. Guidelines 2000 for Cardiopulmonary Resuscitation and Emergency Cardiovascular Care. Part 6: advanced cardiovascular life support: section 3: adjuncts for oxygenation, ventilation and airway control. The American Heart Association in collaboration with the International Committee on Resuscitation. Circulation 2000;102(Suppl 8):I95–104.
14. Pennant JH, White PF. The Laryngeal Mask Airway. Its uses in anesthesiology. Anesthesiology 1993;79:144–63.
15. Jolliffe L, Jackson I. Airway management in the outpatient setting: new devices and techniques. Curr Opin Anaesthesiol 2008;21(6):719–22.
16. Galvin EM, van Doorn M, Blazquez J, et al. A randomized prospective study comparing the Cobra Perilaryngeal Airway and Laryngeal Mask Airway-Classic during controlled ventilation for gynecological laparoscopy. Anesth Analg 2007; 104(1):102–5.
17. Maltby JR, Beriault MT, Watson NC, et al. Gastric distension and ventilation during laparoscopic cholecystectomy: LMA-classic vs. tracheal intubation. Can J Anaesth 2000;47(7):622–6.
18. Bapat PP, Verghese C. Laryngeal mask airway and the incidence of regurgitation during gynecological laparoscopies. Anesth Analg 1997;85(1):139–43.
19. Shafik MT, Bahlman BU, Hall JE, et al. A comparison of the Soft Seal disposable and the Classic re-usable laryngeal mask airway. Anaesthesia 2006;61(2):178–81.
20. Miller DM, Youkhana I, Karunarante WU, et al. Presence of protein deposits on "cleaned" re-usable anaesthetic equipment. Anaesthesia 2001;56(11):1069–72.
21. Cook TM, Lee G, Nolan JP. The ProSeal laryngeal mask airway: a review of the literature. Can J Anaesth 2005;52(7):739–60.
22. Roth H, Genzwuerker V, Rothhaas A, et al. The ProSeal Laryngeal Mask Airway and the Laryngeal Tube Suction™ for ventilation in gynaecological patients undergoing laparoscopic surgery. Eur J Anaesthesiol 2005;22(2):117–22.

23. Cook TM, Cranshaw J. Randomized crossover comparison of ProSeal Laryngeal Mask Airway with Laryngeal Tube Sonda during anaesthesia with controlled ventilation. Br J Anaesth 2005;95(2):261–6.
24. Evans NR, Skowno PJ, Bennett MF, et al. A prospective observational study of the use of the ProSeal™ laryngeal mask airway for postpartum lubal ligation. Int J Obstet Anesth 2005;14(2):90–5.
25. Hohlrieder M, Brimacombe J, Eschertzhuber S, et al. A study of airway management using the ProSeal LMA laryngeal mask airway compared with the tracheal tube on postoperative analgesic requirements following gynaecological laparoscopic surgery. Anaesthesia 2007;62(9):913–8.
26. Agro F, Frass M, Benumof JL, et al. Current status of the Combitube: a review of the literature. J Clin Anesth 2002;14(4):307–14.
27. Frass M, Frenzer R, Zdrahal F, et al. The esophageal tracheal Combitube: preliminary results with new airway for CPR. Ann Emerg Med 1987;16(7):768–72.
28. Bein B, Carstensen M, Gleim L, et al. A comparison of the ProSeal laryngeal mask airway, the laryngeal tube S and the esophageal-tracheal combitube during routine surgical procedures. Eur J Anaesthesiol 2005;22(5):341–6.
29. Oczenski W, Krenn H, Dahaba AA, et al. Complications following the use of the combitube, tracheal tube and laryngeal mask airway. Anaesthesia 1999;54(12):1161–5.
30. Gaitini LA, Vaida SJ, Somri M, et al. A randomized controlled trial comparing the ProSeal Laryngeal Mask Airway with the laryngeal tube suction in mechanically ventilated patients. Anesthesiology 2004;101(2):316–20.
31. Gaitini L, Carmi N, Yanovski B, et al. Comparison of the Cobra PLA (Cobra Perilaryngeal Airway) and the Laryngeal Mask Airway Unique in children under pressure controlled ventilation. Paediatr Anaesth 2008;18(4):313–9.
32. Gaitini L, Yanovski B, Somri M, et al. A comparison between the PLA Cobra and the Laryngeal Mask Airway Unique during spontaneous ventilation: a randomized prospective study. Anesth Analg 2006;102(2):631–6.
33. Hooshangi H, Wong DT. Brief review: the Cobra Perilaryngeal Airway (Cobra PLA) and the Streamlined Liner of Pharyngeal Airway (SLIPA) supraglottic airways. Can J Anaesth 2008;55(3):177–85.
34. Cook TM, Lowe JM. An evaluation of the Cobra Perilaryngeal Airway: study halted after two cases of pulmonary aspiration. Anaesthesia 2005;60(8):791–6.
35. Miller DM, Light D. Laboratory and clinical comparisons of the Streamlined Liner of the Pharynx Airway (SLIPA) with the laryngeal mask airway. Anaesthesia 2003;58(2):136–42.
36. Hein C, Plummer J, Owen H. Evaluation of the SLIPA (Streamlined Liner of the Pharynx Airway), a single use supraglottic airway device, in 60 anaesthetized patients undergoing minor surgical procedures. Anaesth Intensive Care 2005;33(6):756–61.
37. Uppal V, Fletcher G, Kinsella J. Comparison of the i-gel with the cuffed tracheal tube during pressure-controlled ventilation. Br J Anaesth 2009;102(2):264–8.
38. Richez B, Saltel L, Banchereau F, et al. A new single use supraglottic airway device with a noninflatable cuff and an esophageal vent: an observational study of the i-gel. Anesth Analg 2008;106(4):1137–9.
39. Beylacq L, Bordes M, Semjen F, et al. The I-gel, a single-use supraglottic airway device with a noninflatable cuff and an esophageal vent: an observational study in children. Acta Anaesthesiol Scand 2009;53(3):376–9.
40. Gibbison B, Cook TM, Seller C. Case series: protection from aspiration and failure of protection from aspiration with the i-gel airway. Br J Anaesth 2008;100(3):415–7.

Challenges in Pediatric Ambulatory Anesthesia: Kids are Different

Corey E. Collins, DO[a,b], Lucinda L. Everett, MD[b,c,*]

KEYWORDS

• Pediatric anesthesia • Ambulatory surgery • Risks
• Morbidity • OSA • PONV

The care of the child having ambulatory surgery presents a specific set of challenges to the anesthesia provider. This review focuses on areas of clinical distinction that support the additional attention children often require, and on clinical controversies that require providers to have up to date information to guide practice and address parental concerns.

Specifically, this article addresses various categories of risk as applied to children presenting for ambulatory surgery (cardiovascular and respiratory risk, as well as the potential for neurocognitive dysfunction in the very young). The authors consider the role of perioperative anxiety and agitation, the influence these phenomena have on the experience of pediatric patients and their families, and potential strategies to minimize these outcomes. Considering the preponderance of head and neck surgery for pediatric ambulatory surgery, the authors focus on issues that complicate ear, nose, and throat (ENT) cases, including surgical risk, issues related to sleep-disordered breathing, and postoperative nausea and vomiting (PONV). This article discusses guidelines for pediatric anesthesia care and possible future implications for credentialing providers.

RISK IN PEDIATRIC AMBULATORY ANESTHESIA

Many pediatric anesthetics are done on an outpatient basis; although these are minor cases, they may present significant challenges to the clinician. In 2006, the most

[a] Department of Anesthesiology, Pediatric Anesthesia, Massachusetts Eye and Ear Infirmary, 243 Charles Street, Boston, MA 02114, USA
[b] Harvard Medical School, 25 Shattuck Street, Boston, MA 02115, USA
[c] Department of Anesthesiology, Critical Care and Pain Management, Pediatric Anesthesia, Massachusetts General Hospital, 55 Fruit Street, GRB-444, Boston, MA 02114, USA
* Corresponding author. Department of Anesthesiology, Critical Care, and Pain Management, Pediatric Anesthesia, Massachusetts General Hospital, 55 Fruit Street, GRB-444, Boston, MA 02114.
E-mail address: leverett@partners.org

Anesthesiology Clin 28 (2010) 315–328
doi:10.1016/j.anclin.2010.02.005 **anesthesiology.theclinics.com**

common cases in children less than 15 years of age were myringotomy with tube insertion (667,000), tonsillectomy with or without adenoidectomy (530,000), and adenoidectomy alone (132,000).[1]

Information about risk comes from several types of data. Large descriptive series give an overall picture of pediatric anesthesia outcomes, but may be limited in the type and amount of detail, and often come from a single institution; most of these are not specific to outpatients. Incident-reporting studies such as the American Society of Anesthesiologists (ASA) Closed Claims study give more detail on individual serious adverse events, but do not have denominator data to describe the population. Clinical registries gather data prospectively about a given population or problem; the Pediatric Perioperative Cardiac Arrest (POCA) registry has provided valuable information about anesthetic-related cardiac arrest, and in the future more and larger registry efforts should yield more precise outcomes data.

Risk factors associated with serious adverse events in pediatric anesthesia include young age (most frequently <12 months), coexisting disease as reflected by higher ASA status (particularly congenital heart disease), and emergency surgery.[2] A recent large study from France reflects the modern era of anesthetic drugs and monitoring and shows a low overall rate of major morbidity related to anesthesia.[3] In outpatient outcome studies, Fleisher and colleagues[4] analyzed data of 783,558 surgical admissions in New York State, but no pediatric-specific risks were identified. A retrospective survey of outpatient-procedure–related death in Massachusetts between 1995 and 1999 did not report any pediatric deaths.[5] Smaller series of pediatric ambulatory cases primarily detail unanticipated admission rates (0.9%–2%, usually for extensive surgery or protracted vomiting) and the rates of minor complications such as vomiting, cough/croup, and somnolence.[6–8]

The ASA Closed Claims Project reviews claims against anesthesiologists after the cases have reached some conclusion in the legal system. Analysis of patterns of injury from these cases has identified several situations in which anesthesiologists can recognize and decrease risk, such as cardiac arrest in adults having spinal anesthesia. Comparison of pediatric with adult claims in the early era of the Closed Claims Project showed that claims in pediatric patients were more likely to have been precipitated by a respiratory event, and more often deemed preventable by reviewers.[9] Analysis of the more recent pediatric cases in the Closed Claims database found a relative reduction in claims for death/brain damage and for respiratory events, particularly inadequate ventilation and oxygenation. This improvement may be related to the adoption of pulse oximetry and capnography as standards in the early 1990s.[10] Again, younger age and higher ASA status correlated with risk; half of the claims involved patients less than 3 years of age, and one-fifth were ASA 3 to 5.

Cardiac Risk

After the observations in the early Closed Claims series relating cardiac arrest to respiratory events, the POCA Registry was established to study anesthetic-related cardiac arrest in children. The initial results showed a cardiac arrest rate of 1.4 per million anesthetics, with the highest incidence in children less than 1 year of age and ASA 3 to 5. Cardiac arrests described in healthy children were primarily related to respiratory difficulty (laryngospasm or anatomic airway obstruction) and to relative anesthetic overdose (primarily with halothane), the latter accounting for nearly half of cardiac arrests in patients who were ASA 1 to 2.[11] The POCA group published a follow-up analysis in 2008 that showed a significant decline in cardiac arrest related to volatile anesthetic overdose, but a constant proportion of respiratory causes, with laryngospasm still prominent.[12] The other causes of pediatric cardiac arrest identified in healthy patients (hypovolemia from blood loss and hyperkalemia from transfusion of stored blood) are unlikely to be seen in the ambulatory population. There was only 1 cardiac arrest in the 2000 POCA report related to hyperkalemia from succinylcholine in a patient with unrecognized myopathy; case reports of this clinical scenario from the early 1990s resulted in a US Food and Drug Administration (FDA) warning against the routine use of succinylcholine in pediatric patients.[13]

Respiratory Risk

As noted earlier, perioperative respiratory adverse events (PRAE) in children may precipitate serious adverse outcomes. Respiratory events are common in studies of pediatric anesthesia complications; in evaluating these studies, it is important to consider the definitions used, which are frequently not consistent (eg, selection of an oxygen saturation of 95% as the threshold to describe a complication will result in a higher incidence than a threshold of 90% saturation). It is also important to consider the patient population, case type, and anesthetic technique; for example, a series of children with indwelling central venous catheters having propofol anesthetics for diagnostic and therapeutic procedures described a significantly lower incidence of laryngospasm than was seen in many other series.[14]

In a large series of pediatric patients, Murat and colleagues[3] found that respiratory events represented 53% of all intraoperative events, and were more frequent in ENT surgery, with ASA physical classification status 3 to 5, and with tracheal intubation. Mamie and colleagues[15] described an overall 1.57 relative risk increase for PRAE in any child having ENT surgical procedures. Other risks for PRAE included provider experience, younger age, and upper respiratory infection. Although data suggest low overall risks for brief procedures such as myringotomy and ventilation tube (M&T) placement,[12,16] the clinician must consider the risk of upper respiratory infection, potentially difficult mask ventilation, and comorbidities. In 1990, Markowitz-Spence and colleagues[17] reported their experience with 510 children having M&T with 12% minor PRAE and 1.4% serious PRAE. In 2002, Hoffman and colleagues[18] reported a similar series of 3198 children with a 9% adverse-event rate and 1.9% major PRAE. All patients received inhalation induction with halothane, and therefore it is unclear whether the data are applicable to today's practice. Their data included 19/1005 cases of laryngospasm, airway obstruction, or significant desaturation.[18] These investigators and others report that significant comorbidities and concurrent illness, including acute or recent respiratory infection, predicted increase PRAE.[19–21] Both of these series represent data from a pediatric specialty center, and applicability to a general anesthesia practice should be made with caution; available data make it impossible to quantify whether risks are different in other settings. Because most M&T patients are less than 6 years of age, with peak incidence during infancy, an effort should be made to optimize the timing of the procedure and perioperative care to minimize risk.

Neurocognitive Outcomes

Although there is generally a focus on immediate risk in the perioperative period, a growing concern among parents relates to the possibility of adverse neurocognitive outcomes in very young children after anesthesia. In the last several years, the lay press has picked up on some animal and preliminary clinical studies that raise these questions. The initial animal studies involved chronic exposure of pregnant rats to subanesthetic concentrations of halothane, and showed behavioral abnormalities in the rat pups produced. Subsequent studies designed more specifically to study the effects on the brain have found neural degeneration, usually apoptosis (programmed cell death) in a diffuse pattern.[22] Multiple studies have shown this effect, although some have not. Almost all classes of anesthetic and sedative medications have been shown to have adverse effects in laboratory animals (volatile anesthetics, nitrous oxide, benzodiazepines, propofol, barbiturates, ketamine). Opioids generally show minimal effects, and there is some suggestion of mitigation of adverse effects of isoflurane by dexmedetomidine.[23] Some animal data suggest that the adverse effects on neuronal development occur to a more significant extent in the absence of a painful stimulus, and so would be more relevant to sedation/anesthesia for intensive care unit (ICU) care or prolonged procedures. There remains much to learn about the mechanism of the tissue changes seen in animals, as well as how the experimental factors apply to humans (developmental age, duration of exposure and dosages, animal species, and anesthetic management).[22]

Epidemiologic information from human studies has only recently become available. A study from the Mayo Clinic used an existing birth cohort for learning disability, and found that children who had received 2 or more anesthetics before the age of 4 years were at increased risk to develop learning disability.[24] This was a retrospective study and impossible to discern whether this was a causal association or whether anesthesia was a marker for other factors which might cause learning disability; the anesthetics involved also occurred in children born between 1976 and 1982, before the availability of current drugs or monitoring modalities. A retrospective pilot study found more behavioral disturbances in children who had anesthesia/urologic surgery before 24 months of age.[25] Most recently, a twin study showed no differences in learning ability in twin pairs in which 1 was exposed to anesthesia before the age of 3 and 1 was not; these investigators concluded that anesthesia at an early age is a marker of vulnerability for learning disability rather than a causative factor.[26] Several large prospective studies are being designed or are in process to attempt to find a more definitive answer to this question, but conclusive data are likely to be several years away. However, it seems that, if risk for postanesthetic neurocognitive dysfunction exists in human infants, it is greatest in the very premature infant, for prolonged anesthesia/sedation and possibly at very high doses, and in the absence of painful stimuli. All of this should be reassuring to parents of children coming for brief ambulatory procedures.

Preoperative Anxiety and Postoperative Agitation

Predicting and managing anxiety in the child and parents is an important part of creating a safe and pleasant anesthetic experience for the pediatric outpatient. Studies confirm some of our clinical impressions: risk factors for high anxiety at induction include younger age, behavioral problems with previous health care attendances, longer duration of procedure, having more than 5 previous hospital admissions, and anxious parents.[27,28] Kain and colleagues[29,30] have published on several aspects of this issue, showing that midazolam premedication or parental presence decreases anxiety and improves acceptance of a mask induction, with midazolam somewhat more effective than parental presence, but that parental presence does not add to the benefit of premedication. Detailed analysis shows that children who benefit most from parental presence are somewhat older, have lower levels of anxiety at baseline, and have calmer parents who value preparation and coping skills for medical situations.[28] A calm parent did benefit anxious children, whereas overly anxious parents did not confer any benefit. A comprehensive patient preparation program decreased anxiety and improved the quality of induction to a similar degree compared with midazolam, but patients in the preparation program also had decreased incidence of emergence delirium, lower requirements for opioids in the recovery area, and a shorter time to discharge compared with premedication or parent-present induction alone.[31]

Emergence agitation or delirium is a troublesome and poorly understood entity. It occurs most often in children aged 2 to 5 years, and an association has been found between preoperative anxiety in the child and parent, emergence delirium, and maladaptive behaviors (sleep disturbances, and so forth) after discharge.[32] Agitation is more common after volatile anesthetics than after propofol. Although the clinical opinion of many recovery nurses is that delirium is more common after the shorter-acting volatile anesthetics than after halothane or isoflurane, the literature does not strongly support this[33,34]; the occurrence in the early postoperative period with these shorter acting medications may lead to this impression. The rate of emergence does not seem to be responsible for the agitation itself, as comparison between sevoflurane and propofol showed that children emerged at the same rate but there was significantly higher agitation with sevoflurane.[35] Midazolam premedication does not seem to decrease the incidence of emergence agitation, whereas several studies have suggested that ketamine has a favorable effect, perhaps related to duration of sedation. Small doses of propofol or dexmedetomidine near the end of anesthesia have been effective in reducing agitation.[36,37]

In true emergence delirium, children are agitated, unaware of their surroundings, and inconsolable.[38] Several clinical scales have been developed to attempt to quantify the severity of emergence delirium. The clinician faced with such a child needs to determine whether pain is, or could be, a component, in which case analgesics should be titrated if there is no contraindication. For nonpainful procedures, or if pain is believed to have been treated adequately, sedative drugs may be administered. In a monitored setting with appropriate staffing, a small dose of propofol may be used. Some agitation is self-limited; the anesthesia team should assess the need for treatment, weighing the potential for patient injury against risks such as respiratory depression, nausea/vomiting, and delayed discharge.

CHALLENGES IN AMBULATORY ENT ANESTHESIA

As noted earlier, rates of mortality or significant morbidity are low in pediatric ambulatory anesthesia. ENT surgery is routinely cited as the highest-risk surgical area for pediatric outpatients,[3,11,12,39] and anesthetic-related decisions can affect length of stay (LOS), total costs, patient satisfaction, and secondary morbidity.[40,41] Favorable results are reported in many series of outpatient ENT surgery with careful preoperative screening and intraoperative management; Gravningsbräten and colleagues[42] reported an office-based practice of ENT surgery in 1126 children with 90 minutes or less of observation time with 1 reintubation for atelectasis (0.1% immediate complication rate).

Tonsillectomy with or without adenoidectomy confers some specific risks resulting from a shared airway, a surgical site in the pediatric airway, and sequelae from the necessary depth of anesthesia. Bleeding, pain control, oral intake, and oxygenation are the primary early complications following elective pediatric tonsillectomy.[43–45] Most sources support the safety of tonsillectomy as an outpatient procedure in older children who are ASA 1 to 2 at general hospitals,[19,41,44–46] but some literature reports an increase in complications among children less than 3 years of age.[47,48] Other reports recommend application of clinical indicators to recommend safe discharge, even in younger children.[19,48,49] Same-day discharge may be more costly than admission because of increased recovery-room LOS in children less than 3 years of age.[50] Children with obstructive sleep apnea (OSA) may require overnight monitoring, as is discussed in more detail later.

Despite the overall low morbidity associated with ambulatory tonsillectomy in children, there are important rare and ominous risks. In a 2008 review of closed claims in New York State, awards against anesthesiologists were higher than against surgeons ($5 million vs $839,650) and often involved airway complications.[51] The presenting indications for many children undergoing tonsillectomy may include comorbidities that increase risk, such as OSA, obesity, central sleep apnea, or syndromes associated with facial dysmorphisms (eg, trisomy 21 syndrome, CHARGE syndrome). Post-tonsillectomy hemorrhage (PTH) can result in death. Windfuhr and colleagues[52] reported survey data on lethal and near-lethal hemorrhage and concluded that delay in return to the operating room, repeated hemorrhage episodes, and aspiration of blood contributed to mortality. They also concluded that admission status did not affect morbidity. These investigators urge aggressive airway management to prevent the secondary sequelae of aspiration and inability to intubate when faced with significant PTH[53]; immediate volume resuscitation, and transfusion, if indicated, are also important components of care.

Direct vascular injuries can occur, most often during adenoidectomy. Significant vascular branches of the external carotid artery (tonsillectomy) or the facial and maxillary arteries (adenoidectomy) may be injured during surgery and may require proximal carotid control for repair. Other rare complications include atlantoaxial subluxation, mandible condyle fracture, infection, and eustachian tube injury.[54] Myringotomy and tube placement can also be complicated by significant vascular events (intrapetrous internal carotid artery puncture leading to pseudoaneurysm formation or arterial hemorrhage requiring endovascular intervention; profuse venous hemorrhage from injury to an anomalous jugular bulb[55]).

Surgical technique may affect the quality of recovery, with techniques such as radiofrequency ablation of tonsillar tissue having less pain than standard cold tonsillectomy; dissection with electrocautery seems to be associated with the highest degree of postoperative pain. Injection of local anesthesia after tonsillectomy seems to confer a modest reduction in pain, but systematic review suggests that equivalent results can be obtained by topical application using swabs.[56] Rare serious events are reported related to local anesthetic injection (cervical osteomyelitis, Horner syndrome, and airway obstruction due to vocal cord paralysis).

Anesthetic management can also affect the perioperative course. Intubation without muscle relaxant has become more common in pediatric anesthesia because of a lack of appropriately short nondepolarizing muscle relaxants; although adequate depth must be ensured to avoid laryngospasm, this obviates any possible emetogenic effects of reversal agents and the risk of residual muscle weakness.[57] A propofol-based technique offers advantages in minimizing PONV and may be associated with less bleeding during tonsillectomy.[58]

Supraglottic airways are used enthusiastically in tonsillectomy by some providers but are not widely embraced; providers in the United Kingdom report the use of an endotracheal tube in 79% of cases, despite the continued trend to avoid paralytics and the availability of reinforced supraglottic devices.[59] Conversely, a recent Norse report documented 1126 cases of office-based tonsillectomy and adenoidectomy with a supraglottic airway; 0.6% required conversion to endotracheal tube.[42] A letter in response from Xue and colleagues[40] presented a thorough argument for a reinforced supraglottic airway with specific attention to the implications of kinking and dislodgment from the intraoral surgical gag, the mechanical impediment tonsillar hyperplasia can create, and the risk of PRAE without adequate anesthetic depth. Clearly, safe airway management can include a spectrum of techniques, and further study is needed to confirm whether any specific technique is superior.

OSA

The implications of sleep-disordered breathing, OSA, or central sleep apnea are significant and can introduce predictable risk in the care of the pediatric patient. As Lerman[61] states in a 2009 review, there are important pathophysiological, anatomic, and pharmacological considerations and important distinctions between the child with this disease and the adult.[49] In children, this disease affects both genders equally, is associated with all body types, and is primarily a surgically treated entity; in adults, incidence in men exceeds women, obesity is often present, and nonsurgical interventions are first-line therapy (continuous positive airway pressure [CPAP], weight loss). Children and adults can suffer cardiovascular sequelae such as cor pulmonale and pulmonary hypertension. Cognitive impairment, learning disorders, and behavioral problems can complicate both populations.[60] Although children with OSA are recognized as being at increased risk perioperatively, the provider must consider whether extensive preoperative testing (echocardiogram, electrocardiogram, complete blood count, nocturnal somnography) will contribute to decision making about management or plans for admission.[61,62]

A review of adenotonsillectomy for OSA in young children found a significantly higher incidence of respiratory complications before the age of 3 years, and recommended routine admission for those patients.[63] In a survey of anesthesiologists in the United Kingdom, only 36% of respondents considered children for same day discharge after tonsillectomy with adenoidectomy, especially with a history of OSA.[59] Sanders and colleagues[64] documented increased complications after tonsillectomy with adenoidectomy in children with OSA versus those without, but found no effect on LOS.

Several articles have documented enhanced sensitivity to opioids in children with OSA. Brown and colleagues[65] calculated that sleep somnography can predict the risk of sensitivity to parenteral morphine: if the pulse oximetry nadir was less than 85%, a subject requires roughly 50% of the postoperative dose of morphine for analgesia. Hullett and colleagues[66] described equivalent analgesia with less respiratory depression using tramadol compared with morphine in nonobese children with OSA after tonsillectomy with adenoidectomy.

Obesity

Obesity is an important confounder for ambulatory risk. An estimated 16% of the children in the USA meet the definition of obesity. Tait and colleagues[67] reported that obese children are significantly more likely to present for surgery with complicating comorbidities such as asthma, reflux disease, type II diabetes mellitus, and OSA. Obesity increased the risk of complication during anesthesia including higher incidence of difficult mask ventilation, airway obstruction, and PRAE. Four-hundred and two of 1147 subjects underwent ENT surgery. The obese children had significantly less PONV (4.8% vs 16.8%).[67] Ye and colleagues[68] reported an 11.2% PRAE rate following tonsillectomy for OSA; obesity (as well as young age and higher apnea-hypopnea indexes) was identified as a significant risk factor. Nafiu and colleagues[62] correlated obesity with increased risks for PRAE after tonsillectomy, including intraoperative desaturation, difficult laryngoscopy, and airway obstruction in the operating room and the recovery room. A correlation between body mass index (BMI) and LOS was documented.

Outcomes after surgery may be variable. In an article comparing tonsillectomy with tonsillotomy, de la Chaux and colleagues[69] reported complete surgical cure of OSA (apnea-hypopnea index [AHI] 14.9 preoperative to 1.1 postoperative) with significantly less pain and lower PTH rates after CO_2 laser tonsillotomy. Shine and colleagues[70] found a less dramatic effect with tonsilloadenoidectomy in morbidly obese children with OSA; although all subjects benefited from surgery (AHI 20.7 preoperatively to 7.3 postoperatively), only 8 of 18 children no longer needed CPAP management after surgery. They were unable to assign variables for responders to nonresponders to surgery.[70] A 2009 meta-analysis further documented the incomplete benefit of surgery in obese children with OSA.[71] In 2004, Shatz[72] investigated the effectiveness of adenoidectomy in 24 infants with OSA symptoms and reported curative results with no morbidity.

PONV and Pain Management in Tonsillectomy

PONV can be troublesome to patients and families, and is known to delay discharge. General risk factors for PONV in children include age more than 3 years, duration of surgery more than 30 minutes, strabismus surgery, and history of postoperative vomiting in the child or PONV in the parents.[73] PONV after tonsillectomy occurs at rates as high as 50% to 89%, which is believed to be related to swallowed blood, pharyngeal stimulation, and the need for opioid analgesics. Blacoe and colleagues[74] reported their experience with unplanned admissions after ambulatory surgery and found PONV to be the most common reason for admission. General surgery cases were significantly more likely to result in PONV than ENT cases (24% vs 15%). Edler and colleagues[75] studied LOS data after tonsillectomy with adenoidectomy in 2008 and found PONV to be the most significant factor in delayed discharge readiness. Each PONV/retching episode increased LOS by 30 minutes (as did a single Spo_2<95%). Prophylaxis is generally recommended using 1 or more agents including dexamethasone, 5-hydroxytryptamine-3 (5-HT_3) antagonists, droperidol, or promethazine.[76] Dexamethasone, frequently used by the otolaryngologist to decrease swelling and improve oral intake, is also effective in reducing PONV.[77] The usual dose is 0.5 mg/kg, although a prospective dose-response study showed no difference within the range of 0.0625 to 1.0 mg/kg in the outcomes of pain, vomiting, time to oral intake, or voice change.[78] Dexamethasone at 0.5 mg/kg has recently been linked to increased PTH.[79]

Nonsteroidal antiinflammatory drugs (NSAIDS) are used infrequently in tonsillectomy in the United States because of concern for bleeding, but a Cochrane Review concluded that their use significantly decreased PONV without significant effect on PTH.[77] A recent survey of pediatric anesthetists in the United Kingdom revealed that 77% use NSAIDs in the perioperative care of children having tonsillectomy.[59] Acetaminophen is effective when effective loading doses are used, although rectal administration has a slow and variable onset; intravenous propacetamol (not available in the United States at the time of writing) may offer further advantage.[80] Other non-opioid analgesics such as ketamine, tramadol, and dexmedetomidine have shown efficacy and opioid-sparing effects in small studies. Although codeine is frequently prescribed for post-tonsillectomy analgesia, newer understanding of the pharmacogenetic basis of variability of codeine activity and reports of respiratory depression after discharge suggest that a uniformly safe and effective analgesic regimen has yet to be identified.[81]

Although no data currently document the variability in practice among American anesthesia providers, it seems prudent to recommend a tonsillectomy technique that uses dexamethasone and 5-HT_3 antagonists, minimizes opioid doses possibly (including a revisitation of the American acceptance of NSAID use), and uses propofol as a main component of the anesthetic. Cost analysis also supports the use of propofol and multimodal PONV prophylaxis.[82,83] Several groups have described low incidence of complication in outpatient tonsillectomy with appropriate patient selection and clinical protocols designed to manage postoperative pain and decrease PONV.[84,85] Unlike adult patients, there is a requirement to consider the ability of the parent or guardian to understand the discharge risks and instructions, proximity, and potential causes for delay should return to hospital become indicated, and the overall clinical assessment of the surgical team before discharge.[86] Each institution should consider these issues in formulating specific discharge criteria.

CREDENTIALING IN PEDIATRIC ANESTHESIA

Credentialing continues to be an area of controversy in pediatric anesthesia; which patient requires a pediatric anesthesiologist? What is the definition of a pediatric anesthesiologist? There is general consensus that high-risk procedures should not be undertaken on an infrequent basis, but specifics are less clear on what numbers are required for ongoing competency and what situations require specialized care. There is some evidence that adverse events are less common in the hands of experienced pediatric anesthesiologists.[87–89] The 1989 conclusion of the National Confidential Enquiry into Perioperative Deaths recommended that surgeons and anesthetists in the United Kingdom not undertake occasional pediatric practice[90]; in the United Kingdom, specialists care for children younger than 5 years of age, and in Scandinavia, the age is 2 years.

Training programs are accredited by the Accreditation Council for Graduate Medical Education (ACGME); pediatric anesthesia was the first operating room (OR) subspecialty of anesthesiology to have accreditation for fellowship training, beginning in 1997. Anesthesiologists receive board certification through the American Board of Anesthesiology (ABA); at present, subspecialty board certification does not exist for any OR subspecialty of anesthesiology, although it does exist for Pain Management and Critical Care. The Society for Pediatric Anesthesia has proposed "subspecialty certification in advanced pediatric anesthesiology" as part of a tiered system to provide excellent care to high-risk pediatric patients, but, at the time of writing, this proposal remains with the Board of Directors of the ABA.

Until formal requirements, if any, are developed for pediatric anesthesia care, institutions and anesthesiologists should consider their individual practice settings and competencies, and guidelines from several professional organizations. The American Academy of Pediatrics (AAP) Section on Anesthesiology has published *Guidelines for the Pediatric Perioperative Anesthesia Environment*, which suggest that each facility define the spectrum of pediatric patients and cases for which it will provide care, and the number of cases of each required for the facility to maintain its competence. These guidelines also suggest that the institution define which pediatric patients are considered to be at increased risk, and that their anesthesia care should be provided by anesthesiologists who are fellowship trained in pediatric anesthesia or have equivalent experience. Similar recommendations have been made by the ASA and the Society for Pediatric Anesthesia. Some states have also instituted or considered requirements to have anesthesiologists caring for children (of some defined age) meet certain minimal case numbers. The AAP guidelines also include recommendations for appropriately sized airway and monitoring equipment, child-friendly spaces including separate preoperative area for children/families, and age-specific competencies and resuscitation skills for OR and recovery staff.

SUMMARY

Careful patient screening and selection help to minimize the risk of adverse outcomes in pediatric ambulatory surgery, and the overall rates of serious morbidity in the United States remain low. Errors in medication doses and effects, airway management, malfunctioning equipment or alarms, distraction, inexperience, or other human-related issues contribute to many preventable events. The unique physiologic, anatomic, and pharmacologic state of children of various ages challenges the anesthesia provider to remain vigilant during surgery; knowledge of potential complications in common pediatric ENT procedures may help avoid risk. Each institution should continuously review admission criteria, staffing decisions, postoperative management resources, and quality-improvement methods to moderate risk and respond to crises.

REFERENCES

1. Cullen KA, Hall MJ, Golosinskiy A. Ambulatory surgery in the United States, 2006. Natl Health Stat Report 2009;11:1–25.
2. Tiret L, Nivoche Y, Hatton F, et al. Complications related to anaesthesia in infants and children. A prospective survey of 40240 anaesthetics. Br J Anaesth 1988; 61(3):263–9.
3. Murat I, Constant I, Maud'huy H. Perioperative anaesthetic morbidity in children: a database of 24,165 anaesthetics over a 30-month period. Paediatr Anaesth 2004;14(2):158–66.
4. Fleisher LA, Pasternak LR, Lyles A. A novel index of elevated risk of inpatient hospital admission immediately following outpatient surgery. Arch Surg 2007; 142(3):263–8.
5. D'Eramo EM, Bookless SJ, Howard JB. Adverse events with outpatient anesthesia in Massachusetts. J Oral Maxillofac Surg 2003;61(7):793–800 [discussion: 800].
6. Patel RI, Hannallah RS. Anesthetic complications following pediatric ambulatory surgery: a 3-yr study. Anesthesiology 1988;69(6):1009–12.
7. D'Errico C, Voepel-Lewis TD, Siewert M, et al. Prolonged recovery stay and unplanned admission of the pediatric surgical outpatient: an observational study. J Clin Anesth 1998;10(6):482–7.
8. Awad IT, Moore M, Rushe C, et al. Unplanned hospital admission in children undergoing day-case surgery. Eur J Anaesthesiol 2004;21(5):379–83.
9. Morray JP, Geiduschek JM, Caplan RA, et al. A comparison of pediatric and adult anesthesia closed malpractice claims. Anesthesiology 1993;78(3):461–7.
10. Jimenez N, Posner KL, Cheney FW, et al. An update on pediatric anesthesia liability: a closed claims analysis. Anesth Analg 2007;104(1):147–53.
11. Morray JP, Geiduschek JM, Ramamoorthy C, et al. Anesthesia-related cardiac arrest in children: initial findings of the Pediatric Perioperative Cardiac Arrest (POCA) Registry. Anesthesiology 2000;93(1):6–14.
12. Bhananker SM, Ramamoorthy C, Geiduschek JM, et al. Anesthesia-related cardiac arrest in children: update from the Pediatric Perioperative Cardiac Arrest Registry. Anesth Analg 2007;105(2):344–50.
13. Larach MG, Rosenberg H, Gronert GA, et al. Hyperkalemic cardiac arrest during anesthesia in infants and children with occult myopathies. Clin Pediatr (Phila) 1997;36(1):9–16.
14. Burgoyne LL, Anghelescu DL. Intervention steps for treating laryngospasm in pediatric patients. Paediatr Anaesth 2008;18(4):297–302.
15. Mamie C, Habre W, Delhumeau C, et al. Incidence and risk factors of perioperative respiratory adverse events in children undergoing elective surgery. Paediatr Anaesth 2004;14(3):218–24.
16. Pereira MB, Pereira DR, Costa SS. Tympanostomy tube sequelae in children with otitis media with effusion: a three-year follow-up study. Braz J Otorhinolaryngol 2005;71(4):415–20.

17. Markowitz-Spence L, Brodsky L, Syed N, et al. Anesthetic complications of tympanotomy tube placement in children. Arch Otolaryngol Head Neck Surg 1990;116(7):809–12.
18. Hoffmann KK, Thompson GK, Burke BL, et al. Anesthetic complications of tympanostomy tube placement in children. Arch Otolaryngol Head Neck Surg 2002;128(9):1040–3.
19. Postma DS, Folsom F. The case for an outpatient "approach" for all pediatric tonsillectomies and/or adenoidectomies: a 4-year review of 1419 cases at a community hospital. Otolaryngol Head Neck Surg 2002;127(1):101–8.
20. Tait AR, Malviya S. Anesthesia for the child with an upper respiratory tract infection: still a dilemma? Anesth Analg 2005;100(1):59–65.
21. Tait AR, Malviya S, Voepel-Lewis T, et al. Risk factors for perioperative adverse respiratory events in children with upper respiratory tract infections. Anesthesiology 2001;95(2):299–306.
22. Istaphanous GK, Loepke AW. General anesthetics and the developing brain. Curr Opin Anaesthesiol 2009;22(3):368–73.
23. Sanders RD, Xu J, Shu Y, et al. Dexmedetomidine attenuates isoflurane-induced neurocognitive impairment in neonatal rats. Anesthesiology 2009;110(5):1077–85.
24. Wilder RT, Flick RP, Sprung J, et al. Early exposure to anesthesia and learning disabilities in a population-based birth cohort. Anesthesiology 2009;110(4):796–804.
25. Kalkman CJ, Peelen L, Moons KG, et al. Behavior and development in children and age at the time of first anesthetic exposure. Anesthesiology 2009;110(4):805–12.
26. Bartels M, Althoff RR, Boomsma DI. Anesthesia and cognitive performance in children: no evidence for a causal relationship. Twin Res Hum Genet 2009;12(3):246–53.
27. Davidson AJ, Shrivastava PP, Jamsen K, et al. Risk factors for anxiety at induction of anesthesia in children: a prospective cohort study. Paediatr Anaesth 2006;16(9):919–27.
28. Kain ZN, Mayes LC, Caldwell-Andrews AA, et al. Predicting which children benefit most from parental presence during induction of anesthesia. Paediatr Anaesth 2006;16(6):627–34.
29. Kain ZN, Mayes LC, Wang SM, et al. Parental presence during induction of anesthesia versus sedative premedication: which intervention is more effective? Anesthesiology 1998;89(5):1147–56.
30. Kain ZN, Mayes LC, Wang SM, et al. Parental presence and a sedative premedicant for children undergoing surgery: a hierarchical study. Anesthesiology 2000;92(4):939–46.
31. Kain ZN, Caldwell-Andrews AA, Mayes LC, et al. Family-centered preparation for surgery improves perioperative outcomes in children: a randomized controlled trial. Anesthesiology 2007;106(1):65–74.
32. Kain ZN, Caldwell-Andrews AA, Maranets I, et al. Preoperative anxiety and emergence delirium and postoperative maladaptive behaviors. Anesth Analg 2004;99(6):1648–54.
33. Meyer RR, Munster P, Werner C, et al. Isoflurane is associated with a similar incidence of emergence agitation/delirium as sevoflurane in young children–a randomized controlled study. Paediatr Anaesth 2007;17(1):56–60.
34. Kain ZN, Caldwell-Andrews AA, Weinberg ME, et al. Sevoflurane versus halothane: postoperative maladaptive behavioral changes: a randomized, controlled trial. Anesthesiology 2005;102(4):720–6.

35. Cohen IT, Finkel JC, Hannallah RS, et al. Rapid emergence does not explain agitation following sevoflurane anaesthesia in infants and children: a comparison with propofol. Paediatr Anaesth 2003;13(1):63–7.
36. Abu-Shahwan I. Effect of propofol on emergence behavior in children after sevoflurane general anesthesia. Paediatr Anaesth 2008;18(1):55–9.
37. Isik B, Arslan M, Tunga AD, et al. Dexmedetomidine decreases emergence agitation in pediatric patients after sevoflurane anesthesia without surgery. Paediatr Anaesth 2006;16(7):748–53.
38. Vlajkovic GP, Sindjelic RP. Emergence delirium in children: many questions, few answers. Anesth Analg 2007;104(1):84–91.
39. Jones S, Raffles A. Pediatric Peri-Operative Cardiac Arrest (POCA) Registry. Qual Saf Health Care 2002;11(3):210–1.
40. Xue FS, Li TZ, Liao X. Safe use of a laryngeal mask airway in children undergoing a tonsillectomy. Acta Anaesthesiol Scand 2009;53(5):684–5 [author reply: 686].
41. Mills N, Anderson BJ, Barber C, et al. Day stay pediatric tonsillectomy–a safe procedure. Int J Pediatr Otorhinolaryngol 2004;68(11):1367–73.
42. Gravningsbräten R, Nicklasson B, Raeder J. Safety of laryngeal mask airway and short-stay practice in office-based adenotonsillectomy. Acta Anaesthesiol Scand 2009;53(2):218–22.
43. Werle AH, Nicklaus PJ, Kirse DJ, et al. A retrospective study of tonsillectomy in the under 2-year-old child: indications, perioperative management, and complications. Int J Pediatr Otorhinolaryngol 2003;67(5):453–60.
44. Leong AC, Davis JP. Morbidity after adenotonsillectomy for paediatric obstructive sleep apnoea syndrome: waking up to a pragmatic approach. J Laryngol Otol 2007;121(9):809–17.
45. Brown KA, Morin I, Hickey C, et al. Urgent adenotonsillectomy: an analysis of risk factors associated with postoperative respiratory morbidity. Anesthesiology 2003; 99(3):586–95.
46. Brigger MT, Brietzke SE. Outpatient tonsillectomy in children: a systematic review. Otolaryngol Head Neck Surg 2006;135(1):1–7.
47. Ross AT, Kazahaya K, Tom LW. Revisiting outpatient tonsillectomy in young children. Otolaryngol Head Neck Surg 2003;128(3):326–31.
48. Mitchell RB, Pereira KD, Friedman NR, et al. Outpatient adenotonsillectomy. Is it safe in children younger than 3 years? Arch Otolaryngol Head Neck Surg 1997; 123(7):681–3.
49. Lalakea ML, Marquez-Biggs I, Messner AH. Safety of pediatric short-stay tonsillectomy. Arch Otolaryngol Head Neck Surg 1999;125(7):749–52.
50. Shapiro NL, Seid AB, Pransky SM, et al. Adenotonsillectomy in the very young patient: cost analysis of two methods of postoperative care. Int J Pediatr Otorhinolaryngol 1999;48(2):109–15.
51. Morris LG, Lieberman SM, Reitzen SD, et al. Characteristics and outcomes of malpractice claims after tonsillectomy. Otolaryngol Head Neck Surg 2008; 138(3):315–20.
52. Windfuhr JP, Schloendorff G, Baburi D, et al. Lethal outcome of post-tonsillectomy hemorrhage. Eur Arch Otorhinolaryngol 2008;265(12):1527–34.
53. Windfuhr JP, Schloendorff G, Sesterhenn AM, et al. A devastating outcome after adenoidectomy and tonsillectomy: ideas for improved prevention and management. Otolaryngol Head Neck Surg 2009;140(2):191–6.
54. Randall DA, Hoffer ME. Complications of tonsillectomy and adenoidectomy. Otolaryngol Head Neck Surg 1998;118(1):61–8.

55. Brodish BN, Woolley AL. Major vascular injuries in children undergoing myringotomy for tube placement. Am J Otolaryngol 1999;20(1):46–50.
56. Grainger J, Saravanappa N. Local anaesthetic for post-tonsillectomy pain: a systematic review and meta-analysis. Clin Otolaryngol 2008;33(5):411–9.
57. Morton NS. Tracheal intubation without neuromuscular blocking drugs in children. Paediatr Anaesth 2009;19(3):199–201.
58. Okuyucu S, Inanoglu K, Akkurt CO, et al. The effect of anesthetic agents on perioperative bleeding during tonsillectomy: propofol-based versus desflurane-based anesthesia. Otolaryngol Head Neck Surg 2008;138(2):158–61.
59. Allford M, Guruswamy V. A national survey of the anesthetic management of tonsillectomy surgery in children. Paediatr Anaesth 2009;19(2):145–52.
60. Bandla P, Brooks LJ, Trimarchi T, et al. Obstructive sleep apnea syndrome in children. Anesthesiol Clin North America 2005;23(3):535–49, viii.
61. Lerman J. A disquisition on sleep-disordered breathing in children. Paediatr Anaesth 2009;19(Suppl 1):100–8.
62. Nafiu OO, Green GE, Walton S, et al. Obesity and risk of peri-operative complications in children presenting for adenotonsillectomy. Int J Pediatr Otorhinolaryngol 2009;73(1):89–95.
63. Statham MM, Elluru RG, Buncher R, et al. Adenotonsillectomy for obstructive sleep apnea syndrome in young children: prevalence of pulmonary complications. Arch Otolaryngol Head Neck Surg 2006;132(5):476–80.
64. Sanders JC, King MA, Mitchell RB, et al. Perioperative complications of adenotonsillectomy in children with obstructive sleep apnea syndrome. Anesth Analg 2006;103(5):1115–21.
65. Brown KA, Laferriere A, Lakheeram I, et al. Recurrent hypoxemia in children is associated with increased analgesic sensitivity to opiates. Anesthesiology 2006;105(4):665–9.
66. Hullett BJ, Chambers NA, Pascoe EM, et al. Tramadol vs morphine during adenotonsillectomy for obstructive sleep apnea in children. Paediatr Anaesth 2006;16(6):648–53.
67. Tait AR, Voepel-Lewis T, Burke C, et al. Incidence and risk factors for perioperative adverse respiratory events in children who are obese. Anesthesiology 2008;108(3):375–80.
68. Ye J, Liu H, Zhang G, et al. Postoperative respiratory complications of adenotonsillectomy for obstructive sleep apnea syndrome in older children: prevalence, risk factors, and impact on clinical outcome. J Otolaryngol Head Neck Surg 2009;38(1):49–58.
69. de la Chaux R, Klemens C, Patscheider M, et al. Tonsillotomy in the treatment of obstructive sleep apnea syndrome in children: polysomnographic results. Int J Pediatr Otorhinolaryngol 2008;72(9):1411–7.
70. Shine NP, Lannigan FJ, Coates HL, et al. Adenotonsillectomy for obstructive sleep apnea in obese children: effects on respiratory parameters and clinical outcome. Arch Otolaryngol Head Neck Surg 2006;132(10):1123–7.
71. Costa DJ, Mitchell R. Adenotonsillectomy for obstructive sleep apnea in obese children: a meta-analysis. Otolaryngol Head Neck Surg 2009;140(4):455–60.
72. Shatz A. Indications and outcomes of adenoidectomy in infancy. Ann Otol Rhinol Laryngol 2004;113(10):835–8.
73. Eberhart LH, Geldner G, Kranke P, et al. The development and validation of a risk score to predict the probability of postoperative vomiting in pediatric patients. Anesth Analg 2004;99(6):1630–7.

74. Blacoe DA, Cunning E, Bell G. Paediatric day-case surgery: an audit of unplanned hospital admission. Anaesthesia 2008;63(6):610–5.
75. Edler AA, Mariano ER, Golianu B, et al. An analysis of factors influencing postanesthesia recovery after pediatric ambulatory tonsillectomy and adenoidectomy. Anesth Analg 2007;104(4):784–9.
76. Gan TJ, Meyer T, Apfel CC, et al. Consensus guidelines for managing postoperative nausea and vomiting. Anesth Analg 2003;97(1):62–71.
77. Cardwell M, Siviter G, Smith A. Non-steroidal anti-inflammatory drugs and perioperative bleeding in paediatric tonsillectomy. Cochrane Database Syst Rev 2005;(2):CD003591.
78. Kim MS, Cote CJ, Cristoloveanu C, et al. There is no dose-escalation response to dexamethasone (0.0625–1.0 mg/kg) in pediatric tonsillectomy or adenotonsillectomy patients for preventing vomiting, reducing pain, shortening time to first liquid intake, or the incidence of voice change. Anesth Analg 2007;104(5):1052–8.
79. Czarnetzki C, Elia N, Lysakowski C, et al. Dexamethasone and risk of nausea and vomiting and postoperative bleeding after tonsillectomy in children: a randomized trial. JAMA 2008;300(22):2621–30.
80. Alhashemi JA, Daghistani MF. Effects of intraoperative i.v. acetaminophen vs i.m. meperidine on post-tonsillectomy pain in children. Br J Anaesth 2006;96(6):790–5.
81. Ciszkowski C, Madadi P, Phillips MS, et al. Codeine, ultrarapid-metabolism genotype, and postoperative death. N Engl J Med 2009;361(8):827–8.
82. Elliott RA, Payne K, Moore JK, et al. Which anaesthetic agents are cost-effective in day surgery? Literature review, national survey of practice and randomised controlled trial. Health Technol Assess 2002;6(30):1–264.
83. Elliott RA, Payne K, Moore JK, et al. Clinical and economic choices in anaesthesia for day surgery: a prospective randomised controlled trial. Anaesthesia 2003;58(5):412–21.
84. Ewah BN, Robb PJ, Raw M. Postoperative pain, nausea and vomiting following paediatric day-case tonsillectomy. Anaesthesia 2006;61(2):116–22.
85. White MC, Nolan JA. An evaluation of pain and postoperative nausea and vomiting following the introduction of guidelines for tonsillectomy. Paediatr Anaesth 2005;15(8):683–8.
86. Kanerva M, Tarkkila P, Pitkaranta A. Day-case tonsillectomy in children: parental attitudes and consultation rates. Int J Pediatr Otorhinolaryngol 2003;67(7):777–84.
87. Brennan LJ. Modern day-case anaesthesia for children. Br J Anaesth 1999;83(1):91–103.
88. Atwell JD, Spargo PM. The provision of safe surgery for children. Arch Dis Child 1992;67(3):345–9.
89. Hackel A, Badgwell JM, Binding RR, et al. Guidelines for the pediatric perioperative anesthesia environment. American Academy of Pediatrics. Section on Anesthesiology. Pediatrics 1999;103(2):512–5.
90. Campling EA, Devlin HB, Lunn JN. The report of the national confidential enquiry into perioperative deaths 1989. London: Her Majesty's Stationary Office; 1989.

Management by Outcomes: Efficiency and Operational Success in the Ambulatory Surgery Center

Douglas G. Merrill, MD, MBA[a,*], John J. Laur, MD, MS[b]

KEYWORDS

- Ambulatory surgery center • Quality of care
- Systems improvement • Clinical outcome

Quality of care and service in health care can benefit from the use of algorithm-driven care (standard work) that integrates literature assessment and analysis of local outcome and process data to eliminate unnecessary variation that causes error and waste.[1–6] Effective management of an ambulatory surgery center requires that leadership emphasize constant improvement in the processes of care to achieve maximum patient safety and satisfaction, delivered with highest efficiency. Such work is only effective if staff and physicians understand the value of such improvement to patient and family experiences, and if they believe there is a gap between current operations and the ideal. Therefore, leadership needs a method to obtain, evaluate, and share process and outcome measurements in an open, objective, and clear manner.

Measurement and explication of outcomes of operational workflow are of value in directing process improvement efforts in a variety of industries, including health care.[7–10] The seemingly ubiquitous increase in operational improvement models (Six

---

Disclosure: Both authors are members of SAMBA, and DGM is a member of the Board of Directors for SAMBA and the AQI.
Excel is a registered trademark of the Microsoft Corporation.
Toyota Production System (TPS) is a registered trademark of the Toyota Motor Manufacturing Corporation.
The Six Sigma Management System is a registered trademark of Motorola Inc.

[a] Outpatient Surgery, Dartmouth-Hitchcock Medical Center, One Medical Center Way, Lebanon, NH 03753, USA
[b] Ambulatory Surgery, University of Iowa Hospitals and Clinics, 200 Hawkins Drive, 6JCP, Iowa City, IA 52240, USA
* Corresponding author.
E-mail address: douglas.g.merrill@hitchcock.org

Anesthesiology Clin 28 (2010) 329–351
doi:10.1016/j.anclin.2010.02.012 **anesthesiology.theclinics.com**
1932-2275/10/$ – see front matter

Sigma, Toyota Production System, and so forth) reflects their emphasis on reducing waste in workflow and eliciting best practices, efforts that focus on efficient and effective operations. Such activity should be natural for health care providers, as these efforts are an outgrowth of the scientific method, that is, observing, constructing a theory, and gathering data to determine the validity of that theory.[11] Nonetheless, management of sometimes widely disparate attitudes and beliefs among health care providers is often difficult. This can be facilitated and care improved by basing facility and individual practice changes on objective, comparative outcomes assessments and applying "find and implement the best" strategies.[12–14] As James and colleagues[12] note in their seminal work on quality improvement (p. 9): "Two principles are involved in quality improvement: process operators use measurement tools to (1) eliminate inappropriate variation (usually in care process steps) then (2) document continuous improvement (usually in outcomes). 'Find and implement the best' redirects energy from finding fault (and the natural defensive response that it provokes) to finding solutions. It creates a much more positive atmosphere within which to measure, criticize, and improve health care processes."

To garner the commitment to continuing improvement that is required to achieve the highest quality, management must actively integrate all staff and surgeons into creating and maintaining the means of collecting accurate data. To maintain the credibility of the data and management's assignation of importance to it, the assessment and presentation of that data should be routine and repetitive, objectively spotlighting quality gaps and recognizing improvement. A direct link between the present data and the focus of future improvement efforts is necessary to engage the staff in operational improvements.

The attachment of financial remuneration to improved outcomes for an entire center and for the various subunits (administration, postanesthesia care unit [PACU], preoperative, operating room, central supply, and so forth), as well as for individual staff and surgeons can be an effective means of accomplishing steady and significant quality improvement.

Process improvement may be achieved by simple measurement alone (the Hawthorne effect). However, as shown in this article, the authors have successfully used the implementation of regular measurement and open discussion of patients' clinical outcomes and other operational metrics to focus active systems improvement projects in ambulatory surgery centers, with excellent results.

WHAT SHOULD BE MEASURED?

Clinical, operational, and financial metrics are all critical to the success of an ambulatory surgery center, and therefore management should measure all 3 domains and share the results with staff and surgeons. Clinical safety tops patient, family, and surgeon concerns, but postoperative nausea and vomiting (PONV) is as important as major injury to many patients, as is pain management.[15,16] Also, no patient, family, or surgeon will be satisfied if their time spent at the center was 4 hours if they were promised it be only 2 hours, so operational process evaluation (eg, turnover, case cart readiness, and so forth) is also important to customer satisfaction.

The center must operate in a manner that ensures financial success. Whether surgeon-investor, hospital, or corporate ownership is the selected model, most owners expect an ambulatory surgery facility to be a source of considerable income. In the current economic environment, a center must be able to replace current equipment and instruments but also be willing to expend capital on new technology. Providing proof to ownership that staff and leadership are doing all they can to conserve and improve profit is another significant value of the quality improvement process. The authors have found certain metrics to be most valuable in process improvement and they are provided in Appendix 2 (Box 1 lists appropriate financial measures, Box 2 lists operational process measures, and Box 3 contains clinical measures).

WHO SHOULD CHOOSE THE METRICS?

We highly recommend that the choice of metrics be a function of a facility committee of staff, anesthesia providers, surgeons, and management. This use of a group of stakeholders is an important way to involve staff and surgeons in the process improvement program. However, implementation of guidelines requires more than management's commitment. It requires the dedication of all team members and gaining that interest can be a significant challenge.[17] A committee charged to manage the data process not only ensures that the program is measuring the processes and outcomes that are important to a particular facility but also provides leadership for the rest of the staff and surgeons to advance change initiatives that arise from these measurements. Representatives of each of the staffed areas (PACU, operating room, administration, business office) should be solicited to serve on the committee. It has been of value in some instances to include lay representation (a former patient at the facility is an ideal participant) in this process.

HOW SHOULD THE MEASUREMENT BE DONE?

Ideally, all data would be obtained via electronic records, through an automated download of individual data points, thereby distancing practitioners from the measurement and providing objectivity. Of course, any data that is actively keyed in by personnel is subject to bias and error. For instance, a radiofrequency identification (RFID) system that automatically logs a patient into a room by reading a chip embedded in the wristband will generate more objective turnover data than will derive from an electronic health record (EHR) that requires a nurse to physically enter the time of arrival. However, the EHR produces fewer errors than a system wherein the staff writes the time on paper and later a clerk keys that information into a database.

Nonetheless, because electronic health records still do not represent most ambulatory surgery record keeping systems, use of a paper entry that is later translated into a simple database will suffice. The authors have successfully used a single sheet of paper (patient diary; see Appendix 2) as a data collection tool that is attached to the patient's chart and follows the patient throughout the day. Each segment of the diary is used by the appropriate team member to record only the few events that are owned by that area (ie, the preoperative admission clerk, the preoperative nurse, the anesthesia team, the operating room nurse, the PACU nurse, and the call-back clerk). No single staff member has more than a few entries to record, an important point because the diary represents extra work, as most of the data are also required to be entered into the medical record (the diary is a quality improvement document and should not stay with the patient's record once discharge occurs).

HOW DO YOU SHARE THE DATA?

Once collected, data on the processes and outcomes of care are only useful when synthesized into clear reports and shared with all staff and practitioners. A significant value of this data distribution is the sense of local control that it engenders among the staff and surgeons of a small unit (or subunit, such as the eye service team). Staff members can assess trends in their own area and quickly see what solutions (or people) are working and workable, rather than waiting for leadership to declare an identified best way. To facilitate discussion, we have posted data to help staff and physicians evaluate their own and the whole unit's performance over time. Only if they see the need for a redesign, via repeated examination of outcomes, will they support (sometimes radical) redesign. This approach to improved practice has proven to be of value in health care when applied over a prolonged period and in conjunction with local champions.[18]

If you operate within a large organization, you will also have to convince middle management and senior leadership that your group has assessed the data and correctly determined appropriate responses. If your staff are accustomed to viewing all the data regularly, with nothing held back, it will be easier for them to help you redesign your systems and to convince your internal and external managers that you are moving in the right direction. As Kotter[19] notes, leadership must "align information and personnel systems to the vision" to achieve effective and long-term change. This approach of full disclosure and emphasis on self-directed improvement has convinced leadership and external accrediting bodies that our dedication to quality improvement is sincere and effective.

Typically, we have posted monthly and cumulative data (all data associated with each physician and staff, by name and as amalgamated information; eg, by service line) in the staff lounge or the PACU medication room. The chosen areas should be secure from the public, but open to all employees. In addition, each employee and practitioner can receive his or her own data via personal e-mail, and comparisons with the averages for his or her risk group on a monthly or quarterly basis. We also distribute this information to senior management or owners with the notation that our unit's teams also reviewed it and that these data will serve to focus our quality improvement efforts. We set aside time at each weekly all-staff meeting to discuss some aspect of our clinical, operational, or financial performance.

ARE THERE VALID BENCHMARKS WITH WHICH TO COMPARE AN INDIVIDUAL CENTER AND IS THAT COMPARISON OF ANY VALUE?

National benchmarks for performance in ambulatory surgery centers are not readily available, reliable, or risk-adjusted. Various private ambulatory surgery center companies have their own data collections and frequently a corporate quality assurance nurse reports to the individual facilities about their performance comparisons within the company. However, these data collection systems are hampered by variations in employee self-reporting, the terminology and dictionary differences between facilities (eg, what do you mean by "severe" nausea?), and are not usually driven by local leadership, making them less effective as a means to focus improvement strategies. Thus, their applicability to individual centers is also inconsistent and the unit and subunit employees may discount the value of such data, particularly if there is no direct effect on bonuses or increases. Of course, should a financial impact exist, there is the risk that self-reporting will be prejudiced, although such risk exists for any system where the provider data are shared with peers.

Outside corporate and hospital systems, national data registries are gaining in importance. The members of the Ambulatory Surgery Center Association (ASC, http://www.ascassociation.org/medicarequalityreporting/) can participate voluntarily in a reporting and data collection process run by that organization. However, no on-site auditing occurs and there is no way to ensure that the data submitted are accurate or comparable. This is also true for the University Hospitals Consortium (UHC) database, another members-only registry that attempts to risk adjust by facility size and practice type, but which also has no auditing function. The Society for Ambulatory Anesthesia (SAMBA) and the Anesthesia Quality Institute (AQI) are creating registries that, if successful, would be of value to individual practitioners, ASCs, hospitals, and office practices as a means of benchmarking. However, like the other registries, these may not provide much assurance of accuracy if some method of auditing is not adopted as part of their system.

With the advancement of health care reform legislation that (currently) recommends or requires the use of data registries by health care providers, the quality of and participation in national registries may improve, providing a better set of national benchmarks. At this point, however, the best benchmarks available to ambulatory practices are historical comparisons within their own units, which would ideally show steady progressive improvement.

MAKING USE OF THE DATA: CREATING A STANDARD PRACTICE

How Do You Know the Standard Practice that You Design is a Best Practice?

Business school libraries are replete with books and entire institutions exist to describe and foster creation of the best approaches to health care.[20] Consequently, this article concentrates on practical methods of value to outpatient surgery and anesthesia providers that can be implemented with relative ease in any size facility (office, freestanding ambulatory surgery center, or hospital outpatient department). System-wide approbation and implementation of best practices are a means by which institutions can avoid allowing caregivers to provide care to patients based on anecdotal, unproven opinions or beliefs that may induce quality defects and error. Error reduction and safety are the sine qua non of quality. Unnecessary variation in care based on anecdotal experience is often the cause for error and unnecessary expense.[21]

A common pathway for generating a best practice is through systematic review of published health care processes. The actual process of such review is time-consuming and difficult for an individual to complete and often requires a team of people to carry out.

The task of identification and dissemination of best practice is daunting as evidence is usually open to interpretation and anecdotal belief systems that are jeopardized by such evidence are strong barriers. It has been demonstrated that a 17-year time span is necessary to allow new best practice information derived from clinical trials and basic science research to be disseminated and absorbed into clinical practice. Even then, such new practice is adopted by inhomogeneous groups of practitioners and often not widely implemented.[22] When data are eventually synthesized into new practice guidelines, it may not be the best health care for all groups of patients. Woolf and colleagues[23] describe the difficulty in discerning the difference between good medical care and published practice guidelines. Therefore, it is critical to review local outcomes and synthesize the national experience with that of local practitioners (accurately measured) when creating evidence-based guidelines for a local practice. The use of both sources diminishes the negative impact of the bias of each.[24]

Nonetheless, if a new facility does not have sufficient outcome data, a standard practice committee has a good starting point for creation of clinical care algorithms using various professional societies' guidelines and a review of the literature. The Cochrane Collaboration, the US Agency for Healthcare Research and Quality (AHRQ), the UK National Institute for Health and Clinical Excellence (NICE), and the multinational-minded World Health Organization (WHO), as well as several professional societies that publish guidelines of care (eg, the American Society of

Anesthesiologists [ASA], SAMBA, the Society of Pediatric Anesthesia [SPA], and the American Society of Regional Anesthesia and Pain Medicine [ASRA]) all provide reviews or meta-analyses that may prove useful starting points for the committee's work. The committee then collects evidence from peer-reviewed literature, sorts, categorizes, consolidates, and assesses it, using an approved method of evidence-based medicine grading.[25] Once graded, the evidence can be incorporated into the ensuing algorithm, with footnotes for critical steps to explicate the sources of decision point recommendations. A draft of the algorithm is disseminated to the providers and staff for review and comment before implementation. Thereafter, we have laminated the algorithms and attached them to the germane workstations as well as published them by e-mail (**Figs. 1–3**).

Once an algorithm is final, process and outcome metrics are chosen that will best reflect a practitioner's adherence to the chosen practice pattern and consequent outcomes. Results are monitored and reported at appropriate time intervals. The results usually yield 4 groups: those caregivers who follow the algorithms and whose outcomes improve, those caregivers who follow the algorithms with no improvement in outcomes, those practitioners who do not follow the algorithms but whose outcomes are better than average, and those practitioners who ignore the algorithms and practice anecdotal care with poor outcomes. If the second group outweighs the first, then the best practice must be reexamined and amended, then measured again. If the third group is significant in number, or even if one practitioner has stellar outcomes using an anecdotal approach, then his or her technique should be assessed for possible use as a better best practice. If the fourth situation is encountered (refusal to follow the algorithm with poorer than average outcomes), the medical director of the facility should meet individually with the practitioner and review the literature and other supporting evidence for the algorithm. He or she should urge the practitioner to convert his or her practice to meet the tenets of the algorithms to improve outcomes. Depending on the frequency and volume of that provider's work at the facility, 30 to 90 days further measurement should be used to assess the result. If the practitioner still will not alter his or her behavior, then it is reasonable to recommend a reduction in privileges. It is always important to remind practitioners that practice in the facility is reserved for those caregivers whose goals are aligned with those of the patient, family,

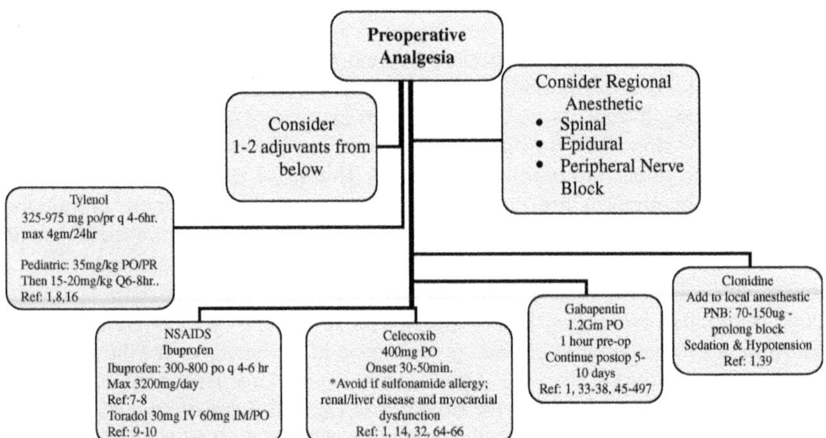

Fig. 1. Algorithm for preoperative best practice regarding multimodal analgesia.

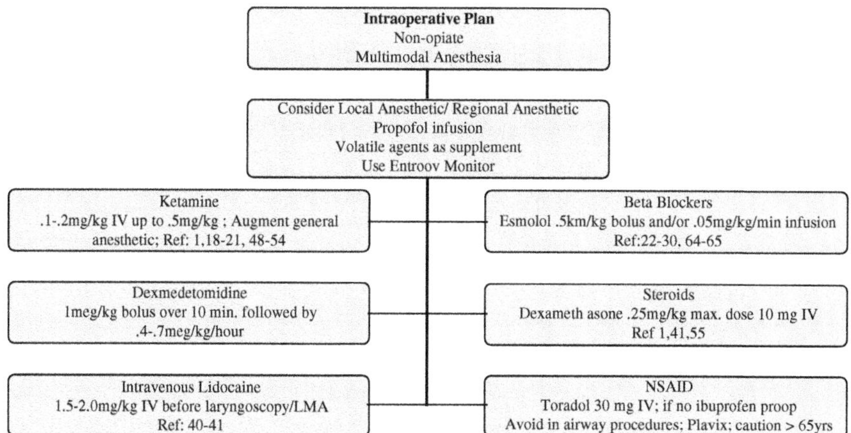

Fig. 2. Algorithm for intraoperative best practice regarding multimodal analgesia. Please note that "Ref" in these figures refer to reference lists developed by the UIHC Standard Work Committee and are not reproduced in this paper.

and surgeons. Thus, if a provider willfully fails to manage patient care in accordance with the facility's recommended practice and the patients, families, or surgeons' goals are therefore not met, then there is no reason for the practitioner to work in the facility.

Even as the group chooses new clinical issues for pathway creation, the completed algorithms are put on a timetable for review (at least annually) to ensure that local practice data and recent literature or society guidelines remain congruent.

It should be noted that evidence-based medicine does not dictate that a set of practitioners accept the tenets of society guidelines or randomized controlled studies. The committee must review each entire algorithm with the appropriate process or outcome metrics assayed to see if in fact a "best practice" is actually "best" at that particular facility. Further iterations are amended in a continuous effort to improve the outcomes important to the organization. Evidence-based medicine is always best determined locally.[25]

How Do You Make Sure You Choose the Right Pieces of Your Practice About Which to Create a Best Practice?

The types of health care processes and outcomes that should be monitored initially are those that can be changed with the least amount of effort and yet have the widest potential positive effect on the most patients or practitioners (or net margin), that is, the proverbial "low hanging fruit". Domains to consider are clinical safety, care quality as discovered by frequently occurring patient-distress outcomes (eg, PONV, pain), efficiency, productivity, cost, and satisfaction of patients, providers, and staff. Items considered important by accreditation bodies such as the Joint Commission (JC), Accreditation Association for Ambulatory Health Care (AAAHC), American Association for Accreditation of Ambulatory Surgery Facilities (AAAASF) that monitor quality outcomes at many segments throughout the health care system are reasonable sources, with the Physician Quality Reporting Initiative (PQRI) metrics for a surgical specialty being of greatest value to the practitioners at the ASC. Common perioperative outcomes are: major morbidity and mortality (although rare in the ambulatory setting), emergency department visits, 7-day and 30-day postoperative hospital admissions, PACU and postdischarge pain scores, patient fast-track times, postoperative/postdischarge nausea and vomiting, patient's care rating (eg, using a Likert

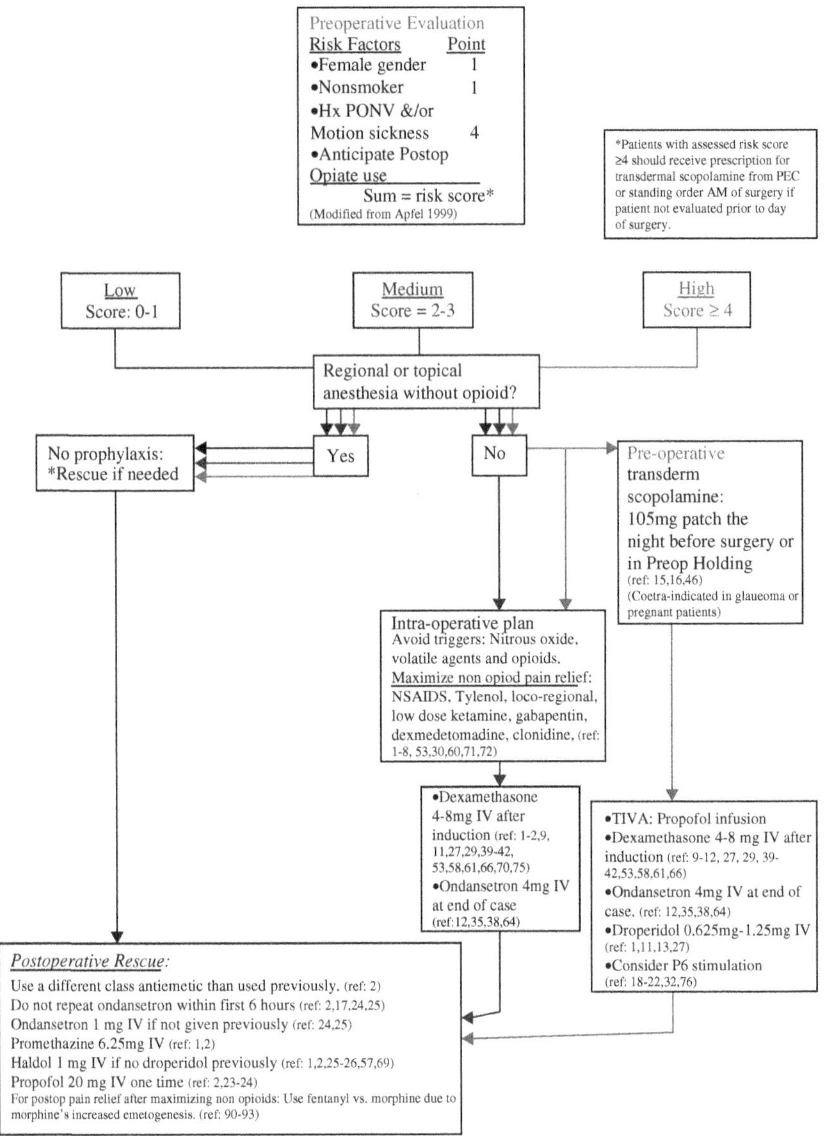

Fig. 3. Algorithm for best practice regarding PONV reduction. Please note that "Ref" in these figures refer to reference lists developed by the UIHC Standard Work Committee and are not reproduced in this paper.

scale).[26–28] Please refer to Boxes 2 and 3 for outcome and process metrics the authors have chosen.

Frequently, constraints of personnel availability prevent an in-depth de novo analysis of the literature by a committee of the facility's staff and faculty, and wherein the facility has not yet measured its own outcomes. In this setting, a reasonable initial step is to adopt existing guidelines generated by national professional societies and to measure process or outcome indicators that are germane to those guidelines. Specialty and subspecialty organizations and societies exist that create standards of practice, algorithms, consensus statements and guidelines with a narrower focus that may better suit the needs of the institution.[29–31]

When Do You Abandon a Metric?

As new knowledge is created and disseminated, evidence in the literature or in local practice outcomes dictate that best practices also change. Sometimes this happens soon after an algorithm or guideline is implemented.[32] One way to determine when to revise or expunge a given algorithm is to monitor the results of its use. As noted earlier, if local practitioners do not follow the algorithm but have equal or better outcomes, that may be the best indicator that an algorithm needs reevaluation. If data on all provider outcomes remain static, that is, if use of a standard practice does not lead to ongoing and continuous improvement, then that may indicate that the committee should seek new evidence and revise the algorithm. A periodic sunsetting of all algorithms is appropriate, with a mandated annual review and updating of the evidence and local outcome data to drive any necessary revision or elimination. A good exercise for the committee or medical director is to review each algorithm in light of these 4 questions:

1. Are the end points we were attempting to change now better or worse?
2. Are trends slowing their rate of improvement and becoming asymptotically flat?
3. Have we achieved benchmarks better than those of our peer institutions (if available)?
4. Is a particular outcome no longer important to patients or surgeons (eg, Centers for Medicare and Medicaid Services plans to sunset PQRI measures when widespread conformity has been achieved)?

The answers to these 4 questions should indicate the current position for any given algorithm's life cycle.

IS THERE PROOF THAT SUCH PROCESS IMPROVEMENT MAKES A DIFFERENCE TO PATIENTS?

Creating standard practice by using systems analysis principles has value to patients in that it reduces error and thereby increases safety.[9] By supporting efforts to improve clinical outcomes (eg, decreased perioperative pain and PONV), such programs are of clear benefit to the patient. This process is of use to organizations because it also reduces expense.[33] Standardization decreases waste and allows for use of economies of scale in purchasing, rather than the smaller boutique purchases necessitated by practitioners who create variation in equipment and supply use in the absence of a single identified best practice. This lesser cost should generate a better profit margin and reinvestment in the facility by management. Upgrading salaries, equipment, and physical plant should all have a salutatory effect on the patient and family experience in the perioperative period.

HOW DO YOU REWARD IMPROVEMENT AND DETER NONCOMPLIANCE?

Most members of an ambulatory surgery facility are motivated by internally driven interests in providing excellent patient care in an expedient manner. Consequently, most facility staff find sufficient reward in evidence of optimal unit performance (it has been our experience that the simple act of sharing this information is a significant impetus for high morale). Not surprisingly, when we have also been able to use these metrics to justify enhancements of staff and practitioner income (eg, salary increases, quarterly or year-end bonuses, or returns on stock) or time off (eg, if efficient, allowing staff to go home when the cases are done, yet still receive a full day's pay), then the daily emphasis on cost-cutting, efficiency improvement, and patient-centered service has been well supported.

Although we have used outcome and process metrics to justify such rewards, we have never seen value in using evidence of under-performance to drive punishment. To garner staff and surgeon support for measurement and for change, it is essential that no one anticipates that these efforts will lead to salary cuts or lay-offs, as long as the employee or physician is making a good-faith effort to follow policy and algorithms. As an example, senior management at the Virginia Mason Clinic (VM) determined that the Toyota Production System (TPS or Lean) was the ideal quality improvement and management system for the institution and adopted it in the early years of this past decade. Part of the new approach was the use of kaizen, a process improvement method in which teams of employees rapidly investigate ways to streamline care processes and eliminate waste. When a kaizen event was successful there would frequently be fewer employees needed for the newly created care process. Early in the adoption of TPS, VM senior leadership publicly announced that no employees would ever be laid off or fired as the result of such improved efficiency, but rather they were always guaranteed another position at the same pay within the organization. As a result, employees did not fear these events and came to embrace them for the best reasons: they saw that these sometimes drastic changes in process benefitted patients and the organization, and therefore they usually supported them.[34] It is absolutely critical not to use measurement and change to punish employees, but rather they should be counseled to model their own behavior on those employees or teams who are creating best practices, and to compete to be the one employee or team that is the example of best practice the next quarter.

REAL-WORLD RESULTS

For the past several years, the authors have served as leaders at 2 academic health care ambulatory surgery centers and have used the patient diary, its outcomes and process assessments, and the model of local team empowerment to drive consistent improvement in care through the identification of best practice and creation of standard algorithms and processes of care. Implementation of the measurements, posting of the findings, and use of the findings to direct education of staff and patients has led to overall improvement in patient care, primarily driven by care team self-assessment rather than lectures or mandates.

The University of Iowa Hospitals and Clinics (UIHC) opened a new ASC on the main campus in March 2007. We implemented the use of a diary to evaluate the processes of patient care and outcomes (see Appendix 1). In the first 6 months, the form was continually refined by nursing and medical leadership, but the general format was operational soon after opening day. A single sheet of paper was printed on both sides with questions covering each stage of a patient's experience. Clerical admission, preoperative nursing preparation, anesthesia preoperative preparation, intraoperative anesthetic management, stage I recovery, stage II recovery, and postdischarge periods were each represented. All stages had a data field for the name of each practitioner participating in the patient's care, start and stop times of each stage, and various patient responses to medical care. The diary was affixed to the patient's chart at the time of admission and then detached on discharge and conveyed to the room where clerks and registered nurses made postoperative calls to the patient the day(s) after discharge. The diary was finalized at the time of that call and then given to a clerk to

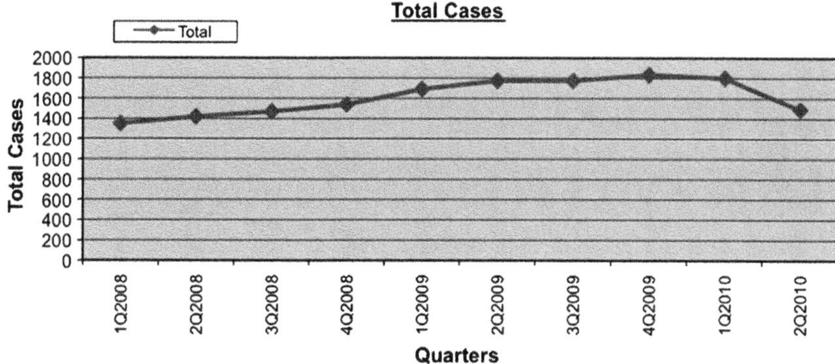

Fig. 4. Total cases done, by fiscal quarter.

transcribe into an Excel spreadsheet. Analysis of data was performed on a quarterly basis and posted in the employee lounge. Data were separated for posting in the following manner: by quarter and year to date, separated by attending surgeon, by attending anesthesiologist, and certified registered nurse anesthetist. At a previous ASC (VM) individual nursing staff members' data were posted.

Senior management of the ASC (medical director, administrator, nursing director) periodically monitored the data. When potential areas for improvement were identified, the medical director met with any affected or involved staff (eg, operating room or pre- or postoperative nursing staff, operating room and central sterilization/supply technical personnel, housekeepers, surgeons, anesthesia providers) to create action plans for improvement. In addition, weekly staff meetings provided opportunities for staff-led discussion of the data and opportunities for improvement.

The diary, its data and reports were overseen by an information technology specialist and were maintained on a secure server with a backup of accumulated data performed

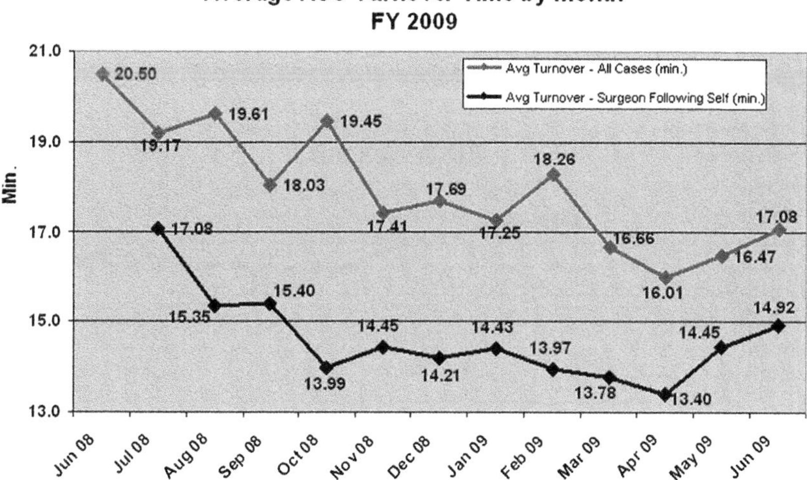

Fig. 5. Average turnover time all cases and for surgeon following self, by month (◆ = average of turnover time for surgeons following themselves; ◆ = average of all turnover times).

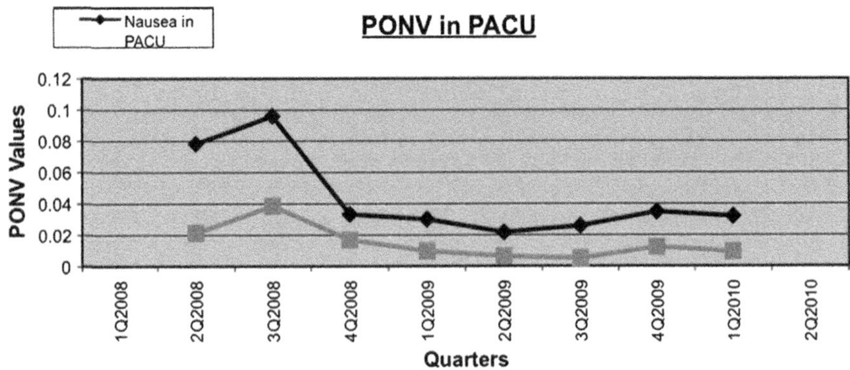

Fig. 6. PONV observed in PACU, by quarter (■ = nausea; ◆ = vomiting).

each evening. Senior management reviewed reports and altered diary questions and reports if new questions arose about care. At the end of the fifth fiscal quarter of the ASC's function, surgeon-specific process and outcome data gathered during the first year were used to establish the amount of incentive payments made to individual surgeons.

Reports were also shared with the ASC Medical Executive Board, chief financial officer, chief operating officer, and chief executive officer, as well as the chief medical officer and vice-president for medical affairs of the University at regular meetings with each. At Iowa, these reports were used in combination with financial data to direct strategic decisions, including the decision to open a seventh and an eighth room, 15 months after the original 6 rooms were put into operation.

Data trends from the first several quarters of operation are portrayed in **Figs. 4–9**. **Fig. 4** simply displays the quarterly volume of cases done at the facility. Although **Fig. 5** notes a general decrease in turnover time, the most valuable posting (not shown here) was turnover time by service line, which allowed each team to gauge their improvement against themselves and by which more marked change was delineated for some groups. Turnover time showed steady improvement until the first fiscal quarter of 2008, the period of the opening of rooms 7 and 8. At that point, several new services were brought on line and new staff and faculty were added, leading to some initial fall back in several measures of efficiency.

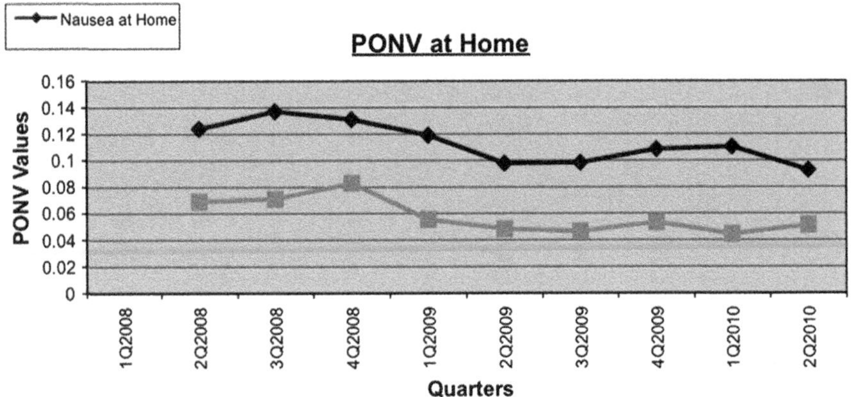

Fig. 7. PONV stated on call back, by quarter (■ = nausea; ◆ = vomiting).

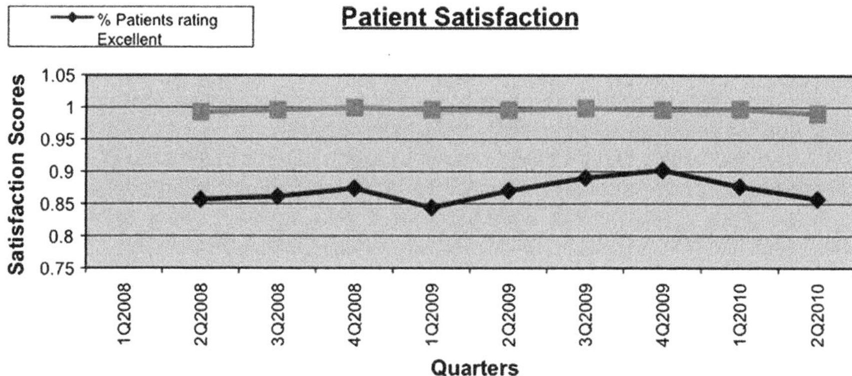

Fig. 8. Overall patient satisfaction (◆ = rating good AND excellent; ■ = only those who ranked excellent), by quarter.

Indices of PONV generally decreased with time (see **Figs. 6** and **7**). We attributed this improvement to a general decrease in the use of opioids outside of the PACU and improved use of prophylactic measures and multimodal analgesia before reaching the PACU, as a result of compliance with the algorithms created by the Standard Practice Committee (see **Figs. 2** and **3**).

Patient satisfaction, measured by 2 postdischarge questions (How would you rate your experience at the ASC? (poor, fair, good, or excellent), Would you refer a friend or loved one to the ASC if they needed a similar procedure?) was at all times high and no trends were noted (see **Fig. 8**). As noted, opioid use by anesthesia providers decreased, yet first pain scores in PACU stayed flat and low (see **Fig. 9**). These seemingly opposed trends (opioid use down, pain low) reflected a concentrated effort to increase the use of multimodal, nonopioid analgesia strategies (eg, regional anesthesia, low-dose ketamine, dexamethasone, nonsteroidal antiinflammatory drugs, and local anesthetic infiltration) in the pre-PACU period.

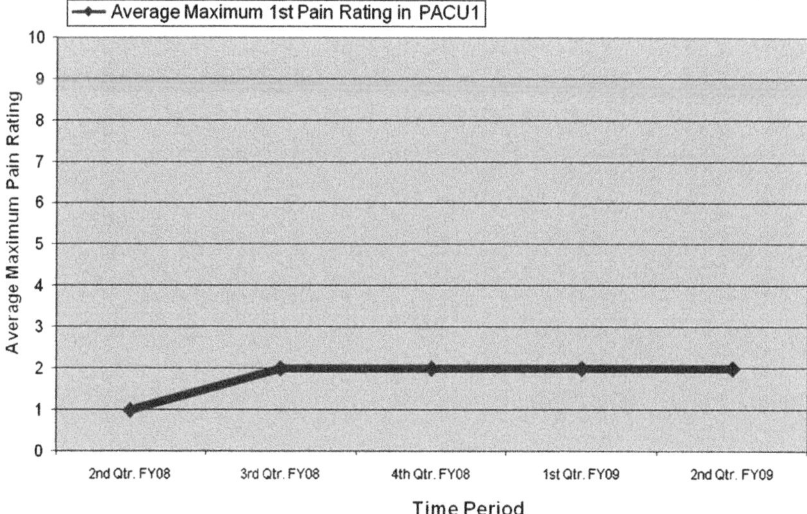

Fig. 9. Average of first pain rating on arrival in PACU (first stage only), by quarter.

Process indices also showed improvement: quality of patient preparation improved, as measured by a diminishing incidence of passport defects (lack of consent, history and physical examination, escort, and so forth); time in preoperative preparation and postoperative time (stage I and stage II) also decreased, evidence that operational delays were increasingly avoided pre- and postoperatively.

Thus, the use of the patient diary was associated with improvements in quality of care processes and outcomes. As with the effort regarding multimodal analgesia use, some of the improvements were associated with vigorous, active improvement efforts in addition to the measurement (eg, regarding PONV improvement, a decrease in opioid use, and an increase in use of prophylaxis were each the subjects of aggressive education for nursing and anesthesia providers). In other cases (eg, turnover), the primary leadership approach was to post data and allow the teams to discuss and implement strategies for improvement, without a top down strategy. It could be argued that measurement alone induced some change and that passage of time, with the probable associated increasing experience of the staff also led to improvements in throughput and outcomes.

One notable active change we implemented was the use of a tabletop photo of a standard layout of anesthesia medications and materials, an idea first used by Dr Robert Caplan at VM to drive decreases in medication error and improve accuracy of hand-offs in the operating room. A photo (**Fig. 10**) was taken of a standard layout of medication and instruments, blown up to full size and then laminated on the top of the anesthesia carts. Each practitioner was instructed to lay out the tray as shown. The practitioners were allowed to add medications if this standard setup did not cover their typical induction process, but this photograph represents the minimum of what was to be prepared before any patient's induction. The value of this approach is that another practitioner providing either a routine break or help in an emergency situation would be immediately certain if one of the medications had already been given. Also, use of certain medication is subtly supported (eg, dexamethasone and ketamine), whereas others tend to decrease (eg, opioids) because they are not in the template. Although underreported and too infrequent in incidence to be certain, syringe swaps could also be prevented by this strategy. Certainly, hand-offs were enhanced, as it is evident at a glance which medications have and have not been

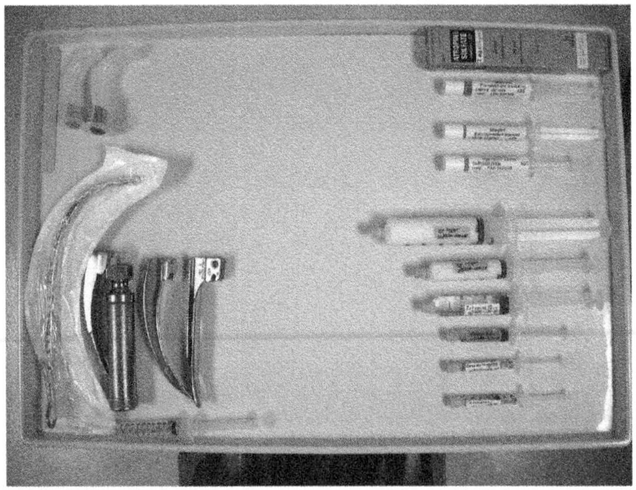

Fig. 10. Table top photo (see text).

given. Potentially, case set-up is made more accurate and speeded up by this practice, but this has not been measured.

SUMMARY

Compared with the day-to-day operations of an inpatient surgical venue, ambulatory surgery facilities are more predictable in the nature of their surgical procedures, processes, patients' health, and work hours. This is certain for those facilities that are of a single discipline (eg, cataract centers, endoscopy centers), but even those that are multidisciplinary in nature are characterized by a smaller range of case types, a smaller number of surgeons and staff, and a higher degree of uniformity in the health of its patients and their goals (ie, to go home today, in safety and comfort).

In view of this homogeneity of practice, the ambulatory surgery arena should be an ideal location for the creation of standard approaches (ie, protocols) to patient care delivery, and management of resources and other operational processes. The use of process and outcome metrics in this setting to support ongoing quality improvement and to improve safety by decreasing variability in practice should be most effective. Staff, surgeons, and anesthesia providers should scrutinize their daily practices to become aware of opportunities to streamline patient care techniques. If 95% of our patients are the same (healthy and motivated to go home) each day, and 95% of our surgical procedures are the same each day, then at least 95% of the processes used to accomplish patients' goals should be the same, no matter who the provider is. Evaluation of each practitioner's practice outcomes to focus systems improvement efforts is most effective in industry where the processes are most uniform. Nowhere in health care should this be more applicable than in the ambulatory surgery center setting. The authors have seen significant success in the application of outcome data-focused process improvement in this setting and recommend it to all caregivers and managers in outpatient surgical facilities.

ACKNOWLEDGMENTS

The authors wish to thank the certified registered nurse anesthetists, nurses, staff, and faculty of the UIHC ASC and the Virginia Mason ASC at Federal Way, whose willingness to make use of the diary and process improvements have been salutatory. The superb quality of patient care, outcomes and very high patient satisfaction at those institutions are because of their dedication to excellence in patient care. These successes are also attributable to the creative programming work of Kristine Ogden, Sarah King, and Swarup Bhattacharya. Quality improvement can only succeed if there is avid administrative support, and we always received just that from Drs Stephen Rupp and Robert Caplan at Virginia Mason, and Eric Bloom and Dr Eric Dickson (Iowa).

APPENDIX 1: USEFUL METRICS FOR A PROCESS IMPROVEMENT PROGRAM

Note that these lists are a menu, and not many programs will be able to follow all the metrics all the time and still sustain focused improvement. Also, many of these are amenable to examination by single service (eg, orthopedics or sports medicine, pediatric ear, nose, and throat, and so forth) with sometimes significant differences in the degree of quality gaps noted. One service may need to focus on a given area, whereas another does not. The more specific the metrics and assessments to a given service line, the more significant will be the potential improvements.

Box 1
Financial measures useful to monitor for quality improvement

Days in accounts receivable

Net profit (gross income less expenditure) by week, by month, by quarter

Cost (total operating expense) per case

Full time equivalent (FTE) per case

Cost per FTE (total operating expense per month/total no. of FTEs per month)

Cases per month (actual vs budgeted)

Gross charges (day, week, month, quarter, year to date)

Collection rate (budgeted vs actual)

Total operating expenses

- Personnel (labor) expense by department (eg, preoperative, PACU, operating room, administration, central supply and processing, housekeeping)
- Nonpersonnel expense
  - Patient supplies (eg, implant costs, instruments, other)
  - Other nonpersonnel supplies (eg, linen, outsourced housekeeping, and so forth)

Projected versus budgeted versus actual net income (monthly projected includes anticipated income based on that month's charges diminished by the historic collection rate adjustment and then compared with actual income at some future point for actual)

Box 2
Operational measures useful to monitor for quality improvement

Operational measures useful to monitor for quality improvement

Cases per room

Cases per day (average)

Turnover time, average, same surgeon following self

Turnover time, average, all cases

Minutes patient in room (MPIR) per room per day

Minutes of operation (MOO) (skin to skin) per room per day

MOO/MPIR

Minutes from skin closure to room exit

Minutes from room entry to skin incision

Use[a] by service or surgeon

Passport defect rate[b]

Case time estimation accuracy: estimates that are either too long or too short (>15% of the actual case time either way is our definition) are deleterious to efficient use of the operating room.

Delayed entry into the operating room, rate: in preoperative room, not associated with passport

Delay rate: room entry to incision

Delay rate: after incision, before closure

Delay rate: after closure to room exit

Delay rate: after ready for discharge

% of patients who would recommend the facility to a friend or family member who needed the same procedure

% of patients who would return to this facility if the surgeon suggested it

% of patients who assessed their care and experience as "excellent"

% of a surgeon's cases captured[c]

[a] Entire books could be written about the theory of the best way in which to measure utilization. An example of one aspect of the controversy is whether or not to include turnover time in the numerator. Should a surgeon's utilization consist of a numerator of first patient in the room to last patient out and a denominator of all the minutes allocated to the surgeon for that day, or should the numerator count only the time of patient in the room, not including turnover?). If turnover time is included in the numerator, then the surgeon or service is credited with a larger amount of utilization, which might really have reflected poor use of time or a surgeon's decision to go to lunch between cases. On the other hand, if the turnover is not included in the utilization numerator, then slow turnovers that are out of the surgeon's control (eg, poor case cart management or an uninspired anesthesia team) are nonetheless counted as a portion of his or her own utilization, when indeed that time should be counted against the facility's team. In this particular case, we have elected to count utilization both ways and present both numbers to surgeons and staff. Any large difference would have implication for turnover efficiency, but in reality we have rarely seen more than a 2% difference between the 2 measures (meaning that longer cases require longer turnover, in general).

[b] The passport or passport to surgery is a term used by many institutions to describe the set of documents and functions that must be accomplished before the patient's entry into the operating room. At this time, our facility requires that a patient have a ride arranged, have an escort on-site while in the facility, have a caregiver set to be on site at home for 24 hours after surgery, that a surgical history and physical were performed by the surgeon within the previous 30 days, an anesthetic update of the history and physical done the morning of surgery, preoperative antibiotic orders and postoperative pain medication and (if appropriate) antibiotic prescriptions ready, the surgical site marked, all implants or instrumentation appropriately ordered (eg, C-arm, cadaver tissue grafts, and so forth) and ready 24 hours in advance, and that an anesthesia consent and a surgical consent are completed. Failure to have any of these conditions met, such that there is a delay of entry into the operating room is termed a passport defect and a great deal of our process improvement efforts are aimed at the surgeon office preoperative process in an effort to decrease this defect rate.

[c] If the outpatient facility is a part of a hospital system, it is possible to measure how many of a surgeon's cases were scheduled in the outpatient facility vs the inpatient operating room. Maximization of that percentage is consonant with ideal use of hospital and ambulatory surgery center resources.

Box 3
Clinical measures useful to monitor for quality improvement

These measures should be attributed on reports to each individual who touched the patient (eg, operating room technicians are partially responsible for turnover but also for first pain and PONV, because we ask them to be the advocates for local anesthetic use intraoperatively)

PONV: in PACU and at call back (PDNV)

Pain: first rating in PACU and highest after discharge, rated at call back

Visit to emergency department or physician in first 24 hours

Visit to emergency department or physician, unscheduled, in first 30 days

Infection at surgical site within 30 days

Near miss:

- Anesthesia
- Operative
- Other

Intraoperative medical event

Intraoperative anesthesia induction failure requiring rescue

Anesthesia plan alteration (intraoperative conversion from regional or Monitored Anesthesia Care general)

Failed intubation

Reintubation in operating room or PACU

Conversion of laparoscopic procedure to open procedure

Perforated viscous

Cardiac arrest

Respiratory arrest

Use of nebulizer treatment in PACU, unplanned

Admission/transfer to hospital or emergency department postoperatively

Hypoxemia in PACU

Transfer to PACU with endotracheal tube or laryngeal mask airway in situ

Use of ventilator in PACU

Laryngospasm

Failure to monitor before induction (blood pressure, electrocardiograph, oximeter)

Evidence of prolonged neurologic dysfunction after surgery or nerve block

Postoperative cognitive alteration or dysfunction

Transfusion

Use of cardioversion, external pacing, or amiodarone

Evidence of embolism

Evidence of transient ischemic attack or cerebrovascular accident on site or within 30 days

Comorbidities for risk adjustment groups (8 suggested) a:

- Obstructive sleep apnea, known difficult airway
- Chronic heart failure, previous myocardial infarction, hypertension
- Reactive airway disease, chronic obstructive pulmonary disease

Insulin-dependent diabetes mellitus, noninsulin-dependent diabetes mellitus, chronic renal failure

Congenital abnormality

Developmental delay, cognitive dysfunction

Body mass index (calculated as weight in kilograms divided by the square of height in meters) >35 kg/m^2, >40 kg/m^2, >45 kg/m^2

Hypoxic PONV or motion sickness

[a] Risk adjustment systems can use presence of comorbidities to apportion risk of postoperative morbidity, but can also simply sort by surgical procedure types or surgeons. The latter approach assumes a proclivity for certain types of surgery by each surgeon. For example, consider 2 ophthalmologists: surgeon A performs pediatric eye muscle surgery whereas surgeon B performs only cataract procedures. It is true that the risk of PONV should be quite different between the 2 surgeons' patient cohorts. Therefore, an anesthesia provider who has done a large number of cases with surgeon A and few with surgeon B would be expected to have a significantly higher PONV rate than one who works exclusively with surgeon A. Each anesthesia provider should rightfully be compared only with other anesthesia providers with a similar profile. This system is quite easy to construct and one need only track which physicians work with each other in and what volumes in order to risk stratify anesthesia providers appropriately

APPENDIX 2: THE PATIENT DIARY

Surgery includes or Procedure is	**Procedure Start**	PLACE PATIENT LABEL HERE
Scalpel incision through skin with		Procedure ____
No injection of local anesthetic/other substance	Time of incision	Admitting Clerk
Injection prior to incision and before prep	Time of incision	Scheduled Arrival __:__
Injection prior to incision, but after prep	Time of injection	
BMT, or airway surgery (e.g., T&A)	Time of table turn	
Intra-ocular eye surgery	Time surgeon first looks into positioned microscope	

I. Pre-Op

Admitting NA ____ Primary Pre Op RN ____

Passport Defects? Yes No, If yes, Specify:

- ☐ Anesthesia Update ☐ Surgical Consent ☐ Surgical H&P
- ☐ Antibiotic Orders ☐ Meds/Equip Orders ☐ Ride/Escort

Was the patient marked at time Nursing Ready for OR? Yes No

Any Other Delays or Problems? ____

24-hour clock

ASC Desk Arrival __:__

Preop Arrival __:__

Nursing Ready for OR __:__

II. ANESTHESIA

Regional Type: (Check all that apply)

- ☐ None
- Brachial plexus
  - ☐ Cervical para-vertebral w/wo catheter/infusion
  - ☐ Infraclavicular w/wo catheter/infusion
  - ☐ Interscalene w/wo catheter/infusion
  - ☐ Axillary w/wo catheter/infusion)
  - ☐ Supraclavicular w/wo catheter/infusion
- ☐ Other peripheral
- ☐ Other
- ☐ Spinal
- ☐ Epidural / Caudal
- ☐ Para-vertebral (Thoraic/Lumbar)
- ☐ Femoral
- ☐ Sciatic
- ☐ Popliteal
- ☐ Saphenous
- ☐ IV Regional (Bier)

Anesthesia Interview Complete __:__

If multiple Regional Blocks, record earliest Start and latest Finish

Regional Start __:__

Regional Finish __:__

Drug(s) Given: (Check all that apply)

☐ None	☐ Ephedrine	☐ Lorazepam	☐ Pancuronium
☐ Alfentanil	☐ Esmolol	☐ Mepivicaine	☐ Phenylephrine
☐ 2-Chloroprocaine	☐ Fentanyl	☐ Meperidine	☐ Procaine
☐ Atracurium	☐ Glycopyrrolate	☐ Metoclopramide	☐ Propofol
☐ Atropine	☐ Heparin	☐ Metoprolol	☐ Rapacuronium
☐ Bupivacaine	☐ Hydralazine	☐ Midazolam	☐ Rocuronium
☐ Desflurane	☐ Isoflurane	☐ Morphine	☐ Ropivacaine
☐ Dexamethasone	☐ Ketamine	☐ N2O	☐ Sevoflurane
☐ Diphenhydramine	☐ Ketorolac	☐ Naloxone	☐ Succinylcholine
☐ Dolasetron	☐ Labetalol	☐ Neostigmine	☐ Thiopental
	☐ Lidocaine	☐ Ondansetron	☐ Vecuronium

☐ Other ____

Induction Start __:__

Anesthetic Technique(s):

- ☐ Local/Topical (no IV meds)
- ☐ MAC
- ☐ Regional Only
- ☐ Regional with sedation
- ☐ Regional with general
- ☐ General Anesthesia only
- ☐ TIVA
- ☐ Volatile Anesthestic

Primary Airway Technique(s)

- ☐ None
- ☐ O2 Nasal Cannula/Mask
- ☐ Oral/Nasal Airway
- ☐ General with Mask
- ☐ LMA
- ☐ Endotracheal

Did anesthesia induction delay surgical start? ☐ Yes ☐ No

Difficult intubation? Yes No If Yes, Recognized Pre-op? Yes No

Intubation Technique	Success	Attempts			
Direct Laryngoscopy	Yes No	☐ 1	☐ 2	☐ 3	☐ 4 or More
Flexible Fiber optic	Yes No	☐ 1	☐ 2	☐ 3	☐ 4 or More
Rigid Fiberoptic	Yes No	☐ 1	☐ 2	☐ 3	☐ 4 or More
Intubating LMA	Yes No	☐ 1	☐ 2	☐ 3	☐ 4 or More

Antibiotic initiated __:__

Antibiotic finished __:__

Describe ANY anesthesia NEAR MISSES:

____

III. OR NURSING

NURSE IV Sedation? Yes No

Circulator RN 1 ____ 2 ____

Scrub Tech 1 ____ 2 ____

Were there delays/Problems? Yes No ☐ Operative ☐ Equipment ☐ Tissue

____

____

Ready for Prep __:__

Prep Complete __:__

Procedure Starts __:__

IV. PACU	Stage I	Stage II	STAGE I
RN Name	______	______	Arrival __:__
Was pt. transported w/O2?	Yes No	Yes No	Ready for Departure __:__
Lowest SPO2 in PACU?	______%	______%	
Unexpected Urinary Cath?	Yes No	Yes No	Actual Departure __:__
First Pain Score	0 1 2 3 4 5 6 7 8 9 10	0 1 2 3 4 5 6 7 8 9 10	
Final Pain Score	0 1 2 3 4 5 6 7 8 9 10	0 1 2 3 4 5 6 7 8 9 10	
Nausea	Yes No	Yes No	
Vomiting	Yes No	Yes No	Regional Start __:__
PADSS Score	**Arrival 1st Stage PACU**	**Arrival 2nd Stage PACU**	
Level of Consciousness	0 1 2	0 1 2	Regional Finish __:__
Physical Activity	0 1 2	0 1 2	
Hemodynamic Stability	0 1 2	0 1 2	
Oxygen Saturation	0 1 2	0 1 2	
Pain	0 1 2	0 1 2	
Emetic Symptoms	0 1 2	0 1 2	

Problems in PACU I? ______

Problems in PACU II? ______

Reason for any delayed discharge from ASC?

☐ Nausea / Vomiting ☐ Hospital (Escort/Bed/Etc.) ☐ Anesthesia Delay
☐ Drowsiness ☐ Pharmacy Delay ☐ Patient needs clothing/Restroom/Etc.)
☐ Urinary Retention ☐ Surgery Delay
☐ Ride ☐ Other: ______

Anesthesia Post-operative Block (PACU):

☐ Brachial plexus ☐ Sciatic ☐ Para-vertebral ☐ Femoral ☐ Other ______

STAGE II
Arrival __:__
Ready for Departure __:__
Actual Departure __:__

V. CALL BACK:

Nurse recording responses: ______
Date of Call Back: __/__/__
Phone #: ______
Message Left 1: __/__/__
Message Left 2: __/__/__

Person spoken to: ☐ Patient ☐ Spouse ☐ Parent ☐ Other: ______

PATIENT OUTCOMES **AFTER DISCHARGE**:

Highest Pain Score? 0 1 2 3 4 5 6 7 8 9 10
Nausea? Yes No
Vomiting? Yes No
Unplanned urinary catheter? Yes No
Unplanned admission to ED or Hospital? Yes No
Problem that required they call the doctor? Yes No

How would you rate how you were treated at check-in?
☐ No opinion ☐ Poor ☐ Fair ☐ Good ☐ Excellent

How would you rate the care you received at the UI ASC?
☐ No opinion ☐ Poor ☐ Fair ☐ Good ☐ Excellent

If the patient had a nerve block, ask: (Circle one)

When did the numbness in your (arm, leg) begin to wear off (XX:XX)? __:__ **Same Day** or **Next Day**

If you have a similar surgery in the future, will you want to have a nerve block again? Yes No

Are there any particular things they would have liked to seen done differently? ______

Was anything or anyone particularly helpful? ______

Would the patient have a procedure done here again if doctor recommended it? Yes No

Would the patient recommend a loved one or friend have a procedure here if their doctor recommended it? Yes No

Was the pain medication strong enough to take care of their pain and did they have enough? Yes No

Any other comments: ______

REFERENCES

1. Blumenthal D. Quality of care – what is it? Part one of six. N Engl J Med 1996;335: 891–4.
2. Manuel DG, Mao Y. Avoidable mortality in the United States and Canada, 1980–1996. Am J Public Health 2002;92(9):1481–4.
3. Berwick DM. The clinical process and the quality process. Qual Manag Health Care 1992;1:1–8.
4. Eitan-Naveh ZS. How quality improvement programs can affect general hospital performance. Available at: http://www.emeraldinsight.com/10.1108/09526860510602532. Accessed April 13, 2010.
5. Brown EC, Kros J. Reducing room turnaround time at a regional hospital. Qual Manag Health Care 2010;19(1):90–100.

6. Carlhed R, Bojestig M. Improved clinical outcome after acute myocardial infarction in hospitals participating in a Swedish quality improvement initiative. Circ Cardiovasc Qual Outcomes 2009;2(3):458–64.
7. Laffel G, Blumenthal D. The case for using industrial quality management science in health care organizations. JAMA 1989;262(20):2869–73.
8. Spear S. Learning to lead at Toyota. Harv Bus Rev 2004;82(5):78–86.
9. Spencer FC. Human error in hospitals and industrial accidents: current concepts. J Am Coll Surg 2000;191(4):410–8.
10. Uhlig P. Interview with a quality leader: Paul Uhlig on transforming healthcare. Interviewer by Jason Trevor Fogg. J Healthc Qual 2009;31(3):5–9.
11. Goldratt E. The goal. 3rd edition. New York (NY): Northriver Press; 2004. p. 378.
12. James BC. Implementing practice guidelines through clinical quality improvement. Front Health Serv Manage 1993;10(1):3–37.
13. Norton SP, Pusic MV, Taha F, et al. Effect of a clinical pathway on the hospitalization rates of children with asthma: a prospective study. Arch Dis Child 2007;92: 60–6.
14. Becher EC, Chassin MR. Improving the quality of health care: who will lead? Health Aff (Millwood) 2001;20(5):164–79.
15. Macario A, Weinger M, Carney S, et al. Which clinical anesthesia outcomes are important to avoid? The perspective of patients. Anesth Analg 1999;89:652–8.
16. Macario A, Weinger M, Truong P, et al. Which clinical anesthesia outcomes are both common and important to avoid? The perspective of a panel of expert anesthesiologists. Anesth Analg 1999;88(5):1085–91.
17. Cretin S, Farley DO, Dolter KJ, et al. Evaluating an integrated approach to clinical quality improvement: clinical guidelines, quality measurement, and supportive system design. Med Care 2001;39(8 Suppl 2):II70–84.
18. Ellis JA, McCleary L, Blouin R, et al. Implementing best practice pain management in a pediatric hospital. J Spec Pediatr Nurs 2007;12(4):264–77.
19. Kotter JP. Leading change. Boston: Harvard Business School Press; 1996. p. 101–15.
20. Bohmer RMJ. Designing care. Aligning the nature and management of health care. Boston: Harvard Business Press; 2009.
21. Gawande A. The cost conundrum. The New Yorker June 1, 2006. Available at: http://www.newyorker.com/reporting/2009/06/01/090601fa_fact_gawande. Accessed January 3, 2009.
22. Closing the quality gap: a critical analysis of quality improvement strategies. Rockville (MD): Agency for Healthcare Research and Quality; March 2004. Fact Sheet. AHRQ Publication No. 04–P014. Available at: http://www.ahrq.gov/clinic/epc/qgapfact.htm. Accessed January 1, 2010.
23. Woolf SH. Do clinical practice guidelines define good medical care? Chest 1998; 113:166S–71S.
24. Sackett DL, Rosenberg WM, Gray JAM, et al. Evidence based medicine: what it is and what it isn't. BMJ 1996;312:71–2.
25. Fletcher RH. Clinical epidemiology: the essentials. Baltimore (MD): Lippincott Williams & Wilkins; 2005. p. 205–21.
26. Bettelli G. High risk patients in day surgery. Minerva Anestesiol 2009;75(5): 259–68.
27. Fleisher LA, Pasternak LR, Herbert R, et al. Inpatient hospital admission and death after outpatient surgery in elderly patients: importance of patient and system characteristics and location of care. Arch Surg 2004;139(1):67–72.

28. Mingus ML, Bodian CA, Bradford CN, et al. Prolonged surgery increases the likelihood of admission of scheduled ambulatory surgery patients. J Clin Anesth 1997;9:446–50.
29. Available at: http://www.asra.com/consensus-statements/. Accessed January 1, 2010.
30. Available at: http://www.sambahq.org/. Accessed January 1, 2010.
31. Available at: http://www.asahq.org/publicationsAndServices/sgstoc.htm. Accessed January 1, 2010.
32. Shojania KG, Sampson M, Ansari MT, et al. How quickly do systematic reviews go out of date? A survival analysis. Ann Intern Med 2007;147:224–33.
33. Lubarsky DA, Glass PS, Ginsberg B, et al. The successful implementation of pharmaceutical practice guidelines: analysis of associated outcomes and cost savings. Anesthesiology 1997;86(5):1145–60.
34. Black C. To build a better hospital, Virginia Mason takes lessons from Toyota plants. Available at: http://www.seattlepi.com/local/355128_lean15.html. Accessed December 23, 2009.

Office-Based Anesthesia: How to Start an Office-Based Practice

Matt M. Kurrek, MD, FRCP(C)[a], Rebecca S. Twersky, MD, MPH[b,*]

KEYWORDS

- Office-based anesthesia (OBA) • Ambulatory anesthesia
- Patient safety • Standards of care

Ambulatory, office-based anesthesia (OBA) has experienced an exponential growth in the last decade. In the United States between 1995 and 2005, there has been a 100% increase in the number of elective procedures performed in offices, to approximately 10 million procedures per year. It is estimated that between 17% and 24% of all elective ambulatory procedures are currently being performed in an office-based setting.[1] With the evolution of newer surgical and anesthetic techniques, ever more invasive procedures will be done outside of hospitals. This tremendous growth is primarily motivated by the perceived economic advantages as well as the personal attention, care, service, aftercare, ease of scheduling, greater privacy, increased efficiency, decreased nosocomial infection, and consistency in nursing personnel associated with OBA.[2]

Despite its appeal, OBA is not for every provider, nor is it appropriate for every patient or procedure. Special considerations must be made when comparing OBA to a hospital setting, particularly with respect to facility and environment, administration, and accreditation. In an OBA setting, an anesthesiologist must often provide care

No conflicts of interest are declared.
Disclaimer: Care has been taken to assure the accuracy of the information presented, however the investigators are not responsible for errors, omissions or for any consequences from application of the information in this article and make no warranty, expressed or implied, with respect to the currency, completeness or accuracy of the contents of this publication. The application of this information in a particular situation remains the professional responsibility of the practitioner, particularly in view of ongoing changes in regulations.

[a] Department of Anesthesia, University of Toronto, 150 College Street, Room 121, Fitzgerald Building, Toronto, ON M5S 3E2, Canada
[b] Department of Anesthesiology and Ambulatory Surgery Unit, SUNY Downstate Medical Center, 450 Clarkson Avenue, Box 6, Brooklyn, NY 11203, USA
* Corresponding author.
E-mail address: Rebecca.Twersky@downstate.edu

Anesthesiology Clin 28 (2010) 353–367
doi:10.1016/j.anclin.2010.02.006 anesthesiology.theclinics.com
1932-2275/10/$ – see front matter

without significant backup resources and support, and needs to ensure personally that established policies and procedures regarding issues such as fire, safety, drugs, emergencies, staffing, training, and unanticipated patient transfer are in place. While office surgery standards vary depending on specific regulatory statutes, it must be continuously emphasized that the standard of anesthesia care in an office is no different than that of a hospital.

PATIENT SAFETY

Triggered by media coverage of tragic mishaps that allegedly occurred due to a lack of the resources usually available in hospitals, the growth of OBA has led to considerable concerns about its safety. Statistics on the morbidity and mortality of OBA are difficult to analyze and compare, because most literature is based on retrospective studies with limited sample sizes. There are no uniform criteria for morbidity and mortality (some studies use 24-hour mortality vs 7-day or 30-day mortality, or exclude cases that are judged to be unrelated to the procedure). The authors have selected 2 of the most prominent publications from the medical literature for a brief review.

One of the most frequently cited studies of adverse events in OBA was published by Vila and colleagues in 2003.[3] Comparing OBA and ambulatory surgical centers (ASCs) in Florida between 2000 and 2002, Vila and colleagues found an increased risk of both adverse events (66 per 100,000 procedures in offices vs 5.3 in ASCs) and death (9.2 deaths per 100,000 procedures in offices vs 0.78 in ASCs) and estimated that the relative risk for injuries and deaths for OBA versus ASC was 12.4 and 11.9, respectively. The data were subsequently reexamined by Venkat and colleagues in 2004,[4] who pointed out the limitations of Vila's data analysis: an overestimation of the OBA adverse event and death rates by using all events (from registered and unregistered offices) as the numerator while using only procedures estimated from registered offices as the denominator. Venkat and colleagues reassessed events and death rates using improved estimates of the numbers of cases performed in these settings. Using Venkat's calculations, the adverse event and death rates were not higher in physicians' offices compared with ASCs.

Fleisher and colleagues[5] reported rates of adverse events after 16 commonly performed outpatient surgeries in elderly Medicare patients for outpatient hospitals, ASCs, and offices between 1994 and 1999. When comparing outcomes of OBA to ASCs and hospitals there was no statistical difference in 7-day mortality rates (expressed per 100,000 procedures: 35 for OBA, 25 for ASC, and 50 for hospitals). The rate of emergency room visits of 0 to 7 days was greatest for hospital ambulatory surgery (expressed per day per 100,000 procedures: 109.9 for OBA, 103.6 for ASCs, and 259.1 for hospitals), while the 0- to 7-day inpatient admissions (expressed per day/per 100,000 procedures) were greater for both offices and hospitals compared with ASCs: 226.5 for OBA, 91.3 for ASCs, and 432.7 for hospitals. In multivariate models, more advanced age, prior inpatient hospital admission within 6 months, surgical performance at a physician's office or outpatient hospital, and invasiveness of surgery identified those patients who were at increased risk of inpatient hospital admission or death within 7 days of surgery at an outpatient facility. These data would support the contention that physicians appropriately perform surgery in patients at the highest risk in the location with the greatest available resources, and that risk was not greater for OBA. However, the investigators correctly recognized that the study only included patients older than 65 years having procedures covered by Medicare, and that only a small fraction of all procedures was performed in physicians' offices (28,199 of 564,267, or 5%). Furthermore, a bias with respect to selecting patients for a certain setting (office vs ASC vs outpatient hospital) or the type of anesthesia could not be excluded.

SOURCES OF INFORMATION FOR THE NOVICE ANESTHESIA PROVIDER

The American Society of Anesthesiology (ASA) has had a long-standing interest in guiding the safety of OBA and, under the auspices of the ASA Committee on Ambulatory Surgical Care and in conjunction with the Society for Ambulatory Anesthesia (SAMBA), in 1999 developed and approved the *Guidelines for Office-Based Anesthesia*, which were subsequently endorsed by the ASA House of Delegates as the nation's most comprehensive medical guidelines for OBA care.[6]

In 2002, because of continued member interest and inquiries, the ASA produced a publication titled *Office-Based Anesthesia: Considerations for Anesthesiologists in Setting up and Maintaining a Safe Office Anesthesia Environment*, which was just recently updated and revised in its second edition.[7] This manual provides "nuts and bolts" advice as well as further resources and references for anesthesiologists who currently practice, or plan to practice, in the office setting.

Interested readers may also consider several available textbook references that are dedicated to OBA.[8–10]

FACILITY ACCREDITATION

Despite the increasing popularity of OBA and the persistent concerns about its safety, there still remains a relative lack of oversight; currently only 25 states in the United States have fully functional guidelines or regulations in place to ensure adequate facility and equipment standards, patient care provider qualification, and proper patient selection. Many states now require accreditation through one of several agencies to evaluate the office-based practice setting. At present there are 3 major accrediting organizations: The Joint Commission (TJC),[11] the Accreditation Association for Ambulatory Health Care (AAAHC),[12] and the American Association for Accreditation of Ambulatory Surgical Facilities (AAAASF)[13]; all of which are deemed to meet Medicare certification requirements, without being subject to an actual Medicare survey and certification process. Whereas the accreditation process includes a comprehensive and detailed survey of a facility's physical layout, environmental safety, administration, patient and personnel records as well as operating room personnel, the anesthesia requirements remain fairly nonspecific. The key differences between the 3 accrediting organizations are shown in **Table 1**.

Anesthesiologists are responsible for ensuring adequate standard of care and are advised to thoroughly inspect facilities, especially in the case of offices that are not accredited, before assuming any responsibility for patients. The most common elements of a basic checklist are listed in **Box 1**.

FACILITY ADMINISTRATION

An appropriate administrative structure includes a medical director who is ultimately responsible for facility as well as personnel, and who must ensure that all applicable local, state, and federal laws, codes, and regulations are observed. A formal policy and procedure manual should be available to address various issues, including provider qualification, records and documentation, quality improvement activities, professional liability, handling of controlled medications, and policies for clinical care issues.

Table 1
Key differences between the 3 accrediting organizations in the United States

	TJC	AAAHC	AAAASF
Number of offices accredited	453	537	1265
Fee in US $ per 3 year cycle (± Medicare certification fee)	$6950	$3800	$3000–$5000
Surgeon qualification	–	–	+
Anesthesia qualifications	LIP	MD/DDS or MD-supervised	Anesthesiologist/ MD-supervised
Perioperative anesthesia care	+	+	+
Operating room personnel	–	–	+
Overnight stays	–	±	+
Patient discharge	–	–	+ LIP
Patient transfer	–	+	+
Peer review	+	+	+
Adverse event reporting	–	–	+

Abbreviations: AAAASF, American Association for Accreditation of Ambulatory Surgical Facilities; AAAHC, Accreditation Association for Ambulatory Health Care; LIP, licensed independent practitioner; TJC, The Joint Commission; +, addressed in standards; –, not addressed in standards; ±, not clearly addressed in standards.

All health care providers should hold a valid license and be qualified to perform their respective services. Maintenance of certification in ACLS (or PALS if providing care to children) should be kept and should comply with local and state regulations. For non-anesthesia and surgical personnel, proficiency in basic CPR is recommended, at a minimum.

Even in an office-based practice there should be a basic written plan to assess, document, and improve outcome of anesthesia care, which is the responsibility of the anesthesiologist (or anesthesia group). It may be practical to form a single quality improvement (QI) unit if the care is provided at multiple facilities. The QI program should include peer review, risk management, and benchmarking (including patient satisfaction) with an at least annual review. A regular inspection of anesthetic and emergency equipment should be included. Note that the QI outside a hospital may not be protected from legal discovery.

A thorough review of liability coverage with the underwriter is strongly advised. It is recommended to ensure that all health care providers are fully credentialed and have appropriate malpractice coverage, as vicarious liability in the office setting is a common and valid concern.

Anesthesiologists need to ensure that the applicable local, state, and federal regulations concerning the use of controlled medications are followed. A separate DEA 223 registration number will be used by offices that dispense their own medications (which they will order using their own DEA 222 form). Alternatively, the anesthesiologist may supply his or her own controlled medications (and transport them between facilities) using his or her own DEA 222. Proper storage (on site: in a double-locked, securely installed narcotic storage safe), drug reconciliation, and inventory must conform to all state and federal laws. Special precautions should be taken during transport of controlled medications between facilities (to avoid loss or theft, which must be reported immediately using form DEA 106) as well as the disposal of expired controlled medications (use of form DEA 41).

Box 1
Common elements of a checklist during an inspection prior to provision of anesthesia services

Administration:

- Qualification (credentialing and licensing of personnel, including cardiopulmonary resuscitation [CPR], advanced cardiac life support [ACLS], and pediatric advanced life support [PALS])
- Accreditation status
- Malpractice coverage
- Anesthesia record, consent, discharge instructions
- Quality improvement, adverse event reporting and peer review
- Patient follow-up
- Policy and procedure manual
- Emergency planning and drills (power outage, fire, evacuation, ACLS, and other disasters)
- Equipment disinfection and handling of biohazardous waste and sharps
- Storage and ordering of controlled and anesthesia drugs
- Hospital transfer agreement

Facility Engineering:

- Patient flow
- Compressed gases and scavenging
- Fire safety (stretcher stair evacuation, sprinkler system?, fire extinguishers)
- Evacuation
- Equipment: inspection, maintenance, testing, and backup
- Help
- Essential electrical systems (backup power and light)
- Telephone for assistance

Equipment Check:

- Suction (and backup) with suction catheters
- Oxygen (and backup)
- Positive pressure ventilating device capable of delivering O_2 (including reliable O_2 source)
- Appropriately sized airways, laryngoscope blades, masks, and laryngeal mask airways (LMAs)
- Standard ASA monitors (blood pressure, electrocardiograph, stethoscope, pulse oximetry, capnograph, temperature)
- Anesthesia machine with scavenging system
- Functioning resuscitation equipment and defibrillator
- Emergency airway equipment
- Medication cart (including routine, ACLS, and other emergency drugs)
- Malignant hyperthermia (MH) supplies (availability of dantrolene as well as other medications and supplies to treat MH when triggering agents are used)

FACILITY SAFETY

Due to several factors, patients in health care facilities are particularly vulnerable; they may not be able to self-evacuate in the event of an emergency (ie, fire) because of being temporarily immobilized (ie, operating room [OR], postanesthesia care unit [PACU]); they may be exposed to electrical hazards, as they are often connected to medical electronic equipment (ie, electrocautery, electrocardiography, and so forth); and they are regularly in close proximity to biomedical hazards and sources of infectious materials (ie, respiratory pathogens, blood, and secretions). Health care providers working in hospitals take for granted the multitude of rules and regulations that pertain to facility engineering standards to address these issues. Most physicians' offices are not built to the same standard, as they are usually not designed for procedures under general anesthesia. The anesthesia provider must be particularly vigilant and should personally inspect facilities before providing care so that he or she is prepared to assume additional responsibilities and ensure patient safety.

Fire Safety

OR fires are not just a theoretical concern. Some estimate there are between 50 and 200 OR fires per year with a significant morbidity and mortality, and a practice advisory for the prevention and management of OR fires has been published by the ASA.[14] High-risk procedures in OBA include laser and cosmetic facial procedures as well as most dental procedures under sedation, particularly if supplemental oxygen is administered. Flammable skin preps should be avoided and be allowed to dry completely before applying any drapes, and those should be positioned to prevent the accumulation of oxygen (ie, tenting of an oxygen-rich environment). Surgical sponges should be moistened when used in close proximity to ignition sources and nitrous oxide should be avoided in high-risk situations. The disposal of waste anesthetic gases should be assessed from an environmental as well as fire code perspective.

Most hospitals have a 2-stage fire alarm, dedicated supervisory staff, sprinkler protection throughout, fire separation of floor areas into 2 zones for horizontal evacuation of patients, wider corridors and stairs, additional requirements for ORs and recovery rooms including fire separations and dedicated/protected air supply, and elevators to accommodate stretchers in a horizontal position. Office buildings may not meet the standards described in the National Fire Protection Association (NFPA) 99 Health Care Facilities document. The anesthesia provider and other staff must have a fire safety plan and frequently rehearse emergency procedures, including safe evacuation.

Ventilation

While the control of temperature and humidity add to the comfort of patients and health care providers, the adequacy of a properly designed ventilation system in hospitals adds multiple levels of safety that may not be present in office buildings, such as a defined number of air exchanges, individualized ducts and exhaust, as well as scavenging, which may be important for infection control and protection against smoke and toxic fumes in the event of a fire.

The NFPA's standards regarding gas supplies may not apply to offices unless stipulated through an accrediting organization. Proper storage, ventilation, and backup supply with alarmed monitoring needs to be ensured by the anesthesia provider. For practice setups involving the transport of compressed or liquefied gases, the provider is referred to various legislations, including the Compressed Gas Association, the Department of Transport, and additional local, state, and federal regulations.

Electrical and Equipment Safety

Most hospitals have a dedicated biomedical engineer to ensure the safety of all equipment. In an office-based practice the responsibility for the inspection and maintenance of equipment rests with the health care provider. All anesthesia equipment should be fully supported by the manufacturer or qualified service personnel, and should not be obsolete. Each practitioner must ensure continuity of electrical power in the event of a power failure, along with emergency lighting, as well as protection against electrical shock hazards (including the adequacy of receptacles, grounding, and ground fault interrupters, if applicable).

Infection Control and Occupational Safety

Cases of hepatitis B and C patient-to-patient transmission have occurred in nonhospital facilities due to the improper reuse of needles and syringes. These occurrences have paralleled the migration of care from acute-care hospitals to nonhospital care settings,[15] and strict adherence to the Centers for Disease Control and Prevention (CDC) guidelines is expected.[16] Medications should never be administered from the same syringe to more than one patient (even if the needle has been changed), and both needle and syringe are considered contaminated after they have entered a patient's IV bag or administration set. Vials should not be entered with a used needle or syringe and, whenever possible, medications packaged as multidose vials should be used for one patient only. Likewise, IV bags and bottles should not be used a common source of supply for more than one patient. Adequate infection control practices must be observed during preparation and injection of medications. Other elements of infection control include air flow and quality monitoring (as well as maintenance), preprocessing, sterilization, and disinfection along with housekeeping and waste management (including adequate handling of sharps). Additional information regarding occupational safety can be found in relevant standards from the United States Department of Labor and the Occupational Safety and Health Administration (OSHA).

PRACTICE MANAGEMENT

Many providers of OBA will enjoy the flexibility and control, along with financial opportunities that have contributed to the rapid growth of out-of-hospital surgery. However, this also means being confronted with the reality of running a personal business (either solo or in a group), interacting with and recruiting clients, managing a schedule (at times with transit between different offices, perhaps even with fully mobile anesthesia equipment), employing staff (eg, other anesthesia providers, PACU nurses with contractual agreements) and making billing arrangements with Medicare and Medicaid, third-party insurance companies, or patients directly (sometimes with payment plans). The potential success of a growing practice may be enhanced by the development of a marketing and business plan, but practitioners' expectations must be realistic enough to accept that not all potential clients evolve into permanent ones. To improve efficiency and control costs, one should keep track of inventory for medication, supplies, and equipment and as the practice grows, consider purchasing consortiums and hiring staff to manage the inventory. There are several state as well as federal regulations that apply to the provision of services and billing, including laws such as Stark II and the "anti-kickback" law, which are intended to avoid conflicts of interest. These laws prohibit offering or providing any "remuneration"—anything of value, not just monetary payments—in exchange for referral of federal health care program patients (Medicare). It may be best to seek legal advice in order to review and consider all issues. To be competitive, anesthesiologists should consider the expertise they offer to OBA by providing a full service package: knowledge of accreditation processes, providing drugs, supplies, and equipment, overseeing the daily OR management, providing quality anesthesia providers and other staff, and participating in continuous quality improvement (CQI).[7]

With perhaps the exception of therapeutic nerve blocks in pain clinics, it is generally unusual for the anesthesia provider to maintain his or her own office facility and invite other health care professionals (ie, surgeons, dentists, gastroenterologists, and so forth) to his or her office. The vast majority of anesthesia providers will have to solicit other health care professionals who own and maintain their offices and who are looking for anesthesia services, and it will have to be decided how the various anesthesia equipment and medications are to be provided and maintained. Some settings (especially for offices who use anesthesia services rarely) lend themselves to a fully mobile anesthesia model, whereas others (where anesthesia is needed frequently) do better with the equipment set up and installed permanently (either by the anesthesia provider or by the facility owner).

Anesthesia providers can either directly (or through a billing service) charge the patient or third-party payers for their services or invoice the facility owner. Participation with Centers for Medicare & Medicaid Services (CMS) and any insurance company should be discussed up front and the implications for the anesthesia provider be taken into consideration (CMS does not pay a facility fee for office settings, but offers a higher professional fee to the surgeon). A thorough review of the various practice management issues in OBA has been published.[17]

PREOPERATIVE CARE: PATIENT AND PROCEDURE SELECTION

Offices should have policies regarding criteria for patient selection that consider the patient's medical conditions and the intrinsic risk or invasiveness of the procedure. Some states define which procedures can be done in offices while others leave such decisions to the health care provider. As a general rule, patients whose preexisting medical conditions or surgical procedure may pose a risk of perioperative complications beyond the office's resources should not have their procedures done in an office-based facility. **Box 2** lists several factors that should be considered when deciding whether a patient should be scheduled for OBA.

A preoperative workup and assessment are required,[18] though interestingly, a recent publication questioned the use of routine preoperative laboratory testing in a hospital outpatient department for healthy patients undergoing ambulatory surgery.[19]

Patients must receive adequate explanations about the nature of the proposed procedure or treatment and its anticipated outcome, as well as the significant risks involved and alternatives available. This information must be such as will allow the patient to reach an informed consent decision, and this dialog should be documented in the chart, which should also include the signed consent form.

INTRAOPERATIVE CARE

Intraoperative monitoring and management are expected to be of hospital standard.[20] Several techniques, ranging from local infiltration with minimal sedation (anxiolysis) to major regional and/or general anesthesia (total intravenous anesthesia, total

Box 2
Factors to consider in selecting patients for OBA

- Nature of surgical procedure and resources of the office for total perioperative care(blood loss, availability of general anesthesia, postoperative management, and so forth)
- Abnormalities of major organ systems, and stability and optimization of any medical illness (including difficult airway, morbid obesity, and/or obstructive sleep apnea)
- Previous adverse response to anesthesia and surgery
- Family history (malignant hyperthermia or other metabolic conditions)
- Current medications as well as drug allergies (including allergy to latex)
- Risk for deep vein thrombosis and presence of prophylactic measures
- Nil by mouth (NPO) status (time and nature of the last oral intake)
- History of substance use or abuse (including alcohol or painkillers) as well as patient's psychological status
- Availability of a responsible person to accompany the patient home from the office and remain in attendance as necessary

intravenous anesthesia (TIVA), or general inhalational anesthesia with LMA or endotracheal tube) may be chosen, depending on the patient, the procedure, and the level of comfort of the clinician. The anesthesia provider, however, must make plans to potentially rescue any patient from deeper levels of sedation than originally intended,[21,22] and to adequately handle untoward events (including inadequate sedation/regional anesthesia or cardiovascular collapse/respiratory arrest), especially considering the limited resources in office-based settings. Although it is assumed that the office will be supplied with adequate anesthesia drugs, supplies, and equipment for intended care, there also needs to be necessary resuscitation equipment to rescue a patient from deeper level of sedation/anesthesia. All offices should have a reliable source of oxygen, suction, self-inflating hand-resuscitator bag capable of delivering positive pressure ventilation, airway devices including oral and nasal airways, laryngoscope blades, and endotracheal tubes appropriately sized for the population served.

A variety of ambulatory anesthetics are suitable for OBA, provided they can be administered safely. Because of the need for a timely discharge of patients, consideration should be given to the use of short-acting anesthetics and the minimization of side effects that otherwise may delay discharge (pain, nausea, and vomiting). This measure can often be accomplished through judicious infiltration of local anesthetics by the surgeon (and the use of regional techniques, where appropriate, by the anesthesia provider), tailored prophylactic multimodal anesthesia regimens, and liberal administration of antiemetics.

To facilitate fast-tracking after office-based surgery, many common office-based procedures can be done under sedation (monitored anesthesia care), thus avoiding the effects of general anesthesia on cardiopulmonary physiology, airway manipulation, and heat redistribution (contributing to hypothermia). Avoiding muscle relaxation permits muscle tone in the extremities, which can reduce deep vein thrombosis and subsequent pulmonary embolus. In general, muscle relaxants and endotracheal intubation are used sparingly, although airway equipment for intubation or to manage a difficult airway must be available during all cases of general anesthesia.[7] The anesthesia provider may choose from a variety of short-acting agents with rapid onset and recovery, and sedative-hypnotic and analgesic properties that have minimal effect on the cardiovascular and respiratory system as well as no postoperative nausea and vomiting. Popular anesthetic agents include propofol (at times mixed with methohexital), midazolam, ketamine, as well as the more recently introduced α_2 agonist, dexmedetomidine.[23] For short procedures these agents can be administered as small bolus injections (and repeated as necessary), whereas longer procedures can employ continuous infusion techniques. Large doses of opioids are often avoided because of the effect on postoperative nausea and vomiting, as well as respiratory depression. Ultra short-acting opioids (remifentanil) have desirable pharmacokinetics, but their use should be combined with long-acting local anesthetics or nonopioid analgesics if significant postoperative pain is expected.

The compact size and portability of an intravenous infusion pump have made TIVA a popular choice for small offices or mobile anesthesia setups, because it minimizes the need for certain anesthetic equipment (anesthesia machine with scavenging and, usually, MH cart) along with reducing the associated costs. Note, however, that the Malignant Hyperthermia Association of the United States (MHAUS) explicitly recommends that MH supplies be on site if succinylcholine is available, even if only for resuscitation. Because TIVA requires the establishment of intravenous access, it may not always be preferred or feasible (ie, pediatrics, special needs and very needle-phobic patients, and so forth). In addition to full-sized stationary anesthesia machines (with integrated monitors), there are now several approved and portable anesthesia systems available for use in small offices or as part of a mobile setup whereby inhalational induction or maintenance may be used. Charcoal canisters that absorb halogenated agents (without using nitrous oxide) may allow the use of inhalational anesthesia in offices without scavenging capabilities. It is important that the equipment and machines used are maintained, tested, and inspected on a regular basis, and not become a repository for obsolete equipment.[7] The use of monitoring devices for the depth of anesthesia (ie, Bispectral Index, BIS monitoring) may allow minimization of the patient's exposure to anesthetic agents, facilitate recovery, and reduce costs.[24]

Many patients after ambulatory surgery fear postoperative nausea and vomiting (PONV) more than pain, and this can significantly delay discharge or lead to unanticipated admissions. A simplified risk score for predicting PONV, based on gender, history of motion sickness or PONV, smoking status, and use of postoperative opioids has been published, and the Society for Ambulatory Anesthesia (SAMBA) has recently made guidelines for the management of PONV available.[25] Depending on patient risk factors, the type of surgery (ie, plastic, dental, ophthalmologic, ear, nose, throat, or gynecologic) and the anesthetics used (volatile agents, use of nitrous oxide or opioids), a combination of prophylactic and therapeutic agents/strategies may be chosen (adequate hydration, prophylactic dexamethasone, 5-hydroxytryptamine$_3$ receptor antagonists, NK-1 antagonists, H_1 receptor blockers, scopolamine patches, or droperidol; consider the black box warning by the FDA).

Adequate management of postoperative pain, where applicable, requires careful planning, including a multimodal analgesia regimen that may be started before the surgical procedure. In addition to single-shot local anesthetic infiltration, certain procedures (especially abdominal, orthopedic, and breast surgeries) may employ patient-controlled continuous infusion devices for local anesthetics that are placed at the end of the procedure and that can be used for several days.

POSTOPERATIVE CARE AND DISCHARGE

The recovery in an office can present challenges, as there may not be a permanent recovery area. Often patients are expected to recover rapidly in the surgical area or in an adjacent procedure room or holding area. Regardless of the location, applicable standards apply.[26] There should be policies and procedures that specify monitoring, staff qualifications, responsibilities, documentation, and a formal discharge protocol (including predefined anesthesia discharge criteria for "street-fitness").[27–29] Patients should receive detailed written instructions for routine and emergency follow-up, and personnel trained in basic life support/ACLS should be present until the last patient leaves the facility.

SPECIAL CONSIDERATIONS: LIPOSUCTION

Liposuction, one of the most common cosmetic procedures, consists of the surgical removal of subcutaneous fat. There are several different surgical techniques in use, but the more common ones now include so-called tumescent and superwet liposuction, during which the area for surgery is injected with large volumes of a dilute solution of local anesthetic, usually crystalloid and lidocaine with epinephrine (1 mL for each mL of planned adipose removal; in some cases 2–3 times the volume of anticipated adipose resection).[30] Lidocaine doses of 35 mg/kg are accepted during tumescent liposuction, but epinephrine should not exceed 0.07 mg/kg. Even though these doses of lidocaine exceed the recommended maximum, the resulting plasma levels may be below the levels considered safe.[31] Due to the length of the procedure, active warming devices should be considered to avoid the development of hypothermia, as the large volumes of injectate are usually not warmed. In addition, significant volumes of the injectate may be absorbed and significant hypervolemia may result unless fluid management is planned accordingly.

Patients during prolonged cosmetic procedures are at increased risk of deep venous thrombosis, and a policy for thromboprophylaxis should be in place.[32] Due to the increased risk of adverse events, it is not recommended to perform large volume liposuction (>5000 mL of total aspirate, or more than 2000 mL for liposuction as an adjunct procedure) or to combine liposuction with certain other procedures, such as abdominoplasty, in the office-based setting.

SPECIAL CONSIDERATIONS: PEDIATRICS

The most important consideration for pediatric OBA is the presence of adequately qualified staff, confident in caring for the child, as well as the availability of a selection of age-appropriate monitoring and equipment. Even though a minimum age in OBA for an otherwise healthy infant has not been established, it has been suggested to restrict the selection to infants older than approximately 6 months and to exclude ex-premature infants due to the increased risk of apnea. Most children require general anesthesia via inhalational induction, making the presence of an anesthesia machine necessary. If TIVA is chosen, topical analgesia may be applied for performing a venipuncture.

SPECIAL CONSIDERATIONS: DENTAL

The American Dental Association (ADA) has issued guidelines that define educational requirements for dentists to provide anesthesia, and qualified dentists have to apply for state board issued anesthesia permits. In some states, physician anesthesiologists are also required to obtain dental anesthesia permits from their respective dental state board. In general, the state medical board requires an inspection of the facility instead of a formal accreditation.

The majority of dental facilities are not specifically designed for the administration of anesthesia, and this may pose particular challenges for the anesthesia provider: the treatment room may be significantly smaller than a normal operating room and the patient usually rests on a dental treatment chair with only limited positioning (especially for airway management) compared with normal OR tables. Often the anesthesia provider is required to bring his or her own equipment for temporary setup (fully mobile OBA model) and should be aware that many of the usual features present in hospital ORs may not be present (scavenging, backup power, dedicated suction, and so forth). He or she should ensure that this does not compromise safety.

Due to the nature of the surgical intervention (mostly restorative dentistry), and despite the significant anxiety experienced by many dental patients, intravenous sedation (together with local anesthesia administered by the dentist) is often sufficient. Intravenous sedation provides adequate operating conditions for dental providers, especially because they are accustomed to working on "awake" patients. The majority of adult patients tolerate this technique as long as some degree of amnesia is assured.

The anesthesia provider should be ready to provide short-acting supplemental sedation required for brief periods of increased surgical stimulation, which is a frequent occurrence during dentistry. Also, dental and anesthesia provider both "share" the airway, and changes in ventilation and the ability to clear blood, secretions, or water from any drills along with any interference from foreign material (gauzes or instruments) must be considered.[7]

Patients for dental procedures outside the hospital usually have only a minimal understanding of anesthesia and its implications, and may not take preparation (including NPO status) or postoperative instructions seriously. Patients should receive instructions about expectations for preoperative care and the intraoperative period, as well as postoperative instructions.

EMERGENCIES AND TRANSFERS

Due to the limited resources of office-based facilities as compared with hospitals, the management of emergencies requires a detailed policy and procedure for careful planning and preparation, along with regular rehearsals and drills. The goal of handling an emergency in the office is to stabilize the patient and promptly transfer the patient to an acute-care facility with personnel and resources more suited to handle the emergency. Medications and equipment in the office-based setting should be no different than that for a hospital, and additional resources for determining drug dosages, usage, and protocols (ACLS, difficult airway algorithm, Emergency Therapy for Malignant Hyperthermia, Guidelines for the Management of Severe Local Anesthetic Toxicity) should be immediately available.[7] Emergency planning should include a clear understanding of assigned responsibilities to available staff (including surgeon/dentist, assistants, nurses, and so forth), taking into account their qualifications. Means for urgent evacuation of immobilized patients (from the OR or PACU) in the event of a disaster (ie, fire) should be ensured.

In the case of a patient transfer to an acute-care facility, he or she needs to be stable enough to be transferred safely. It is the responsibility of the anesthesia provider to verify that a written transfer agreement is in place (or that the surgeon has admitting privileges at an appropriate facility in close proximity). Although in most areas the emergency transport via 911 is acceptable, some areas without 911 coverage require special arrangements for ambulance transportation.

SUMMARY

OBA continues to grow due to the popularity among patients and health care providers alike. Increasing regulation will ensure that patient safety remains the primary focus. In the meantime, the anesthesia provider must take adequate steps to ensure that the quality of care is comparable to that in a hospital.

REFERENCES

1. American Hospital Association (AHA). Trendwatch chartbook 2007: trends affecting hospital and health systems, April 2007 chapter 2, organization trends. Available at: http://www.aha.org/aha/trendwatch/chartbook/2007/07chapter2.ppt#265. 8, Chart 2.5: percent of outpatient surgeries by facility type, 1981–2005. Accessed September 20, 2009.
2. Byrd HS, Barton FE, Orenstein HH, et al. Safety and efficacy in an accredited outpatient plastic surgery facility: a review of 5316 consecutive cases. Plast Reconstr Surg 2003;112(2):636–41.
3. Vila H Jr, Soto R, Cantor AB, et al. Comparative outcomes analysis of procedures performed in physician offices and ambulatory surgery centers. Arch Surg 2003; 138(9):991–5.
4. Venkat AP, Coldiron B, Balakrishnan R, et al. Lower adverse event and mortality rates in physician offices compared with ambulatory surgery centers: a reappraisal of Florida adverse event data. Dermatol Surg 2004;30(12):1444–51.
5. Fleisher LA, Pasternak L, Herbert R, et al. Inpatient hospital admission and death after outpatient surgery in elderly patients. Arch Surg 2004;139(1):67–72.
6. American Society of Anesthesiologists (ASA). Guidelines for office-based anesthesia. Available at: http://www.asahq.org/publicationsAndServices/standards/12.pdf. Approved by the ASA House of Delegates on October 13, 1999, and last affirmed on October 21, 2009. Accessed December 28, 2009.
7. American Society of Anesthesiologists (ASA). Office-based anesthesia: considerations for anesthesiologists in setting up and maintaining a safe office anesthesia environment. Available at: http://www2.asahq.org/publications/ps-319-2-office-based-anesthesia-considerations-for-anesthesiologists-in-setting-up-and-main taining-a-safe-office-anesthesia-environment-2nd-edition-november-2008.aspx. Accessed September 20, 2009.
8. Shapiro FE. Manual of office-based anesthesia procedures. Philadelphia: Lippincott Williams & Wilkins; 2007. p. 1–200.
9. Hausman L, Rosenblatt M. Office-based anesthesia. In: Barash PG, Cullen BF, Stoelting RK, editors. Clinical anesthesia. 6th edition. Philadelphia: Lippincott-Williams & Wilkins; 2008. p. 1345–57.
10. Vila H, Desai MS, Miguel RV, et al. In: Twersky RS, Philip BK, editors. Handbook of ambulatory anesthesia. 2nd edition. New York: Springer; 2008. p. 283–324.
11. The Joint Commission (TJC). One Renaissance Blvd, Oakbrooke Terrace, IL 60181, Tel: (630) 792-5000, Email: First letter of person's first name plus entire last name@jointcommission.org. Available at: http://www.jointcommission.org/. Accessed March 23, 2010.
12. Accreditation Association for Ambulatory Health Care (AAAHC). 5250 Old Orchard Road, Suite 200, Skokie, IL 60077, Tel (847) 853-6060, Email: info@aaahc.org (Source for Accreditation Handbook of Ambulatory Health Care). Available at: http://www.aaahc.org/. Accessed March 23, 2010.
13. American Association for Accreditation of Ambulatory Surgical Facilities (AAAASF). Manual for accreditation of ambulatory surgical facilities. 1998. P.O. Box 9500, Gurnee, IL 60031, or 5101 Washington St, Suite 2F, Gurnee, IL 60031, Tel: (888) 542-5222, Email: infor@aaaasf.org. Available at: http://www.aaaasf.org/. Accessed March 23, 2010.

14. American Society of Anesthesiologists (ASA) Task Force on Operating Room Fires. Practice advisory for the prevention and management of operating room fires. Anesthesiology 2008;108(5):786–801.
15. Thompson ND, Perz JF, Moorman AC, et al. Nonhospital health care-associated hepatitis B and C virus transmission: United States, 1998–2008. Ann Intern Med 2009;150:33–9.
16. Center for Disease Control and Prevention (CDC). Infection control in health care settings. Available at: http://www.cdc.gov/ncidod/dhqp/index.html. Accessed September 23, 2009.
17. Galati M. Practice management issues in office-based anesthesiology. Semin Anesth Perioperat Med Pain 2006;25(1):32–9.
18. American Society of Anesthesiologists (ASA). ASA basic standards for preanesthesia care. Available at: http://www.asahq.org/publicationsAndServices/standards/03.pdf. Approved by the ASA House of Delegates on October 14, 1987, and amended on October 25, 2005. Accessed September 23, 2009.
19. Chung F, Yuan H, Yin L, et al. Elimination of preoperative testing in ambulatory surgery. Anesth Analg 2009;108(2):467–75.
20. American Society of Anesthesiologists (ASA). Standards for basic anesthetic monitoring. Available at: http://www.asahq.org/publicationsAndServices/standards/02.pdf. Approved by the ASA House of Delegates on October 21, 1986, and last amended on October 25, 2005. Accessed September 23, 2009.
21. American Society of Anesthesiologists (ASA). Continuum of depth of sedation: definition of general anesthesia and levels of sedation/analgesia. Available at: http://www.asahq.org/publicationsAndServices/standards/20.pdf. Approved by the ASA House of Delegates on October 27, 2004, and last affirmed on October 21, 2009. Accessed December 28, 2009.
22. American Society of Anesthesiologists (ASA). Practice guidelines for sedation and analgesia by non-anesthesiologists. Available at: http://www2.asahq.org/publications/pc-180-4-practice-guidelines-for-sedation-and-analgesia-by-non-anesthesiologists.aspx. Accessed September 23, 2009.
23. Urman RD, Shapiro FE. Choosing anesthetic agents. Which one? In: Shapiro FE, editor. Manual of office-based anesthesia procedures. Philadelphia: Lippincott Williams & Wilkins; 2007. p. 58–74.
24. Gan TJ, Glass PS, Windsor A, et al. Bispectral Index monitoring allows faster emergence and improved recovery from propofol, alfentanil, and nitrous oxide anesthesia. Anesthesiology 1997;87(4):808–15.
25. Gan T, Meyer T, Apfel C, et al. Society of ambulatory anesthesia guidelines for the Management of postoperative nausea and vomiting. Anesth Analg 2007;105: 1615–28.
26. American Society of Anesthesiologists (ASA). Standards for postanesthetic care. Available at: http://www.asahq.org/publicationsAndServices/standards/36.pdf. Approved by the ASA House of Delegates on October 27, 2004, and last affirmed on October 21, 2009. Accessed December 28, 2009.
27. Aldrete JA, Kroulik D. A postanesthetic recovery score. Anesth Analg 1970;49(6): 924–34.
28. White PF, Song D. New criteria for fast-tracking after outpatient anesthesia: a comparison with the modified Aldrete's scoring system. Anesth Analg 1999; 88:1069–72.
29. Awad IT, Chung F. Factors affecting recovery and discharge following ambulatory surgery. Can J Anaesth 2006;53(9):858–72.

30. Iverson RE, Lynch DJ, ASPS Committee on Patient Safety. Practice advisory on liposuction. Plast Reconstr Surg 2004;113(5):1478–90.
31. Ramon Y, Barak Y, Ullmann Y, et al. Pharmacokinetics of high-dose diluted lidocaine in local anesthesia for facelift procedures. Ther Drug Monit 2007;29(5):644–7.
32. Iverson RE, ASPS Task Force on Patient Safety in Office-based Surgery Facilities. Patient safety in office-Based surgery facilities: I. Procedures in the office-based surgery setting. Plast Reconstr Surg 2002;110:1337–42.

Office Based—Is My Anesthetic Care Any Different? Assessment and Management

Shireen Ahmad, MD

KEYWORDS

- Office-based anesthesia • Ambulatory anesthesia
- Patient safety

Office-based anesthesia (OBA) involves the conduct of anesthesia in a location that is integrated into a physician's office. The first published report of OBA in the United States appeared almost a century ago, when Ralph Waters described his practice in Sioux City, Iowa: "a modest office equipped with a waiting room and a small operating room with an adjoining room containing a cot on which the patient could lie down after his anesthetic."[1] In the United Kingdom, John Snow had already published his experience with dental anesthesia with nitrous oxide or chloroform much earlier.[2] Advancements in medical technology have led to an increase in the complexity and often the duration of office-based surgery (OBS) procedures, resulting in the need for deeper sedation and analgesia and often general anesthesia. Currently, OBA is one of the fastest growing subspecialties in anesthesia. In the 1980s, less than 5% of all surgeries in the United States were performed in surgeons' offices and by 2005, this number had increased to 17%.[3] Payers, private and public, favor OBS for economic reasons, because procedures performed in an office may cost as much as 70% less than a similar procedure performed in a hospital.[4] Patients find OBS less anxiety provoking and prefer the personalized care provided by familiar staff along with the privacy and convenience of the office. Surgeons choose an office for the increased efficiency, consistency, and convenience.[5] For anesthesiologists, however, an office is a unique practice venue that differs fundamentally from a hospital or ambulatory center paradigm and requires a distinctly different set of clinical and professional skills for safe and effective outcomes.

SAFETY OF OBS

The lack of oversight and regulation is one of the fundamental differences between an OBS facility and a hospital or ambulatory surgery center (ASC). It is for this reason that

Department of Anesthesiology, Northwestern University Feinberg School of Medicine, 251 East Huron Street, F5-704, Chicago, IL 60611, USA
E-mail address: sah704@northwestern.edu

Anesthesiology Clin 28 (2010) 369–384
doi:10.1016/j.anclin.2010.02.008 **anesthesiology.theclinics.com**

OBS has been referred to as the "wild, wild west of health care."[6] There are reports of surgeons performing procedures without adequate training and certification, inadequate supervision of patients due to insufficient or inadequately trained ancillary staff, and inadequate or obsolete equipment. There are reports of surgeons without formal training in anesthesia providing anesthetic care and of procedures performed in areas that do not have a sterile environment. Use of outdated and malfunctioning anesthetic equipment has resulted in serious injuries.[6] Unfortunately, reports of deaths and serious adverse events are usually reported in the lay press rather than in the medical journals, but this has led to an increased awareness regarding the need for the institution of standards in office settings similar to those in hospitals and ASCs.[7] The data regarding the safety of OBS is conflicting. A study of adverse events in Florida (2000–2002) reported a death rate of 9.2 per 100,000 and an adverse incident rate of 66 per 100,000 for OBS compared with 0.78 per 100,000 and 5.3 per 100,000 in ASCs.[8] Other investigators who compared OBS and surgery conducted in ASCs in Florida between 2000 and 2003 reported an estimated mortality rate of 0.4 per 100,000 in offices compared with 0.9 per 100,000 in ASCs. The estimated adverse event rate was 2.1 per 100,000 in offices versus 4.6 in ASCs.[9] Further examination of the Florida data over 7 years revealed that 58% of OBS-related deaths were associated with cosmetic plastic surgery procedures, especially liposuction, performed under general anesthesia, and 13.6% were associated with gastroenterology procedures.[10] The accuracy of the data presented in these studies is questionable, however, because there is no standard method of recording office surgery procedures or of reporting adverse events or mortality related to OBS.

Liposuction is a common cosmetic procedure performed by dermatologic and plastic surgeons. A report of 496,245 procedures revealed 95 deaths, with 47.7% occurring in an office setting compared with 16.9% in hospital-based settings, the major cause being pulmonary embolism.[11] A later review of 66,570 liposuction procedures performed by dermatologic surgeons in 2001, however, revealed that there were no deaths but 45 serious adverse events, and the incidence was higher among inpatients and patients in ASCs than in office settings.[12] They also found that the adverse event rates were higher when intravenous (IV) or intramuscular sedation was used in addition to tumescent anesthesia.

A prospective study of 34,391 patients who underwent oral-maxillofacial surgery in 58 offices between January and December of 2001 reported a complication rate of 1.3%.[13] Patients in this study received local anesthesia (12.6%), conscious sedation (15.5%), and deep sedation or general anesthesia (71.9%). The majority of patients (96.7%) were ranked American Society of Anesthesiologists (ASA) physical status I or II. An oral surgeon was the primary anesthesia provider in 95.5% of procedures. In the majority of locations (>98%), introperative monitoring included blood pressure, heart rate, and oxygen saturation. Respiratory monitoring was used in 95.4% of cases and consisted of visual assessment (49.2%), precordial stethoscope (18.3%), pretracheal stethoscope (20.7%), and capnography (1.5%). The complications included vomiting during induction (0.1%) and recovery (0.3%); laryngospasm, bronchospasm, and other respiratory complications (0.3%); cardiac arrhythmias (0.1%); syncope (0.1%); seizures (<0.1%); neurologic impairment (<0.1%); prolonged recovery (0.2%); peripheral vascular injuries or complications (0.2%); and other complications (0.1%). The reported risk of hospitalization was 5.8 per 100,000 procedures.

The ASA Closed Claims Project data regarding anesthesia malpractice claims revealed that of the 5480 claims in the database, there were 14 (0.25%) claims relating to OBA and 753 (13.7%) relating to procedures in ASCs.[14] The patients in both groups were similar with regard to age, medical status, and type of procedures. However,

64% of the OBA claims were associated with perioperative mortality, whereas 21% of ASC claims were related to death. In the OBA group, the most common cause of injury was a respiratory (50%) or drug-related (25%) event and most events occurred during the course of the anesthetic. The respiratory events included airway obstruction, bronchospasm, inadequate ventilation, and esophageal intubation. Drug-related events were due to the wrong drug or dosage, allergic reaction, or malignant hyperthermia. The most striking finding was that in 50% of the OBA claims the care was judged substandard and 46% of the events could potentially have been prevented with improved monitoring. Furthermore, in 36% of the cases where the care met the accepted standards, the postoperative care after discharge was deemed substandard. Plaintiffs were awarded payments in 92% of OBA claims; the amounts ranged from $10,000 to $2,000,000. There is a need for improvement in the perioperative care of patients undergoing surgery in an office location.

Several patients undergoing office-based procedures are children and although these children are healthier than those who undergo inpatient surgeries, a review of sedation-related adverse events revealed that permanent neurologic damage or death occurred more frequently in an office setting than in hospitals.[15] Eighty percent of events were respiratory in nature and were due to inadequate equipment or monitoring, inadequate presedation evaluation and postoperative recovery procedures, and medication errors. In many cases, the provider was an oral surgeon, periodontist, or nurse anesthetist supervised by the dentist. The investigators concluded that health care providers who sedate children should have training in airway management and resuscitation of children.

FACILITY AND SURGEON CONSIDERATIONS

One of the challenges faced in OBA is creating a safe practice environment in collaboration with a surgeon or proceduralist. In the United States, there are 3 accrediting bodies that inspect OBS locations and at the present time, accreditation is voluntary. These organizations are the American Association for Accreditation of Ambulatory Surgical Facilities (AAAASF), the Accreditation Association for Ambulatory Health Care, and the Joint Commission for Accreditation of Healthcare Organizations (JCAHO). These organizations have standard guidelines for the health care providers, the facility, and patient care that must be fulfilled in order for the facility to be accredited. JCAHO has been involved in accreditation since 1951 and provides education in addition to checking facility compliance with their standards. The AAAASF limits accreditation to facilities owned or operated by board-certified surgeons. Information regarding the accreditation status of facilities is available on the Internet Web sites of these organizations and should be verified by anesthesiologists before they enter into an agreement to provide anesthesia in the facility.

Pressure from the media and the lay public has resulted in an increased awareness of the need for state regulation of OBS; however, there are still many states that lack any type of oversight of these practices and the regulations that do exist vary significantly from state to state. New Jersey was the first state to institute regulations governing the care of patients in office settings in 1998, followed by California, Pennsylvania, Rhode Island, Texas (1999), and Florida (2000). Several other states have also started to regulate the offices where surgeries are performed and office-based anesthesiologists need to be familiar with these state regulations, which vary considerably from state to state, because violations can have serious legal consequences, including revocation of medical license and criminal charges. Although it is important to have a cordial relationship with the surgeon or proceduralist, an anesthesiologist must personally confirm that an office has all the perquisites for the safe administration of anesthesia. The creation of policies covering perioperative patient care, handling of controlled substances, maintenance of supplies and equipment, and management of emergencies that are approved and signed by the anesthesiologist and surgeon/proceduralist before providing anesthetic care in an office establishes the ground rules for a good working relationship (**Box 1**).

Anesthesiologists must confirm that the surgeon or proceduralist has a valid medical license, is board eligible or certified, and has privileges to perform the proposed procedures in a local hospital and that all the nurses involved in patient care are licensed and at minimum have basic life support certification. Surgeons and facilities must have adequate liability insurance. Anesthesiologists must inspect offices to determine that space and equipment are adequate for surgical procedures and recovery of patients. It is essential that anesthesiologists have unobstructed

Box 1
States with regulations regarding OBS and OBA in December 2009

Alabama
Arizona
California
Colorado
Connecticut
Washington, DC
Florida
Illinois
Indiana
Kansas
Kentucky
Louisiana
Massachusetts
Mississippi
New Jersey
New York
North Carolina
Ohio
Oklahoma
Oregon
Pennsylvania
Rhode Island
South Carolina
Tennessee
Texas
Washington

access to patients at all times and that office exits and elevators have adequate clearance to accommodate patients on a stretcher in the event of an emergent transfer. Facilities must be in compliance with local building and fire codes and there must be adequate electrical support for all equipment with an alternate backup electrical source for at least 1.5 hours in case of a power failure. The ability to scavenge waste gases must be available if inhaled anesthetic agents are used. Adequate compressed oxygen must be available even in the presence of pipeline supply and storage of tanks must be in compliance with local laws (**Box 2**).

Functioning resuscitation equipment, cardiac defibrillator and emergency drugs must be readily available in the event of an emergency. The equipment must be age and size appropriate and maintained in accordance with the manufacturer's instructions and emergency drugs must be checked regularly for expiration dates and replaced as needed. If triggering agents are used, dantrolene must be readily available. To assure adequate supplies and adequately trained staff, some office-based anesthesiologists choose to provide all the necessary supplies and staff in the locations where they practice (**Box 3**).

PATIENT AND PROCEDURE CONSIDERATIONS

Although a thorough preanesthetic assessment of patients who are scheduled for OBS is essential, initial screening is often performed by a surgeon/proceduralist. To prevent the scheduling of inappropriate patients, it is necessary to establish clear guidelines regarding the types of patients who are acceptable. Having patients complete a health history questionnaire that can be screened by an anesthesiologist

Box 2
Suggested equipment and supplies for OBA

Physiologic monitors with capnography

EKG patches, temperature strips

Syringe pumps

Oxygen tanks, wrench

Ambu bags, masks

Emergency cart, defibrillator, defibrillator patches

Suction apparatus, Yankaur cannula, suction tubing

Laryngoscope handles with C batteries: Macintosh blades, Miller blades

Endotracheal tubes, stylets, tongue blades

Oral airways, nasal airways

Nasal cannula with capnograph tubing, oxygen masks with tubing

Laryngeal mask airways

IV fluids: lactated Ringer solution 100-mL bags, IV tubing, IV extension tubing

Normal saline (100 mL)

IV catheters, Hep-Locks

Power strip

Latex-free, nonsterile gloves

Flashlight, scissors, hypoallergenic tape, alcohol wipes, gauze 4 $\times$ 4

Box 3
Suggested OBA emergency drugs

Lidocaine
Adenosine
Amiodarone
Atropine
Benadryl
Calcium chloride
Digoxin
Ephedrine
Epinephrine
Esmolol
Flumazenil
Hydralazine
Hydrocortisone
Labetalol
Lasix
Narcan
Nitrostat
Phenylephrine
Procainamide
Propranolol
Sodium bicarbonate
Verapamil

several days before surgery prevents unnecessary cancellations on the day of a procedure. In addition to reviewing screening questionnaires, anesthesiologists should contact patients by telephone before the day of surgery to verify patient history, alleviate any concerns, and formulate an anesthetic plan. The ASA recommends that patients who are American Society for Anesthesiologists Physical Status (ASAPS) I and II are suitable candidates for OBA and that patients who are ASAPS III have a face-to-face consultation with the anesthesiologist before the day of the procedure to determine suitability.[16]

Advances in surgical technology have resulted in an increase in the complexity and duration of the procedures that may be performed in an office setting. The American Society of Plastic Surgeons recommends that procedures performed in an office should not exceed 6 hours in duration and should be completed by 3:00 PM, to ensure adequate recovery time.[17] Procedures that are associated with significant blood loss or fluid shifts or that might result in hypothermia were considered unsuitable for an office setting. It is also recommended that procedures likely to result in significant postoperative pain or immobility be performed in a hospital facility (**Table 1**).[17]

Table 1
Patients not suitable for OBS

Cardiac conditions: Activity level: <4 METS Unstable angina MI: 0–3 months MI: 3–6 months: must have evaluation by cardiologist before surgery Severe cardiomyopathy Poorly controlled hypertension Internal defibrillator or pacemaker Heart transplant recipient/candidate	Pulmonary conditions: Obstructive sleep apnea: PSG+, STOP questionnaire[a] + Severe chronic obstructive pulmonary disease Airway abnormality Previous difficult intubation Asthma: <6 months since last emergency department visit/acute exacerbation Lung transplant recipient/ candidate	Central nervous system: Multiple sclerosis Cerebrovascular accident <3 months Paraplegia/quadriplegia Seizure disorder Psychologically unstable: acute anxiety, rage, or anger Dementia: disoriented
Renal: Significant renal disease: Creatinine >2 mg/dL End-stage renal disease: on dialysis On special diet because of renal disease Kidney transplant candidate	Hepatic: Significant liver disease: Elevated bilirubin/ transaminases Liver transplant candidate	Endocrine: Morbid obesity: body mass index $\geq$35 Poorly controlled diabetes mellitus: HbA1c >8 Type 1 diabetes mellitus
Hematologic: Sickle cell disease Anticoagulant therapy von Willebrand disease Hemophilia	Musculoskeletal: H/O malignant hyperthermia Myasthenia gravis Muscular dystrophy or myopathy	Other: Alcohol/substance overuse No adult escort

Abbreviations: HBAIc, Hemoglobin A1c; H/O, History of; METS, metabolic equivalents; MI, myocardial infarction; PSG, polysomnogram; +, positive.

[a] Chung F, Yegneswaran B, Liao P, et al. STOP questionnaire: a tool to screen patients for obstructive sleep apnea. Anesthesiology 2008;108(5):812–21.

ANESTHETIC CONSIDERATIONS FOR COMMON PROCEDURES

The types of surgeries performed in office locations are not usually encountered in hospital or ASC practices and anesthesiologists are required to deliver an anesthetic with a quick-onset, rapid recovery and minimal postoperative side effects if they are to maintain an efficient office practice. General anesthesia, regional anesthesia, and sedation/analgesia have all been used successfully. The choice of anesthetic is based on the type of patient and nature of surgery to be performed. Moderate to deep sedation/analgesia, frequently referred to as monitored anesthesia care, and propofol-based total IV anesthesia are probably the techniques most commonly used in office locations because they obviate an anesthesia machine and scavenging capabilities. In addition, the development of short-acting anesthetic agents that are easily titratable and the availability of programmable infusion devices that are simple to use have popularized these techniques.

Plastic Surgery

The majority of plastic surgery procedures are performed in office locations and liposuction is the most commonly performed plastic surgery in the United States.[18] The current tumescent technique involves the instillation of 3 to 4 mL of tumescent solution for each mL of anticipated fat that is aspirated. The tumescent solution is usually comprised of lactated Ringer solution (1000 mL) to which lidocaine (200–1000 mg) and epinephrine (0.25–1 mg of) have been added. The acceptable dose range for lidocaine in this situation is 35 to 55 mg/kg.[18] The vasoconstrictor results in improved hemostasis and blood loss varies between 4% and 30% of the aspirate. These procedures can be extensive, resulting in the absorption of a fair amount of the tumescent solution and IV fluids must be carefully titrated. The local anesthetic provides analgesia and small volume liposuction can be performed with minimal sedation analgesia; however, in the case of extensive procedures, moderate to deep sedation is necessary. Propofol may be used alone or in combination with opioid analgesics, such as fentanyl, to increase patient comfort when a local anesthetic is not adequate. The addition of a low-dose ketamine infusion decreases the perioperative opioid dose requirements without adverse psychomimetic effects.

Augmentation mammoplasty involves the placement of an implant through a small inframammary or axillary incision. The procedure is performed with local anesthesia combined with moderate to deep sedation/analgesia, and, in some cases, general anesthesia may be necessary. Reduction mammoplasty consists of removal of breast tissue and may be combined with liposuction. This surgery is usually performed with propofol-based total IV anesthesia, which has been shown to result in a lower incidence of postoperative nausea and vomiting (PONV) and allows patients to bypass the labor-intensive phase I recovery area due to rapid emergence.[19] It has also been reported that patients who receive propofol anesthesia may have less postoperative pain.[20,21]

Rhytidectomies and facelifts are usually performed with local anesthesia and sedation. The intraoperative use of opioid analgesics often results in respiratory depression and need for supplemental oxygen; however, the use of electrocautery during the procedure creates a fire hazard. The use of low-dose ketamine to provide analgesia reduces the need for opioids and also improves postoperative analgesia.[22] The intraoperative use of dexmedetomidine, a highly selective α_2-adrenergic receptor agonist with sedative and analgesic actions, has been described and may be another useful drug in these situations.[23]

There is a growing number of nonsurgical facial and scalp cosmetic procedures, such as hair transplant, dermabrasion, and chemical peels, that are performed with topical local anesthesia, local anesthetic infiltration, or nerve blocks, with or without minimal sedation. The use of propofol as the sole agent for procedural sedation may require significantly large doses and deeper levels of sedation with resultant delayed recovery. The addition of a small IV dose of midazolam (20 μg/kg) does not prolong recovery time with propofol sedation; however, doses larger than 2 mg have been found to increase postoperative cognitive impairment.[24,25]

Gastrointestinal Endoscopy

Upper gastrointestinal endoscopic procedures include esophagogastroduodenoscopy and endoscopic retrograde cholangiopancreatography and are usually performed with topical anesthesia and sedation. The most commonly used topical anesthetic is Cetacaine spray, a mixture of 14% benzocaine and 2% tetracaine hydrochloride. It has a rapid onset (1–2 minutes) and short duration of action (15–20 minutes), and overdosage is associated with methemoglobinemia.[26] Each 1-second spray delivers 28 mg of benzocaine and the maximum recommended dose is 2 seconds of spray; however, methemoglobinemia may occur with even small doses in susceptible individuals.[27] Another option is use of a lidocaine lollipop.[28] Endoscopic procedures are short and propofol is usually used for sedation because of its rapid onset of action and short contact sensitive half-life.[29] Endoscopy may be stimulating, necessitating opioid analgesics during the procedure; however, there is not much postprocedure discomfort and remifentanil is an ideal analgesic for these procedures. Patients who receive remifentanil during gastroscopy require less propofol and recover faster than those who receive fentanyl. There is a higher incidence of bradycardia in the patients who receive remifentanil, but the incidence of hypotension is higher in those who receive fentanyl.[30] The complication rate for upper gastrointestinal endoscopy ranges from 0.13% to 0.08%, with a mortality rate of 0.7 to 1 per 10,000 patients and cardiorespiratory events accounting for 50% of complications and 65% of deaths.[31] It is essential that the sedation for these procedures is administered by practitioners who are trained in emergency resuscitation and airway management.

Colorectal cancer screening has led to a dramatic increase in the number of colonoscopies performed in an office setting. Patients who receive propofol alone for sedation during colonoscopy have longer recoveries than those who receive propofol with fentanyl or midazolam.[32] A comparison of remifentanil and propofol revealed that although early recovery was faster with remifentanil, respiratory depression was more frequent and patient satisfaction was lower.[33] Patient-controlled sedation with propofol for colonoscopy results in the use of less drug, less sedation, fewer desaturation episodes, and quicker discharge in comparison with anesthesiologist administration. A comparison of propofol and remifentanil with midazolam and fentanyl using patient-controlled sedation found that the remifentanil and propofol group achieved adequate sedation levels quicker and also ambulated sooner after the procedure, but the combination resulted in more respiratory depression.[34] The rate of complications for colonoscopies is 0.86% and a rate of serious adverse events in the range of 13 per 8129 procedures. The involvement of anesthesia providers reduces the rate of adverse events.[35]

Dental Surgery

Dentists may seek the help of anesthesiologists for deep sedation in cases involving extraction of impacted third molars, root canal therapy, periodontal procedures, and insertion of implants. Communication between patient, dental surgeon, and anesthesiologist is essential so that all have the same expectations and patient safety is not compromised. Dental surgeons must use low-volume irrigation or a rubber drape to prevent aspiration. The procedures are usually performed with a combination of local anesthetic blocks and IV sedation. The combination of midazolam, fentanyl, and propofol infusion has been compared with midazolam, remifentanil, and propofol in patients undergoing third molar extractions. The patients in the remifentanil group required less propofol and had a shorter recovery time.[36] Small doses of ketamine (10–20 mg) provide additional analgesia without respiratory depression or psychomimetic effects.

Orthopedic and Podiatric surgery

Improvements in surgical techniques and the increased use of regional anesthesia have resulted in many arthroscopic orthopedic procedures transitioned to office locations. The majority of podiatric surgeries are also conducted with regional blocks or local infiltration. Surgery involving bone and periostial structures causes more pain than simple superficial surgeries.[37] A multimodal approach to perioperative analgesia decreases the potential adverse side effects of the individual drugs and improves overall efficacy. In addition to regional anesthesia, nonsteroidal anti-inflammatory drugs, cyclooxygenase-2 inhibitors, acetaminophen, and *N*-methyl-D-aspartate antagonists may be used.[38]

Gynecologic and Genitourinary Surgery

Minor gynecologic and genitourinary procedures have historically been performed in the office, but advances in instrumentation have led to the evolution of more complex office gynecologic procedures. Currently, hysteroscopic surgery for diagnosis and treatment of menorrhagia or sterilization comprises the vast majority of office gynecologic procedures. The procedures are performed with paracervical block and deep sedation due to the significant visceral stimulation during the surgery; however, there is minimal postoperative pain. In a small group of patients who received propofol titrated to a bispectral index of 60 to 80 in addition to remifentanil or fentanyl, the 2 drugs were equally effective.[39] In patients undergoing minor gynecologic surgery, alfentanil (10–20 μg/kg) had similar efficacy to remifentanil (0.2–0.4 μg/kg) when combined with propofol.[40] The addition of a small dose of ketamine (10–20 mg) is a useful adjunct and does not result in psychomimetic effects. Oocyte retrieval procedures are usually performed in infertility clinics and patients who receive remifentanil during the procedure had a higher pregnancy rate compared with those who receive general anesthesia.[41]

Transrectal ultrasound-guided prostate biopsy is one of the most common office urologic procedures for investigation of abnormalities of prostate-specific antigen or its derivatives. The procedure is performed with local anesthesia and moderate sedation, and administration of IV ketorolac significantly reduces the pain during the procedure.[42] Yearly, 500,000 American men undergo vasectomy. This procedure is also performed under local anesthesia with or without IV sedation/analgesia. Refinements in lithotripters have allowed extracorporeal shockwave lithotripsy (ESWL) to be performed in office settings. Despite the noninvasive nature of the procedure it is painful and usually requires sedation with propofol and opioid analgesic agents. Predictive factors for pain during ESWL include younger age, anxiety or depression, previous ESWL, and rib projected or homogenous stones.[43]

Ophthalmologic and Otolaryngologic Surgery

The majority of ophthalmologic surgeries are performed in hospital or ambulatory centers due to costly equipment needs. Refractive surgery, which is painful, is routinely performed, however, in an ophthalmologist's office with local anesthesia and minimal oral preoperative sedation. Pain during the procedure is related to eyelid manipulation and resolves with supplemental local anesthesia.

Improvements in endoscopic instruments have led to an expansion in office otolaryngology procedures. Endoscopic sinus surgery, septoplasty, and myringotomy are performed in offices with local anesthesia and minimal sedation. Laryngeal laser surgery conducted in an office setting has been described using the potassium-titanyl-phosphate laser.[44] It is usually used to treat epithelial diseases, such as dysplasia and papillomatosis. The procedures are tolerated well with extensive topical anesthesia. The main impediment to the extensive use of the technique is the cost of the technology (**Tables 2** and **3**).

POSTPROCEDURE CONSIDERATIONS

Limitations related to staffing and space for recovery after office-based procedures make it essential that the anesthetic techniques promote a rapid emergence and safe transition of the patients to the home setting. In many instances, patients are expected to transfer themselves to a chair immediately after surgery and ambulate shortly thereafter. Prevention of PONV and pain is essential in the OBA setting and to provide a smooth recovery and timely discharge. Because PONV is multifactorial,

Table 2
Pharmacokinetics of sedatives and analgesics commonly used in OBA

Drug	Elimination Halflife (h)	Volume of Distribution (L/kg)	Clearance (mL/kg/min)
Propofol	0.5–1.5	3.5–4.5	30–60
Methohexital	3.9	2.2	10.9
Midazolam	1–4	1.0–1.5	6–8
Ketamine	2–3	2.5–3.5	16–18
Dexmedetomidine	2–3	1.5	9
Remifentanil	0.17–0.33	30	4000
Alfentanil	1.4–1.5	27	238
Fentanyl	3.1–6.6	335	1530

all patients at moderate to high risk for PONV should receive multimodal, prophylactic antiemetic therapy. In addition, many patients may also experience postdischarge nausea and vomiting, and the use of the oral disintegration tablet of ondansetron or scopolamine patch prevents postoperative dehydration and delayed resumption of normal activity that is associated with this complication.[45–48] The use of total IV anesthesia with propofol has also been shown to be effective for prevention of PONV.[49]

Postoperative pain continues to be a major problem after ambulatory surgery.[50] Procedures that might be associated with moderate to severe postoperative pain are usually not performed in an office location; however, there is significant variability in individual levels of pain experienced. Although alfentanil and remifentanil are used in OBS because of their short duration, in the case of procedures that may be associated with significant postoperative pain, it is necessary to administer additional analgesics before the end of surgery. Traditionally narcotics are used to relieve postoperative pain. Small doses of fentanyl (25–50 μg) provide a rapid onset of analgesia and allow patients to transition to oral analgesics before discharge from the facility. The longer-acting opioids, such as morphine or hydromorphone, are best avoided because the sedation and respiratory depression associated with these drugs also lasts for a longer duration.

A multimodal approach to analgesic therapy that incorporates the use of local anesthetic injections, opioid and nonopioid analgesics, maximizes analgesia and minimizes adverse side effects that prolong recovery and delay discharge.[51] The use of nonopioid analgesics, such as nonsteroidal anti-inflammatory agents or cyclooxygenase-2 inhibitors, is effective for mild to moderate pain and should be considered in all patients unless contraindications exist.[52] Other agents, including dexmedetomidine, gabapentin, and dexamethasone, may be useful analgesics but have not been evaluated in office populations.

Table 3
Dosages of sedative and analgesic agents commonly used in OBA

	Initial Bolus	Infusion	Additional Bolus
Propofol	250–500 μ/kg	25–75 μ/kg/min	150 μ/kg
Remifentanil	0.1–0.5 μ/kg	0.02–0.05 μ/kg/min	0.15 μ/kg
Alfentanil	5–10 μ/kg	0.25–1.0 μ/kg/min	1.5 μ/kg
Ketamine	0.3–0.6 mg/kg	5–10 μ/kg/min	0.15 μ/kg
Dexmedetomidine	1 μ/kg over 10 min	0.2–1.5 μ/kg/h	

The use of simple and clear objective discharge criteria allows timely discharge and prevents postoperative complications and hospital admissions associated with premature discharge. The postanesthesia discharge scoring system is used to determine home readiness.[53] Patients must have a responsible adult companion at the time of discharge and should receive clear, written discharge instructions because they may not have complete recovery of cognitive function at the time of discharge. The success of OBS depends on careful planning, attention to detail, and cooperation by all the health care team members (**Tables 4** and **5**).

PROVIDER CONSIDERATIONS

The challenge in OBA is to be able to provide efficient and effective anesthetic care without compromising patient safety. Several subspecialty societies, including the ASA, have published practice guidelines in an attempt to establish minimum standards of care and improve safety.[16,52–55] The recommendations cover all aspects of office-based practice from facility and staffing requirements to anesthetic supplies and drugs, perioperative care, quality assurance, and risk management processes and provide an excellent resource for anesthesiologists setting up an office-based practice.

Many anesthesiologists who embark on office-based practices have no training or prior experience in that type of environment. With the economic restraints on health care, the volume of OBS will continue to grow and it is essential for chairs of academic anesthesiology programs to explore suitable venues in their institutions where residents can be trained in OBA. Anesthesiologists must be taught how to evaluate the safety of an office-based practice and must have knowledge regarding the regulatory and accreditation requirements of particular states; the rules that apply to the physical design, equipment, and supplies; and the protocols for emergencies and quality improvement. Residency programs need to develop OBA curriculum guidelines that incorporate the Accreditation Council for Graduate Medical Education core competencies so that anesthesiologists are trained to be efficient without compromising patient safety. The Society for Ambulatory Anesthesia has established OBA curriculum guidelines, which are available on the Society's Internet Web site (http://www.sambahq.org). Anesthesiology residency program directors will find these guidelines useful for designing institution-specific rotations.

Although clinical and didactic experience is essential, complications occur infrequently and most trainees have limited experience in managing critical life-threatening situations during their OBA rotations. Simulation can be used to recreate complex crisis situations and to train anesthesiologists in the management of these scenarios.

Table 4
Dosages of postoperative analgesic agents

Drug	Suggested Dose	Peak Effect (min)	Duration of Action (h)
Fentanyl	25–50 μg	5–15	0.5–1
Morphine	2–10 mg	5–20	2–7
Hydromorphone	0.2–1	5–20	2–4
Ketorolac	30 mg IV	15–45	4–6
Naproxen	500 mg by mouth	60	6–8
Celecoxib	400 mg	45–60	4–8
Acetominophen/ hydrocodone	325 mg/5 mg	30	4–6

Table 5
Modified postanesthesia discharge scoring system

Vital signs	Within 20% of preoperative value	2
	20%–40% of preoperative value	1
	40% of preoperative value	0
Ambulation	Steady gait/no dizziness	2
	With assistance	1
	None/dizziness	0
Nausea/vomiting	Minimal	2
	Moderate	1
	Severe	0
Pain	Minimal	2
	Moderate	1
	Severe	0
Surgical bleeding	Minimal	2
	Moderate	1
	Severe	0

(Discharge criteria: a score of ≥ 9)

The advantage of simulation is that trainees can be exposed to uncommon critical scenarios without fear of harm to patients. Errors can be permitted to reach their conclusion and the results of decisions and actions become obvious to trainees. Furthermore, an actual office environment can be recreated and interpersonal interactions, communication, and leadership skills can be developed. With respect to the acquisition of critical assessment and management skills, students who participate in simulation training scenarios perform better than those who are trained with problem-based learning sessions.[56] Effective communication between team members is of the utmost importance in an office setting and it has been demonstrated that simulation can be used to improve these nontechnical skills as well.[57]

Research in OBA must be fostered so that the practice can be based on the same type of scientific evidence as the other fields of anesthesiology. Anesthesiology societies and foundations must establish grants specifically designated for investigators in OBA in order for them to develop large multicenter outcomes research projects to generate this type of evidence.

SUMMARY

OBA is a unique and challenging venue, and, although the clinical outcomes have not been evaluated extensively, existing data indicate that there is need for increased regulation and additional education. Outcomes in OBA can be improved by education not only of anesthesiologists but of surgeons, proceduralists, and nursing staff. Legislators must be educated so that appropriate regulations are instituted governing the practice of OBS and the lay public must be educated to make wise, informed decisions about their choice of surgery location. The leadership of societies along with support from the membership must play a key role in this educational process; only then can OBA become as safe as the anesthesia care in traditional venues.

REFERENCES

1. Waters RM. The downtown anesthesia clinic. Am J Surg 1919;33:71–3.
2. Snow J. On chloroform and other anaesthetics. London: John Churchill; 1858. p. 314–5.

3. American Hospital Association TRENDWATCH. The migration of care to non-hospital settings: have regulatory structures kept pace with changes in care delivery. 2006. Available at: www.aha.org/aha/trendwatch/2006/twjuly2006migration.pdf. Accessed December 2, 2009.
4. Bartamian M, Meyer DR. Site of service, anesthesia and postoperative practice patterns for oculoplastic and orbital surgeries. Ophthalmology 1996;103:1628.
5. Byrd HS, Barton FE, Orenstein HH, et al. Safety and efficacy in an accredited outpatient plastic surgery facility: a review of 5316 consecutive cases. Plast Reconstr Surg 2003;112:636–41.
6. Quattrone MS. Is the physician office the wild, Wild West of health care? J Ambul Care Manage 2000;23:64.
7. Landro L. Seeking a safer surgery: some states crack down on doctors who perform unregulated outpatient procedures. Wall Street Journal. July 20, 2009.
8. Vila H, Soto R, Cantor AB, et al. Comparative outcomes analysis of procedures performed in physicians' offices and ambulatory surgery centers. Arch Surg 2003;138:991–5.
9. Venkat AP, Coldiron B, Balkrishnan R, et al. Lower adverse event and mortality rates in physician offices compared with ambulatory surgery centers: a reappraisal of Florida adverse event data. Dermatol Surg 2004;30:1444–53.
10. Coldiron BM, Healy C, Bene NI. Office surgery incidents: what seven years of Florida data show us. Dermatol Surg 2008;34:285–91.
11. Grazer FM, de Jong RH. Fatal outcomes from liposuction: census survey of cosmetic surgeons. Plast Reconstr Surg 2000;105:436–46.
12. Housman TS, Lawrence N, Melen BG, et al. The safety of liposuction: results of a national survey. Dermatol Surg 2002;28:971–8.
13. Perrott DH, Yuen JP, Andresen RV, et al. Office-based ambulatory anesthesia: outcomes of clinical practice of oral and maxillofacial surgeons. J Oral Maxillofac Surg 2003;61:983–95.
14. Domino KB. Office-based anesthesia: lessons learned from the closed claims project. ASA Newsl 2001;65:9–15.
15. Coté CJ, Notterman DA, Karl HW, et al. Adverse sedation events in pediatrics: a critical incident analysis of contributing factors. Pediatrics 2000;105:805–14.
16. Office-Based Anesthesia. Considerations for anesthesiologists in setting up and maintaining a safe office anesthesia environment. 2nd edition. Park Ridge, IL: American Society of Anesthesiologists; 2008. Available at: http://www2.asahq.org/publications/p-319-office-based-anesthesia-considerations-for-anesthesiologists-in-setting-up-and-maintaining-a-safe-office-anesthesia-environment-2nd-edition-november-2008.aspx. Accessed February 16, 2010.
17. Iverson RE. ASPS task force on patient safety in office-based surgery facilities: patient safety in office based surgery facilities. I. Procedures in the office based surgery setting. Plast Reconstr Surg 2002;110:1337–43.
18. Iverson RE, Lynch DJ. Practice advisory on liposuction. Plast Reconstr Surg 2004;113:1478–90.
19. Tang J, Chen L, White PF, et al. Recovery profile, cost, and patient satisfaction with propofol and sevoflurane for fast-track office-based anesthesia. Anesthesiology 1999;91:253–61.
20. Tan T, Bhinder R, Carey M, et al. Day–surgery patients anesthetized with propofol have less postoperative pain than those anesthetized with sevoflurane. Anesth Analg 2009. [Epub ahead of print].

21. Cheng SS, Yeh J, Flood P. Anesthesia matters: patients anesthetized with propofol have less postoperative pain than those anesthetized with isoflurane. Anesth Analg 2008;106:264–9.
22. Mortero RF, Clark LD, Tolan MM, et al. The effects of small-dose ketamine on propofol sedation: respiration, postoperative mood, perception, cognition and pain. Anesth Analg 2001;92:1465–9.
23. Arain SR, Ebert TJ. The efficacy, side effects, and recovery characteristics of dexmedetomidine versus propofol when used for intraoperative sedation. Anesth Analg 2002;95:461–6.
24. Seifert H, Schmitt TH, Gültekin T, et al. Sedation with propofol plus midazolam versus propofol alone for interventional endoscopic procedures: a prospective randomized study. Aliment Pharmacol Ther 2000;14:1207–14.
25. Fanti L, Agostoni M, Arcidiacono PG, et al. Target-controlled infusion during monitored anesthesia care in patients undergoing EUS: propofol alone versus midazolam plus propofol. A prospective, double-blind randomized controlled trial. Dig Liver Dis 2007;39:81–6.
26. Severinghaus JW, Xu FD, Spellman MJ. Benzocaine and methemoglobinemia: recommended actions. Anesthesiology 1991;74:385–6.
27. Guay J. Methemoglobinemia related to local anesthetics: a summary of 242 episodes. Anesth Analg 2009;108:837–45.
28. Ayoub C, Skoury A, Abul-baki H, et al. Lidocaine lollipop as single agent anesthesia in upper GI endoscopy. Gastrointest Endosc 2007;66:786–93.
29. Hughes MA, Glass PSA, Jacobs JR. Context-sensitive half-time in multicompartment pharmacokinetic models for intravenous anesthetic drugs. Anesthesiology 1992;76:334–41.
30. Xu ZY, Wang X, Si YY, et al. Intravenous remifentanil and propofol for gastroscopy. J Clin Anesth 2008;20:352–5.
31. Thompson AM, Wright DJ, Murray W, et al. Analysis of 153 deaths after upper gastrointestinal endoscopy: room for improvement? Surg Endosc 2004;18:22–5.
32. VanNatta ME, Rex DK. Propofol alone titrated to deep sedation versus propofol in combination with opioids and /or benzodiazepines and titrated to deep sedation versus propofol in combination with opioids and/or benzodizepines and titrated to moderate sedation for colonoscopy. Am J Gastroenterol 2006;101:2209–17.
33. Moerman AT, Foubert LA, Herrgods LL, et al. Propofol versus remifentanil for monitored anesthesia care during colonoscopy. Eur J Anaesthesiol 2003;20:461–6.
34. Mandel JE, Tanner JW, Lichtenstein GR, et al. A randomized, controlled, double-blind trial of patient-controlled sedation with propofol/remifentanil versus midazolam/fentanyl for colonoscopy. Anesth Analg 2008;106:434–9.
35. Vargo JJ, Holub JL, Faigel DO, et al. Risk factors for cardiopulmonary events during propofol-mediated upper endoscopy and colonoscopy. Aliment Pharmacol Ther 2006;24:955–63.
36. Lacombe GF, Leake JL, Clokie CML, et al. Comparison of remifentanil with fentanyl for deep sedation in oral surgery. J Oral Maxillofac Surg 2006;64:215–22.
37. Bardiau FM, Taviaux NF, Albert A, et al. An intervention study to enhance postoperative pain management. Anesth Analg 2003;96:179–85.
38. Buvanendran A, Kroin JS. Multimodal analgesia for controlling acute postoperative pain. Curr Opin Anaesthesiol 2009;22:588–93.
39. Ryu JH, Kim JH, Park KS, et al. Remifentanil-propofol versus fentanyl-propofol for monitored anesthesia care during hysteroscopy. J Clin Anesth 2008;20:328–32.

40. Dogru K, Madenoglu H, Yildiz K, et al. Sedation for outpatient endometrial biopsy: comparison of remifentanil-propofol and alfentanil-propofol. J Int Med Res 2003;31:31–5.
41. Wilhelm W, Hammadeh ME, White PF, et al. General anesthesia versus monitored anesthesia care with remifentanil for assisted reproductive technologies: effect on pregnancy rate. J Clin Anesth 2002;14:1–5.
42. Mireku-Boateng AO. Intravenous ketorolac significantly reduces the pain of office transrectal ultrasound and prostate biopsy. Urol Int 2004;73:123–4.
43. Vergnolles M, Wallerand H, Gadrat F, et al. Predictive risk factors for pain during extracorporeal shockwave lithotripsy. J Endourol 2009;23:2021–7.
44. Zeitels SM, Burns JA. Office-based laryngeal laser surgery with the 532-nm pulsed-potassium-titanyl-phosphate laser. Curr Opin Otolaryngol Head Neck Surg 2007;15:394–400.
45. Gan TJ, Sinha AC, Kovac AL, et al. A randomized, double-blind, multi-center trial comparing transdermal scopolamine plus ondansetron to ondansetron alone for prevention of postoperative nausea and vomiting in the outpatient setting. Anesth Analg 2009;108:1498–504.
46. Gan TJ, Franiak R, Reeves J. Ondansetron orally disintegrating tablet versus placebo for prevention of postdischarge nausea and vomiting after ambulatory surgery. Anesth Analg 2002;94:1199–200.
47. Gan TJ, Ginsberg B, Grant AP, et al. Double-blind randomized comparison of ondansetron and intraoperative propofol to prevent postoperative nausea and vomiting. Anesthesiology 1996;85:1036–42.
48. McGrath B, Elgendy H, Chung F, et al. Thirty percent of patients have moderate to severe pain 24 hours after ambulatory surgery: a survey of 5,703 patients. Can J Anaesth 2004;51:886–91.
49. Kehlet H, Dahl JB. The value of "multimodal" or "balanced analgesia" in postoperative pain treatment. Anesth Analg 1993;77:1048–56.
50. White PF, Kehlet H, Neal JM, et al. The role of the anesthesiologist in fast-track surgery: from multimodal analgesia to perioperative medical care. Anesth Analg 2007;104:1380–96.
51. Chung F, Chan VWS, Ong D. A post-anesthetic discharge scoring system for home readiness after ambulatory surgery. J Clin Anesth 1995;6:500–6.
52. Iverson RE. ASPS Task Force on Patient Safety in Office-Based Surgery Facilities. Patient safety in office-based surgery facilities: I. Procedures in the office-based setting. Plast Reconstr Surg 2002;110:1337–42.
53. Iverson RE, Lynch DJ, ASPS Task Force on Patient Safety in Office-Based Surgery Facilities. Patient safety in office-based surgery facilities: II. Patient selection. Plast Reconstr Surg 2002;110:1785–90.
54. American Medical Association. Office-based surgery core principles. Chicago (IL): American Medical Association, 2003. Available at: www.ama-assn.org/ama/pub/category/11807.html. Accessed February 18, 2010.
55. ASA Guidelines for office-based anesthesia. Park Ridge (IL): ASA; 1999, affirmed 2004. Available at: www.asahq.org/publicationsandServices/standards/12.pdf. Accessed February 18, 2010.
56. Steadman RH, Coates WC, Huang YM, et al. Simulation-based training is superior to problem-based learning for acquisition of critical assessment and management skills. Crit Care Med 2006;34:151–7.
57. Yee B, Naik VN, Joo HS, et al. Nontechnical skills in anesthesia crisis management with repeated exposure to simulation-based education. Anesthesiology 2005;103:241–8.

Index

Note: Page numbers of article titles are in **boldface** type.

Anesthesiology Clin 28 (2010) 385–395
doi:10.1016/S1932-2275(10)00048-0 anesthesiology.theclinics.com
1932-2275/10/$ – see front matter

Q

R

S

T

U

V

Printed and bound by CPI Group (UK) Ltd, Croydon, CR0 4YY

03/10/2024

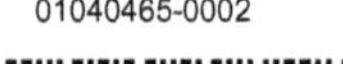

01040465-0002